Food Selection & Preparation

Food Selection & Preparation

JEAN STILL

Macmillan Publishing Co., Inc.
NEW YORK
Collier Macmillan Publishers
LONDON

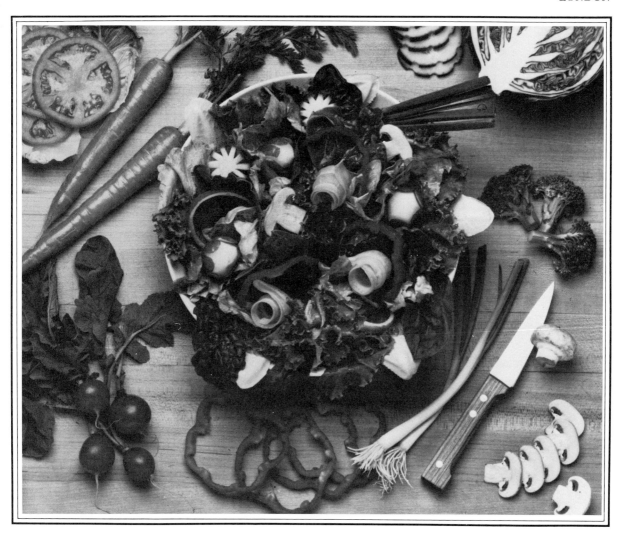

Cover photograph by Preston Lyon, New York City.

Printed in the United States of America

Macmillan Publishing Co., Inc.
866 Third Avenue, New York, New York 10022

Collier Macmillan Canada, Ltd.

Library of Congress Cataloging in Publication Data

Still, Jean.
    Food selection and preparation.

    Bibliography: p.
    Includes index.
    1. Food. 2. Nutrition. 3. Cookery.
I. Title.
TX354.S85   641   80–14368
ISBN 0-02-417510-2

Printing: 1 2 3 4 5 6 7 8   Year: 1 2 3 4 5 6 7 8

Preface

This introductory foods text is designed to meet the needs of the current generation of students who may wish to learn a career, or to change to a new one, or simply to broaden their interests and enrich their lives. Although the sequence of chapters have been chosen for the beginning student, the text as a whole covers a broad scope of subjects that will also interest those who have acquired some prior food experience and wish to upgrade or deepen their knowledge of basic food selection and preparation. Its format permits the instructor to develop learning modules for students desiring to progress at a different pace than their fellow students, and it presents materials that meet individual needs in a group situation. The text has been written without difficult technical terminology or scientific analyses.

Many factors must be considered when learning about food selection and preparation. The student need not only learn how food is properly cooked but also must understand the interrelated factors of nutrition, food storage, safety, food purchasing, equipment, time management, and even social and cultural influences. Each chapter in this text discusses these specific points.

Of basic importance to those learning about food are the factors affecting food selection and purchasing and nutrition. In the introductory chapter the major nutrients, their functions in the body, and their food sources are discussed together with the nutrient needs of specific age groups. Each of the following chapters emphasizes the nutrient contributions of the specific food discussed in the chapter. Each food chapter demonstrates how the food can be used in menu planning to create meals that are nutritionally balanced and aesthetically pleasing to the eye and palate.

The proper selection, use, and care of equipment together with the use of proper measurement techniques are necessary to achieve quality in food preparation. In addition it is necessary for the student to understand both the standard and metric measuring systems. These topics are discussed in Chapter 2.

Another important aspect of food preparation is food safety. Preparing and serving food that is safe to eat is vital to all. Also important to this area of study are the governmental agencies that help to protect our food supply. This information is presented in Chapter 3 and re-emphasized throughout the text.

Techniques and methods of food preparation are constantly changing, with new food products and new equipment appearing on the market daily. *Food Selection and Preparation* provides the most up-to-date methods of food preparation in an easily understood format. Each chapter covers a specific food, and available convenience forms of that food are discussed. Since microwave cooking is becoming a popular method for food preparation, each chapter discusses methods for using the microwave oven and many of the recipes give microwave cooking directions.

Each chapter contains learning activities and review questions and those chapters that discuss specific foods contain recipes in both standard and metric measurements. Learning activities and recipes have been selected to meet the varying abilities of students within a class. The inclusion of learning activities, review questions, and recipes allows the text to be used as a combination text and laboratory manual and for the student as a beginning cookbook.

After taking a basic food course, many individuals may wish to pursue food selection and preparation in depth; to this end a list of reference books is provided near the conclusion of this book. It should also be noted that the extensive index at the very end of the book has been divided into a recipe index and a subject index for easier reference.

Many individuals have worked with me in the writing of this text. I wish to thank the reviewers from Florida State University, Iowa State University, and the University of Illinois at Urbana-Champaign for their constructive comments; also the staff of Macmillan Publishing Company for their direction and advice, particularly my editor, John Beck, my production editor, Hurd Hutchins, and Ellen Gordon, who copyedited the manuscript; the food industry businesses that contributed many of the photos used in this text; Bob Strode for his excellent photography; and my husband, Bob, and children Joe and Jacey, for their continued support and encouragement in writing this text.

Tacoma, Washington   Jean Still

Contents

1

Introduction to Food Preparation

Food is an intrinsic part of life. It is consumed for the growth and maintenance of the life system and for many individuals throughout the world the primary work of the day is to find food for survival. In contrast, others select and eat food that is influenced by other factors including their life-style, psychological and physiological needs, social and cultural needs, time, and economics. Foods are also selected on the basis of smell, taste, texture, and eye appeal. If an individual is knowledgeable of food nutrients, he or she will select food for its nutritional quality.

This introductory chapter discusses factors that influence the selection and purchase of food, the nutrients present in food and their function in the body, and the nutrient needs of specific age groups. Guides that can be used for selecting nutrients and the chemical changes that occur in food preparation are also discussed.

Influences of Food Selection and Preparation

All food eaten, whether it be a snack, breakfast, lunch, or dinner is considered a meal. In contrast to 100 years ago, when nearly all meals were prepared and eaten in the home at a family gathering, a meal today may be eaten in a restaurant, at a fast-food outlet, be selected from a vending machine, or be a frozen meal heated in the oven. Many meals are eaten away from the family, or as in the case of single people, may be eaten alone. Approximately 25 percent of the money value spent on food for a household averaging 3.1 members is spent for food eaten away from home including meals and snacks. Figure 1–1 shows the average amount of money spent on meals eaten at and away from home according to geographical region.

Over the past two decades the money spent for food eaten away from home has changed

1

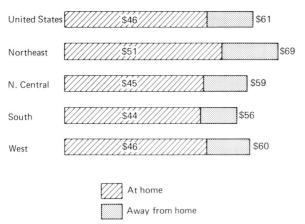

Figure 1–1.

Cost of food at home and away per household per week by region in Spring 1977. (USDA Nation-wide Food Consumption Survey, Spring 1977, Preliminary.)

from that of food being served, as in a restaurant, to that of purchasing prepared food, namely refreshment places or fast-food outlets as shown in Table 1–1.

The food selected for the approximately 75 percent of meals that are prepared from

Table 1–1

Shares of Away-from-Home Food Market Sales 1955–75

Type of Seller	1955	1965	1975
	Per Cent		
Restaurants, lunchrooms, cafeterias	57.0	50.2	41.0
Refreshment places, ice cream and frozen custard stands	5.3	12.1	27.8
Hotels and motels	6.4	6.3	5.7
Schools and colleges[1]	7.0	10.0	7.6
Stores and bars	13.0	7.9	6.1
Recreational places	2.4	2.3	2.2
Others[2]	8.9	11.2	9.6

[1] Excludes child nutrition subsidies.
[2] Includes military outlets.
U.S. Food Expenditures, 1954–78. U.S. Department of Agriculture. Agricultural Economic Report No. 431.

home food supplies are either selected from a range of 8,000 to 10,000 items in a large market or from a small neighborhood store with limited food selection. From the vast array of food items available today, an increasing percentage of foods are commercially prepared mixes such as frozen dinners, and dry cake, pudding, and casserole mixes. Yet the consumer still spends the majority of the food dollar for fresh foods including meats, vegetables, fruits, and dairy products. This information indicates the importance of learning the skills and techniques of food selection and preparation.

According to *Supermarketing's* 32nd Annual Consumer Expenditures Study, the average household's total grocery budget per week during 1978 was $41.14. Of this amount $20.95 was spent on perishable food items and approximately one third of the money designated for food was spent on nonedible items at the supermarket. A further analysis of how the money was spent is shown in Table 1–2.

The lower the income, the higher is the percentage spent on food, but as income rises, the amount spent on food does not increase. However, the trend is to purchase more expensive foods with a higher income. For some low-income peoples, the federal government Food Stamp Program and the various school feeding programs have helped to ease the burden of food purchasing. Figure 1–2 shows the percentage of income spent on food for various income levels.

Food Availability

Food selection and preparation are affected by geographical location and by the season of the year. Certain foods that are available throughout the year may also be very expensive. For example, certain fresh fruits, such as melons and berries, may be available but the price will also be very high.

Table 1-2

How the Average Shopper Spent the Weekly Supermarket Budget*

	1978	1977	1976
Perishables			
Baked goods, snacks	$ 2.49	$ 2.33	$ 2.13
Dairy section	3.08	2.97	2.74
Frozen foods	1.97	1.89	1.76
Fresh meat and provisions	7.63	6.71	6.72
Fresh fish	.34	.29	.27
Fresh poultry	.99	.87	.84
Produce	4.45	4.14	3.77
Total for perishables	$20.95	$19.20	$18.23
Dry Groceries			
Beer	$ 1.85	$ 1.76	$ 1.67
Wine and liquor	.23	.21	.19
Baby food, excluding cereals, formulas	.14	.14	.13
Cereals and rice	.62	.58	.55
Candy and chewing gum	.44	.41	.38
Canned foods			
Fruits	.33	.32	.30
Juices and drinks	.24	.23	.22
Meat and poultry	.42	.40	.39
Seafood	.32	.30	.26
Soups	.25	.24	.22
Vegetables	.56	.55	.52
Milk	.08	.08	.08
Coffee and tea	1.53	1.61	1.19
Dried foods	.48	.47	.44
Jams, jellies, preserves	.15	.15	.14
Macaroni, spaghetti, noodles	.16	.16	.15
Desserts	.06	.06	.06
Soft drinks	1.03	.98	.92
Sugar	.34	.32	.24
All other edibles	1.72	1.64	1.67
Total for dry groceries	$10.95	$10.61	$ 9.72
Total for Foods	$31.90	$29.81	$27.95
Other Groceries			
Paper goods	$ 1.16	$1.03	$ .93
Soaps, detergents	.76	.71	.66
Other household supplies	.89	.85	.81
Pet foods	.66	.63	.58
Tobacco products	1.44	1.38	1.26
Groceries, not edible	.26	.23	.21
Total for other groceries	$ 5.17	$ 4.83	$ 4.45

(Continued)

	1978	1977	1976
General Merchandise			
Health and beauty aids (nonprescription)	$ 1.50	$ 1.40	$ 1.30
Prescriptions	.20	.19	.17
Housewares	.50	.45	.41
All other general merchandise	1.88	1.76	1.58
Total for general merchandise	4.08	3.80	3.46
Grand Total	$41.15	$38.44	$35.86

*Includes one-person households
Supermarketing. 32nd Annual Consumer Expenditure Study, 1979.

Food Advertising

Food advertising can be a very influential factor on the type of food selected. Approximately 69 percent of all food advertising is done through newspapers. Weekly ads in local

Figure 1-2.

Cost of food at home and away per household per week by income in Spring 1977. (USDA Nationwide Food Consumption Survey, 48 States, Spring 1977, Preliminary.)

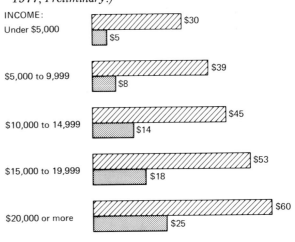

INCOME:		
Under $5,000	$30	$5
$5,000 to 9,999	$39	$8
$10,000 to 14,999	$45	$14
$15,000 to 19,999	$53	$18
$20,000 or more	$60	$25

Table 1-3

Fast-Food Prices: At Franchised Outlets and at Home

Food	Fast-Food Franchise Outlet		At-Home Equivalent					
	Average Weight[1] ounces	Price[2] cents	Serving size	Total Price[3]	Meat	Cheese cents	Bread	Other[4]
Hamburger	3.5	.42	2 oz. patty	.31	.19		.10	.02
with cheese	4.0	.47	1/4 oz. sl.	.36	.19	.09	.10	.02
Special Hamburger	5.7	.90	4 oz. patty	.51	.37		.12	.05
with cheese	6.8	1.00	1 oz. sl.	.64	.37	.10	.12	.05
Fish Sandwich	4.6	.70	3 oz. port.	.44	.31		.10	.03
French fries	2.5	.41	4 oz.	.17				
Soft drink	8 fl. oz.	.39	8 fl. oz.	.12				

[1] Based on a study conducted by WARF Institute, Madison, Wis., "Nutritional Analysis of Food Served at McDonald's Restaurants," 1977.
[2] Prices observed at franchise outlets in Washington, D.C., area, February 1979.
[3] Prices observed at Washington, D.C., area supermarkets, February 1979.
[4] Includes lettuce and tomato, garnish, and condiments.
National Food Review, USDA Summer 1979.

newspapers typically offer three to six items at a reduced price, offer "off-cents" coupons, and inform the consumer of what fresh produce is in good supply. It is important for the consumer to know prices, because some items advertised are not on sale and nothing is a bargain if it cannot be used. If additional travel is involved in purchasing a sale item, usually nothing is saved.

Fast-Food Outlets

In recent years this nation has seen a tremendous growth in the number of fast-food outlets. Of the approximate 25 percent of food money spent for eating outside the home in the average household, 20 percent is spent at fast-food outlets. The working family and single individuals with increased leisure time, transportation mobility, and busy time schedules have probably accounted most for the growth and popularity of these establishments. The foods offered at fast food outlets, such as hamburgers, French fries, and milk shakes have comparative nutritive value to home-cooked products, but because of the limitation in foods available, it is important to learn the nutrients needed daily to ensure good health. Table 1-3 shows the comparative cost for some foods purchased at a fast-food outlet versus home preparation. When analyzing this chart, it must be remembered that food portions, usually meat, may be somewhat smaller when the meal is prepared outside the home. On the other hand, preparation at home includes purchasing, preparing, serving, and cleaning up.

Types of Food Markets

Five basic types of stores sell food and though all five types may not be available in any one locality, there is usually a choice of more than one. The supermarket is a self-service store offering a complete line of food and some general merchandise and health/beauty aids. Food accounts for approximately 75 percent of supermarket sales. A supermarket is defined as a store having $1 million sales or more per year with sales adjusted annually to account for inflation. Supermarkets may be chain-operated or independently owned.

Supermarkets offer the widest selection of products and often have the best prices, because they can buy in quantity and turn their inventory quickly. Supermarkets usually provide several quality and brand variations for one product; some stores will have their own brand label on many products at a lesser cost than some national brands. In addition, there may be speciality sections for gourmet items, cultural foods, and fresh bakery foods.

Another type of store is the "warehouse" or "U-mark" store. This type of store has a minimum of overhead because it is usually located in a low-rent area, and has a limited number of store fixtures and a minimum of customer services. Marking the price on the container, as well as loading the groceries are performed by the customer. Some food items can be purchased at a substantial saving of approximately 6 to 10 per cent of the regular supermarket price. However, warehouse grocery shopping is more time-consuming, and for the single individual purchasing small amounts of food at any one time, the money that can be saved is usually not enough to make this kind of shopping worthwhile.

The smaller grocery store, usually independently owned and commonly called the "mom and pop" store, is most often located in a heavily populated neighborhood of large cities or in rural areas. These stores handle groceries, fresh meat, and produce with a limited variety of selections. The cost of food items in the small store may be higher than that of the supermarket, but the convenience of shopping there may outweigh this factor. These stores often cater to the cultural food needs of a specific area.

The "convenience" store, which is often chain-owned, has experienced a tremendous growth in the past decade. This type of store is usually open on a 24-hour-a-day basis and sells only those items of which a household is commonly in short supply. The cost of these items can be considerably higher than for the same items purchased at a regular market. The convenience store is now offering more fast-food items, such as hot sandwiches, to meet the needs of working individuals.

Some large department stores have a separate section at which grocery items are sold. The kind of grocery items sold in department stores depends upon the buying power of the store's clientele. For example, a department store selling to higher-income customers will sell specialty and gourmet foods, whereas the store selling to low- and middle-income customers will sell more commonly used food items, many of which will be offered at a discount price. However, all items will not be a bargain and it is important to know and compare prices.

Several interesting trends have emerged over the past decade in the types of stores at which food can be purchased. The chain-operated supermarkets and convenience stores have grown considerably, while the independently owned and home delivery services for bread and milk have decreased sharply. This is indicated in Table 1–4, which shows from what sources food purchases were made. Another interesting growth trend, which is seen in specialty food stores, can be partially accounted for by the customer's demand for more services in an inflationary trend.

All stores are organized to meet the needs of their customers; many markets play background music to make shopping a pleasant experience. In addition to weekly sale items, stores set up food displays at strategic points.

Table 1-4
Sales of Food for Home Use, 1955–75

Type of Seller	1955	1960	1965	1970	1975
			Per Cent		
Supermarkets	27.4	37.2	44.5	50.2	55.9
Convenience stores	.1	.6	.9	2.4	4.5
Other grocery stores	43.0	36.8	32.6	27.3	21.7
Other food stores	11.1	9.9	8.4	8.6	8.8
Other stores	5.9	5.1	5.2	5.1	4.7
Home delivered	8.3	6.5	4.6	3.2	1.7
Farmers, processors, wholesalers, other	4.2	3.9	3.8	3.2	2.7

U.S. Food Expenditures, 1954-78. U.S. Department of Agriculture. Agricultural Economic Report No. 431.

The foods displayed are usually not on sale and should not be purchased unless they are needed items.

Some markets provide unit pricing, which tells the consumer the price per unit of measure, such as the price per pound, ounce, quart, or count. Unit pricing is shown below the food item and is helpful when comparing similar items, such as canned fruit juices. Unit pricing, however, cannot be used to compare unlike items, such as fruit juice with soft drink beverages.

Approximately 10,000 food items now have imprinted on the label the Universal Product Code numbering system. The UPC is a symbol consisting of lines, bars, and numbers which identify both the food manufacturer and the food item. The UPC operates with a computer, which once the bar-code symbol is passed over the scanner, looks up the price of the food and prints the price and describes the food on a detailed cash register receipt. The UPC system has proven to be a great saving to the supermarket not only by increasing the speed of check-out and eliminating error at check-out but also by providing a means of controlling inventory. Figure 1–3 shows the UPC system in operation at the check out stand of a market.

Food should always be purchased on a cost per serving basis. This is determined by dividing the number of servings into the retail price. For example, if a can of green beans costs .28 and the label states that the can contains four servings, the cost is $.07 cents per serving. This cost could then be compared to frozen green beans and fresh green beans, if available, to determine the best buy. Since the price is not printed on the can in stores that have converted to the UPC system, the consumer must train himself or herself to read the price information provided below the can.

An average serving for fruits and vegetables is 1/2 cup, whereas for meats, poultry, and fish, it is 2-1/2 to 3-1/2 ounces, cooked. However, other factors including the particular brand, the time involved in preparation, the age of family members, and personal likes and dislikes also influence the specific kind of food purchased.

As with other goods and services, food costs have risen over the past decade. The high cost of food does not happen at the market but is attributed to the long chain of events that happen before the food reaches the market, including transactions in which the farmer, processor, packer, transporter, and others are involved in the distribution of food in the United States. Involved in each of these stages in food distribution are other factors including weather, labor conditions, export demands, spoilage, and the status of the dollar abroad.

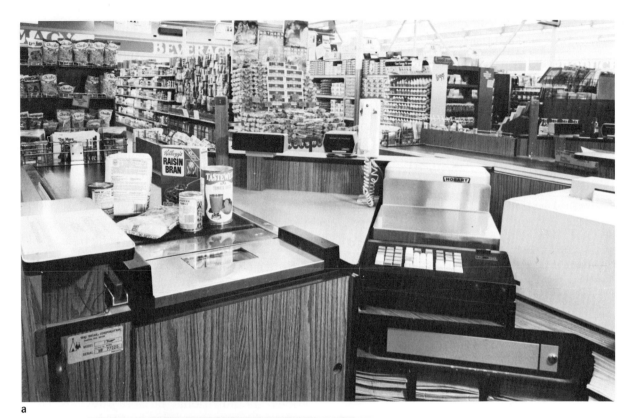

a

b

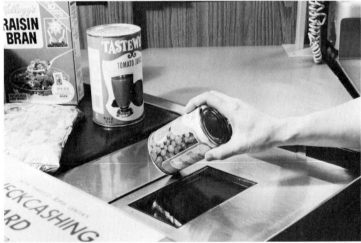

= 12345–67890
(Note: First 5 digits
assigned by UPCC,
Inc.; second 5 by
manufacturer)

c

Figure 1–3.

(a) Supermarkets using the Universal Product Code system have a modernized check-out stand that includes a computer terminal, scale, and display unit providing name of item and price. (b) The bar code symbol on the can or package is passed over the scanner which registers the item and price and records it in inventory. (c) Illustration of how the UPC can be used on a product.

Table 1-5
Breakdown of the Food Dollar

Labor	32.1
Farmers	30.8
Packaging	8.7
Transportation	5.4
Other*	8.4
Profits before federal income tax	4.6
State and local business taxes	2.7
Depreciation	2.0
Rent	1.8
Advertising	1.4
Repairs, bad debt, contributions	1.1
Interest	.9
	100.0

*"Other" expenses include fuel, utilities, insurance, customer service, and losses from spoilage, spillage, and pilferage.
USDA, 1977

Table 1-5, as calculated by the USDA, provides the breakdown of the food dollar and how it is distributed.

Organization for Shopping

How well prepared an individual is for shopping is the single most important factor in food purchasing. This involves planning for meals between shopping intervals, checking for needed food items, and making a list prior to shopping. Individuals who shop without a list are easily influenced by display "pick-up" items, and often spend much money for them. These individuals also tend to forget essential items, requiring them to make an additional shopping trip.

The following are some suggestions to help prepare a shopping list.

1. Plan meals prior to shopping.
2. Plan for sufficient food to last until the next shopping trip.
3. Buy advertised specials and use money-saving coupons if the food will be used.

4. Plan to buy seasonal fresh foods; avoid fresh food that is decayed and bruised.
5. Learn to read labels and know the meaning of various grades.
6. Do not buy damaged cans and packages.
7. Buy the quality of food needed for specific preparations.
8. Buy foods only in amounts that can be stored and used within a safe period of time.
9. Use convenience foods when cost and time warrant their use.
10. Buy foods on a cost per serving basis.

Each chapter in this text dealing with specific foods has a section on food purchasing and available convenience forms of that food, to assist in becoming familiar with the many factors influencing food purchasing.

Nutritional Factors to Consider

Foods are nutritional because they are composed of nutrients needed by the body to keep it nourished. These nutrients are carbohydrate, fat, protein, vitamins, minerals, and water. The basic functions of nutrients are to supply energy to support growth and body maintenance, and to keep the body functioning effectively. Because foods contain varying amounts of nutrients, and some nutrients are needed in larger amounts than others, the consumption of a wide variety of foods is vital to maintaining good health.

Nutrition is the study of food and how it is utilized by the body. As this subject has become one of major interest to the American public, a vast amount of nutrition literature has become available. As nutritional information is read and studied, it is important that there be an understanding of nutrition as based on proven scientific evidence of the specific functions of nutrients. It is of vital importance that food be selected on the basis of its nutrient quality. No single food or nutrient can perform miracles and prevent or cure all ailments. The bibliography at the end of this text provides a list of current books on nutrition. Many of these books will provide the reader with more in-depth information on nutrition.

Carbohydrates

Carbohydrate is the major, energy-providing nutrient in the American diet, with approximately 50 to 60 per cent of all calories consumed coming from foods that are high in carbohydrate. Carbohydrates are found in plants and are commonly called sugars, starches, and cellulose. With the exception of milk, animal foods contain, if any, only a minimal amount of carbohydrate.

One way to classify carbohydrates is by the terms *monosaccharides*, *disaccharides*, and *polysaccharides*. Monosaccharides are the simple sugars and occur as fructose in honey and glucose in ripe fruits. Sucrose, maltose, and lactose are disaccharides, which means that they can be broken into two monosaccharides upon hydrolysis or the addition of water. Sucrose is mainly found in cane or beet sugar; lactose is the sugar present in milk; and maltose is derived from germinating cereals. Since all carbohydrate with the exception of cellulose is broken down to the simple sugar, glucose, during the digestive process to be absorbed into the system, there is no advantage to consuming honey over other forms of carbohydrate. Both monosaccharides and disaccharides taste sweet and are water-soluble.

Polysaccharides are found in foods including cereals, breads, legumes, pastas, and vegetables that are high in starch. Root, tuber, and seed vegetables such as carrots, potatoes, and corn are higher in starch than the leafy and stalk type vegetables such as lettuce and celery. Upon hydrolysis a polysaccharide is broken

into three or more monosaccharides. Cellulose, which forms the structural walls for grains, fruits, and vegetables, is found mainly in the bran of grains and in leafy and stalk vegetables. The human body lacks the necessary enzyme to digest cellulose, but cellulose is important for providing bulk to the diet and moving food through the digestive system.

Because the source of carbohydrates is plants, they are the least expensive source of energy. Protein and carbohydrate are the lowest-calorie sources of energy for the body. Carbohydrate and protein each furnish 4 calories per gram. Carbohydrate is called a "protein-sparer" nutrient, for the reason that if enough carbohydrate is present in the diet to provide energy, the body will not have to convert protein to energy, so that protein is allowed to do its primary function. Another important function of carbohydrate is in the proper utilization of fat.

For a nutritionally balanced diet, carbohydrate foods should be selected that contain other nutrients such as protein, vitamins, and minerals. These foods can be selected from fruits, vegetables, cereal grains or products made from cereal grains. Foods such as soft drinks, candies, most desserts, and frosting contain mainly sugar and should be eaten only when other nutrient requirements have been met. There is no nutritional advantage to consuming raw sugar, blackstrap molasses, or unbleached flour.

Fat

Fat is the second major energy-provider, contributing 40 to 50 per cent of the total calorie content of the American diet. However, it is recommended by many members of the medical profession, and by nutritionists as well, that this amount be reduced to 30 to 35 per cent. One of the reasons for the American diet being so high in fat is the increased consumption of foods fried in deep fat such as french

Table 1-6

Total Meat Consumption in the United States
  (Beef, Veal, Pork, Lamb, and Mutton)

Year	All Meat Consumption Per Capita Pounds
1920	136
1940	142.4
1960[1]	160.9
1970	186.3
1971	191.8
1972	189.0
1973	175.7
1974	188.0
1975	181.1
1976	193.4
1977	193.0
1978*	186.1

[1] Data for 50 states beginning in 1960.
* Preliminary.
Meatfacts. A Statistical Summary about America's
Largest Food Industry. American Meat Institute,
June 1979.

fries, chicken, and seafood. Other contributing factors to the increased consumption of fat are the eating of many foods served with rich cream sauces and the high consumption of meat in most American diets, as shown in Table 1-6.

Lipid is the common term used to encompass all fats, oils, and fatlike substances. A fat is a combination of fatty acids and glycerol and is further classified as saturated, unsaturated, or polyunsaturated, depending on the chemical composition of the fat. Saturated fats are animal fats, including the fat in meat, whole milk, butter, cheese and ice cream. The major sources of polyunsaturated and unsaturated fats are plant foods and include vegetable oils, margarine, and nuts.

Fats have almost twice the energy value of either protein or carbohydrate, with 1 gram of fat furnishing 9 calories. Thus, with a small amount of fat present in the diet the body can more efficiently utilize the protein and carbo-

hydrate. However, an excess of fat will be stored in the body. In addition to the energy contribution that fats make to the diet, they may be important for the absorption of the fat-soluble vitamins A, D, E, and K and in some cases are important carriers of these vitamins. Fats provide a cushion for body organs, form part of the structure of cells, and act as protein-sparers. Because fats take longer to digest than protein or carbohydrate, they provide a longer satiety value. Fats also make food more tender and flavorful.

Cholesterol, a fat-related compound, is found in foods of animal origin such as eggs, meats, and dairy products. Cholesterol is essential to certain body processes and is also synthesized by the body.

Protein

Protein is the nutrient responsible for the growth, maintenance, and repair of body tissue and for the regulation of body processes. The body is also capable of converting protein into energy if enough fat and carbohydrate are not present to meet the body's energy needs. One gram of protein yields an average of 4 calories. If protein is not needed by the body, it is stored as body fat. Protein contributes approximately 10 to 15 per cent of the total calorie content of the American diet. Protein malnutrition still exists in this country because of the expense of purchasing high quality protein foods and ignorance in food selection.

Proteins are composed of amino acids. To date, 22 amino acids have been isolated. Nine amino acids are considered "essential," meaning they cannot be synthesized by the body.[1] Other amino acids can be synthesized by the body providing the essential nine are present. Foods that contain the nine essential amino acids are called "complete" proteins. Animal

[1] Corine H. Robinson, *Fundamentals of Normal Nutrition*, 3rd ed. Macmillan Publishing Co., 1978.

foods are all complete proteins with the exception of gelatin, which is incomplete.

"Partially complete" proteins can maintain body processes but can not promote growth. "Incomplete" proteins, such as those found in plants, cannot promote either maintenance or growth. These two categories of protein are found in the plant and cereal food groups. Incomplete and partially complete protein foods can be made complete by combining them with a small amount of a complete protein. For example, cereal can be combined with milk, spaghetti with a meat sauce, or lima beans with ham. It is also possible to combine two incomplete proteins, which lack differing amino acids, and make a complete protein food.

Vitamins

Vitamins are organic substances found in foods that, although they do not provide energy, are essential for the release of energy from carbohydrates, fats, and proteins. Vitamins are also essential to growth and to the maintenance of proper body functioning, and also aid in the prevention of certain illnesses and diseases. However, there is no miracle cure from vitamins alone. The body must have adequate supplies of the other major nutrients provided by food to promote and maintain a healthy status. Usually, there is no need to buy and take additional vitamin supplements, because vitamins are needed in such minute amounts. Exceptions to this are certain diseases and diets that require special vitamin supplementation. In these cases vitamins should be taken only when prescribed by a doctor.

Vitamins are classified as water-soluble and fat-soluble. Water-soluble vitamins are the B vitamins and vitamin C, ascorbic acid. Water soluble may be readily lost during cooking. For this reason it is important to save and use the juices in which meats, fruits, and vegetables are cooked. Fat-soluble vitamins are not soluble in water, and excesses of these vitamins can be stored in the body.

The following discussion of specific vitamins and their functions and food sources, only highlights some of the major roles that vitamins play in a well-balanced diet.

Water-Soluble Vitamins. Thiamine (vitamin B_1) is important for the proper utilization of carbohydrate and for the maintenance of a healthy nervous system. It is particularly needed by individuals consuming high calorie diets, such as young people and those doing heavy physical work. Some major sources of thiamine include meats, milk, and enriched or whole-grain breads and cereals.

Riboflavin (vitamin B_2) functions to maintain healthy eyes and the tissues of the lips and mouth. It is important in the body's proper metabolism of protein, fat, and carbohydrate. Sources of riboflavin include milk, meats, green leafy vegetables, eggs, and enriched breads and cereals.

Niacin (vitamin B_3) also aids in the metabolism of the major nutrients, and in the healthy functioning of the digestive tract and the nervous system. The major sources of niacin are meat, poultry, fish, and whole-grain or enriched breads and cereals.

Other important B vitamins that are essential in the functioning of a healthy system include folacin, pantothenic acid, pyridoxine (vitamin B_6), and cobalamin (vitamin B_{12}).

Ascorbic acid (vitamin C) is important for the normal healing of wounds, the prevention of infection, the strengthening of the walls of blood vessels, and the proper utilization of iron. Its main food sources are citrus fruits, cabbage, tomatoes, potatoes, raw leafy vegetables, strawberries, and melons.

The Fat-Soluble Vitamins. Vitamin A helps to maintain a healthy condition of many tissues in the body, promotes skeletal growth, and is essential to healthy eye conditions. Animal foods in which vitamin A is highly concentrated include fish liver oils, liver, butter and egg yolk. Plant sources also contain a precursor to vitamin A, called *carotene*, which is converted to vitamin A in the body. Deep-green and yellow vegetables are good sources of carotene, including leafy green vegetables, corn, sweet potatoes, and carrots.

Vitamin D aids in the proper absorption of calcium and phosphorus; the best food source of this vitamin is milk, fortified, with vitamin D. The vitamin can also be obtained by exposure to sunshine.

Vitamin E is important in the control of several blood disorders, such as certain anemias in infants, and serves to prevent the oxidative breakdown of unsaturated fatty acids. The richest source of vitamin E is vegetable oils.

Vitamin K is necessary for the formation of prothrombin, which is the clotting agent of blood. Good sources of vitamin K include green leafy vegetables and vegetable oils.

Minerals

Minerals are inorganic substances that must be furnished by food. Found in both the hard and soft tissues of the body, minerals are important for the formation of healthy bones and teeth, the regulation of body processes, and the functioning of nerves and muscles. Since minerals are found in many foods and are needed in only minute amounts, the intake of only three of these minerals may be inadequate. The following discussion relates to these three minerals.

Calcium is important for the proper growth and maintenance of bones and muscles, the clotting of blood, and a healthy nervous system. The main source of calcium is milk and other dairy products; other good sources of calcium include dark green leafy vegetables, such as collards or mustard greens, and dried beans.

Iron is important for the formulation of red blood cells and hemoglobin, which carries oxygen to the cells. It is the one mineral that is difficult for women and children to receive an adequate amount of unless sufficient servings of meat, particularly organ meats, egg yolk, and green vegetables are eaten.

Iodine is needed to produce thyroxine, a hormone in the thyroid gland, which regulates the metabolic processes of the body. Some areas of the country have a low incidence of iodine in the soil; in these areas it is advisable to always purchase iodized salt. Other good sources of iodine are saltwater fish and shellfish.

Water

It is difficult to single out one nutrient that is needed more than another, but without water in the diet, death will occur within a few days. Fortunately, water is available in all foods that are eaten, in addition to the various liquids which are drunk. The average adult needs to consume five to six glasses of liquid per day; the balance of the body's need for water is met by consuming solid foods.

The principal functions of water are to act as a transport for carrying the various other nutrients to the cells, to aid in the digestion of nutrients, to serve as a lubricant, and to regulate body temperature. Water is also an important component of all cell structures.

Calorie

A calorie is a method of measurement for determining the amount of energy or heat that is available in a food. Some foods yield more energy than others. Fats produce almost twice as much energy as protein or carbohydrate. Vitamins and minerals produce no energy but are necessary for the proper production of energy from fat, carbohydrate, and protein. The terms *calorie* and *kilocalorie* may be used synonymously.

Nutrient Needs of Specific Individuals

All individuals, including the unborn child, have a need for each of the nutrients just discussed. However, the age, activity, body size, sex, and various growth stages of an individual help to determine specific amounts.

Pregnancy. One of the most important factors that has a bearing on a healthy pregnancy is the nutritional state of the mother prior to conception. In other words, body health and nutrient reserves cannot be built at the onset of pregnancy. This is of particular concern to the teenager, who often has a poor diet and whose own body has not completed its final growth. Because the unborn child depends completely on the mother for its food supply, it is vital that all nutrients be furnished each day. Calcium and iron are the two nutrients that must be consumed during pregnancy in greater amounts than during other periods of life. Calcium intake is easily met by consuming three or more glasses of milk per day, but the iron needs of 18 milligrams per day can barely be met if the diet is well balanced with two servings of meat, four or more servings of fruits and vegetables, and four servings of whole-grain or enriched breads and cereals. Because liver is an excellent source of iron, it should be included often in the diet of a pregnant woman.

During the last part of pregnancy, there may be a need to increase the diet by 200 calories per day to assure continued health of both mother and child. The average weight gain of the mother during pregnancy is 24 pounds.

Nursing Mothers. Nursing mothers have an increased need for protein to produce the milk needed by the infant. This is easily met by the consumption of four to six glasses of milk per day and two generous servings of meat, plus one egg daily. Other dietary requirements are easily met by following the diet pattern of pregnancy.

Infants. The first year of life is the fastest growing period of a human life and careful attention must be paid to nutrients the infant receives. During the first six months of infancy, the principal food is milk. In technologically developed countries such as the United States infants grow and thrive on several different dietary programs. The infant may be breast fed or be fed with a formula of cow's milk, evaporated milk, or a milk or soy-based commercially prepared formula.

While there is some controversy regarding the need to supplement the diet of an exclusively breast-fed infant, it is generally recommended that these infants be provided with a daily supplementation of 400 I. U.'s of vitamin D. It is also recommended that the infant who is fed human milk receive 7 milligrams of iron daily and 0.25 milligrams of fluoride per day. During the initial few days of life a vitamin K supplement is also recommended. These supplements must be physician prescribed.

If the infant is fed a commercially prepared iron-fortified formula, supplements of other vitamins and minerals are generally not recommended. If recommended, they must be prescribed by a physician.

Infants less than six months of age may be fed a formula made with evaporated milk. Infants receiving these formulas may need supplements of vitamin C and iron. Supplements must be prescribed by a physician.

At six months of age infants can be fed homogenized vitamin D fortified milk if they are receiving an amount of strained food equivalent to 1.5 jars of a commercially prepared strained infant food. These infants need either a supplement or a food source of vitamin C and iron. Food sources of vitamin C for the infant include strained fruits or juice. The food source for iron can be a fortified infant dry cereal which is diluted with milk when served or cooked egg yolk.

Research today indicates there is no benefit to introducing solid foods before six months of age. However, many infants are introduced to solid foods as early as the first four to six weeks of life.

Preschool. At the start of the second year, the infant's growth rate begins to slow down and its food consumption sharply drops. During the preschool years, basic food habits and attitudes toward food develop as the child's independence increases. Foods need to be carefully selected and planned for preschoolers. They consume smaller portions of food at any one time, but may need to eat more often. Snacks should be provided that help meet their nutrient needs. Some good snacks for this age group include milk, cheese, crackers, fruits, and vegetables. Because the teeth develop at varying stages, some preschoolers may not have full chewing capacity, and it is most important to avoid foods such as popcorn, nuts, and large pieces of firm fruits and vegetables on which they may choke.

School to Teen. In these formative years, breakfast, lunch, and dinner become very important parts of the dietary pattern. The child no longer is in a situation in which food is readily available throughout the day. School-age children need breakfast to perform at a satisfactory level throughout the day. It has been demonstrated that children who do not eat breakfast are apathetic during school hours. Many times lunch is a hurried and an interrupted meal in a lunchroom setting. Most

children need nutritious, well-planned snacks after school. If good snacks are not available, children will ease their hunger by consuming "empty-calorie" foods.

Teen Years. Second only to the infant, this is the fastest growth stage of human development. Unless teenagers have developed sound food habits in their younger years, nutritional deficiencies may occur between the ages of 13 and 18. Teenage girls are particularly vulnerable to poor eating patterns, probably as a result of the continued emphasis on being slim. Teenage boys have a slightly better food consumption pattern, but teenagers of both sexes are prone to fill their hunger needs with empty-calorie and convenience foods. This can in part account for the deficiency of calcium, ascorbic acid, and vitamin A found in many teenage diets. Most teenage girls have an inadequate intake of iron.

Adult Years. Adult status is reached somewhere between the ages of 18 and 21, when the body stops growing. Throughout the adult years the body's activity also slows down. For some individuals, this may mean an increase in weight, unless the food portions eaten become smaller. The body still needs all of the important nutrients required during the growing years for maintenance, repair, and good health. Adults do need to watch the intake of saturated fats, as well as the calories consumed in snacks and cocktails. Many adults tend to eliminate milk from the diet, but the body needs an adequate supply of calcium and phosporus, which can be met by consuming one or two glasses of milk a day. Women need to watch carefully their iron intake and consume foods that meet this requirement.

The senior adult may experience eating problems different from the younger person. Dietary changes often have to be made by the older person because of health problems. Some "seniors" experience chewing difficulty because of the loss of teeth, whereas others may lose interest in eating for psychological and social reasons. However, the nutrient needs do not change. Many senior adults prefer to eat smaller meals and eat more often.

Guides to Selecting Nutrients

Several guides have been developed by nutritional experts to aid both the professional and the lay person to select foods that will assure adequate nutritional status for the individual. An understanding of the basic principles of nutrition will also enhance the individual's selection and consumption of food and thus provide additional assurance that the individual will receive adequate nourishment.

Dietary Guidelines for Americans

In February 1980, the U.S. Department of Agriculture and the U.S. Department of Health, Education and Welfare issued seven dietary guidelines for healthy people to help them maintain their state of well-being. These guidelines are not intended for use by those individuals who need special diets because of disease or conditions that interfere with normal nutrition. These people need special diets and instructions from dietitians in consultation with their physician.

1. *Eat a variety of food.* If foods are selected from a variety of food sources including fruits and vegetables; whole grain and enriched breads, cereals, and grain products; milk, cheese, and yogurt; meats, poultry, fish, and eggs; and, legumes, there is seldom a need to take a vitamin or mineral supplement. The exceptions to this general statement include women who are in the childbearing years who may

need to take an iron supplement to replace iron lost with menstrual bleeding; women who are pregnant or who are breastfeeding who may need additional nutrients such as iron, folic acid, vitamin A, calcium, and the major nutrients; elderly or inactive people who eat little food; and infants, depending on the type of nourishment they are receiving.

2. *Maintain ideal weight.* For most people the ideal weight that should be maintained throughout a lifetime, is that which the individual weighs between the ages of 20 to 25 years of age. This would not be the ideal weight for the individual who was underweight or overweight during this time period. Overweight is associated with such health problems as high blood pressure, increased levels of blood fats, increased levels of cholesterol, common types of diabetes, and the increased risks of heart attacks and strokes.

If weight needs to be lost, it is recommended that a steady loss of 1 to 2 pounds per week be achieved by a better eating program and increased physical activity. A better eating program consists of eating foods that contain the needed nutrients in a caloric range of more than 800 calories per day, eating slowly, eating smaller portions and avoiding seconds. The specific calorie needs of an individual attempting to lose weight are determined by such factors as age, sex, metabolic needs and physical activity. Diets under 800 calories per day can prove to be hazardous to one's health. Usually a diet that provides 1200 to 1500 calories per day allows the individual to successfully lose 1 to 2 pounds per week.

3. *Avoid too much fat, saturated fat, and cholesterol.* The diets of many individuals in the United States have tended to be high in foods that contain saturated fats

and cholesterol. Many of these individuals exhibit a greater chance of heart attack. The American diet can be improved by selecting lean meat, fish, poultry, dry beans and peas and by moderating the use of eggs and organ meats such as liver. The intake of butter, cream, hydrogenated margarines, shortening, coconut oil, and foods made from such products should also be limited. Frying as a cooking medium should be substituted by broiling, baking, or boiling whenever possible. Reading labels can help one determine the amount and type of fat that a food contains.

4. *Eat foods with adequate starch and fiber.* As the fat portion of the diet is decreased, more energy can be provided by increasing carbohydrate consumption. Carbohydrates should be selected that contain other nutrients plus calories. These include foods such as whole grain and enriched breads and cereals, beans, peas, nuts, seeds, fruits, and vegetables. As these foods are increased in the daily diet, the consumption of needed dietary fiber also increases. Carbohydrates such as sugars contain little more than calories.

5. *Avoid too much sugar.* It is estimated that the individual American consumes more than 130 pounds of sugars and sweeteners per year. Sugar is a major cause of tooth decay and its consumption can also be a factor in obesity. It is important for good health that the consumption of foods that contain sugar as a major ingredient be watched closely. Foods high in sugar include jams, jellies, candies, cookies, soft drinks, cakes, pies, sugar coated cereals, catsup, flavored milks, and ice cream.

6. *Avoid too much sodium.* Sodium is a major ingredient in table salt, potato chips, pretzels, salted nuts, soy sauce, specially flavored salts, cheese, pickled foods, and cured meats. Americans consume much more sodium than is needed; it is one of the factors affecting high blood pressure. Intake can be reduced by using less table salt and restricting the intake of foods known to be high in sodium.

7. *If you drink alcohol, do so in moderation.* Although one or two drinks do not appear to cause harm to adults, alcoholic beverages are high in calories and low in other nutrients. Heavy drinkers may not consume foods with necessary nutrients in the appropriate amounts and the alcohol may limit the body's proper absorption and utilization of some essential nutrients. Pregnant women should consume no more than 2 ounces of alcohol per day.

The Recommended Daily Dietary Allowances (RDA), set by the Food and Nutrition Board of the National Academy of Sciences, is used as a guide to safeguard the health of the nation. The RDA serves as a resource base in the establishment of government nutrition programs, research in food-product development, and the amounts of food needed by different portions of the population. The RDA provides the average amount of specific nutrients needed by normal Americans to promote growth in children and to maintain good health for all. The RDA is revised approximately every 5 years to include current research findings and to adjust to changing living patterns. Although the RDA can be used by all individuals, nutrient calculations and evaluations are time consuming and need to be evaluated by a professional who is knowledgeable in the science of nutrition. The RDA is thus most often used by people in this field. Table 1-7 is the revised RDA, 1980.

In addition to the Recommended Daily Dietary Allowance, Revised 1980, the 9th revised edition also includes a table showing the ranges of estimated safe and adequate intakes for 12 additional nutrients and a table showing the recommended energy intakes relative to mean heights and weights for individuals.

The U.S. Recommended Daily Allowances (U.S. RDA), which is based on the Recommended Daily Dietary Allowance, is directed by the Food and Drug Administration. The U.S. RDA is used in nutrition labeling and is further discussed in Chapter 3, "Food Safety."

Other nutritional guides have been developed to help the individual determine what foods provide the needed nutrients. The two most commonly used guides are the Basic 4 Food Groups and the Basic 7. The Basic 4 food groups include milk, meat, vegetables and fruits, and breads and cereals. The Basic 7 are similar to the Basic 4 except that the vegetable and fruit group is separated into citrus fruits, green and yellow vegetables, and other fruits and vegetables, and it includes an additional group for fats, including butter, margarine, and oils.

In 1979, the USDA added a fifth group to the Basic 4, which is commonly called the "Fats-Sweets-Alcohol" group.[1] This group encompasses foods, which are commonly eaten by individuals, that contain mainly calories and few, if any, nutrients. The following is a discussion of the Basic 5 food groups, which are illustrated in Figure 1-4.

Milk. The milk group includes all milk and dairy products, including various forms of milk, cheese, and ice cream. The milk group is an excellent source of high-quality protein, calcium, and riboflavin. Whole milk is a good source of vitamin A, and many forms of milk are fortified with both vitamin A and vitamin D. The calorie intake from milk can be decreased by consuming nonfat milk. The recom-

mended consumption for milk is: for children under 9, two to three glasses a day; for children 9 to 12 and pregnant mothers, three or more glasses a day; teenagers and nursing mothers, four or more glasses a day; and for adults, two or more glasses per day. The calcium equivalent of milk can be met by substituting 1-1/4 ounces of cheddar cheese for a glass of milk; 1/2 cup of creamed cottage cheese for 1/3 glass of milk, or 1/2 cup ice cream for 1/4 glass of milk.

Meat. The meat group includes meats, fish, poultry, eggs, legumes, and nuts. These are all high-quality protein foods, but legumes and nuts contain only about 30 per cent of the protein available from animal foods. Other important nutrients are the B vitamins and iron. It is recommended that all people receive two or more servings daily from this group. This need can be met with a 3- to 4-ounce serving of cooked lean meat, poultry, or fish; 1 cup of cooked dry beans, dry peas, or lentils; 1/4 cup peanut butter or 1 egg. One-quarter cup to 1/2 cut of sesame seeds or sunflower seeds can be counted as 1 ounce of meat, poultry, or fish.

Vegetables and Fruits. Deep-green and yellow vegetables are excellent sources of vitamin A, and it is recommended that a serving be included in the diet every other day. A citrus fruit or another fruit or vegetables high in vitamin C should be eaten each day. Other fruits and vegetables may be used to complete the recommended four servings daily from this group. Fruits and vegetables as a group add important amounts of the B vitamins, many minerals and carbohydrates, and also adds important bulk, dietary fiber, to the diet. An average serving is 1/2 cup.

Breads and Cereals. Four or more servings of whole-grain or enriched breads and cereals

---

[1] Henrietta Fleck, *Introduction to Nutrition.* 4th ed. New York: Macmillan Pub. Co., 1981.

Table 1–7
Recommended Daily Dietary Allowances,[a] Revised 1980

	Age (years)	Weight (kg)	Weight (lbs)	Height (cm)	Height (in)	Protein (g)	Fat-Soluble Vitamins Vitamin A (µg R.E.)[b]	Vitamin D (µg)[c]	Vitamin E (mg α T.E.)[d]
Infants	0.0–0.5	6	13	60	24	kg × 2.2	420	10	3
	0.5–1.0	9	20	71	28	kg × 2.0	400	10	4
Children	1–3	13	29	90	35	23	400	10	5
	4–6	20	44	112	44	30	500	10	6
	7–10	28	62	132	52	34	700	10	7
Males	11–14	45	99	157	62	45	1000	10	8
	15–18	66	145	176	69	56	1000	10	10
	19–22	70	154	177	70	56	1000	7.5	10
	23–50	70	154	178	70	56	1000	5	10
	51+	70	154	178	70	56	1000	5	10
Females	11–14	46	101	157	62	46	800	10	8
	15–18	55	120	163	64	46	800	10	8
	19–22	55	120	163	64	44	800	7.5	8
	23–50	55	120	163	64	44	800	5	8
	51+	55	120	163	64	44	800	5	8
Pregnant						+30	+200	+5	+2
Lactating						+20	+400	+5	+3

[a] The allowances are intended to provide for individual variations among most normal persons as they live in the United States under usual environmental stresses. Diets should be based on a variety of common foods in order to provide other nutrients for which human requirements have been less well defined.

[b] Retinol equivalents. 1 Retinol equivalent = 1 µg retinol or 6 µg β carotene. See text for calculation of vitamin A activity of diets as retinol equivalents.

[c] As cholecalciferol. 10 µg cholecalciferol = 400 I.U. vitamin D.

[d] α-tocopherol equivalents. 1 mg d-α-tocopherol.

[e] 1 N.E. (niacin equivalent) is equal to 1 mg of niacin or 60 mg of dietary tryptophan.

[f] The folacin allowances refer to dietary sources as determined by *Lactobacillus casei* assay after treatment with enzymes ("conjugases") to make polyglutamyl forms of the vitamin available to the test organism.

Water-Soluble Vitamins							Minerals					
Vitamin C (mg)	Thiamin (mg)	Riboflavin (mg)	Niacin (mg N.E.)[e]	Vitamin B_6 (mg)	Folacin[f] (µg)	Vitamin B_{12} (µg)	Calcium (mg)	Phosphorus (mg)	Magnesium (mg)	Iron (mg)	Zinc (mg)	Iodine (ug)
35	0.3	0.4	6	0.3	30	0.5[g]	360	240	50	10	3	40
35	0.5	0.6	8	0.6	45	1.5	540	360	70	15	5	50
45	0.7	0.8	9	0.9	100	2.0	800	800	150	15	10	70
45	0.9	1.0	11	1.3	200	2.5	800	800	200	10	10	90
45	1.2	1.4	16	1.6	300	3.0	800	800	250	10	10	120
50	1.4	1.6	18	1.8	400	3.0	1200	1200	350	18	15	150
60	1.4	1.7	18	2.0	400	3.0	1200	1200	400	18	15	150
60	1.5	1.7	19	2.2	400	3.0	800	800	350	10	15	150
60	1.4	1.6	18	2.2	400	3.0	800	800	350	10	15	150
60	1.2	1.4	16	2.2	400	3.0	800	800	350	10	15	150
50	1.1	1.3	15	1.8	400	3.0	1200	1200	300	18	15	150
60	1.1	1.3	14	2.0	400	3.0	1200	1200	300	18	15	150
60	1.1	1.3	14	2.0	400	3.0	800	800	300	18	15	150
60	1.0	1.2	13	2.0	400	3.0	800	800	300	18	15	150
60	1.0	1.2	13	2.0	400	3.0	800	800	300	10	15	150
+20	+0.4	+0.3	+2	+0.6	+400	+1.0	+400	+400	+150	h	+5	+25
+40	+0.5	+0.5	+5	+0.5	+100	+1.0	+400	+400	+150	h	+10	+50

[g] The RDA for vitamin B_{12} in infants is based on average concentration of the vitamin in human milk. The allowances after weaning are based on energy intake (as recommended by the American Academy of Pediatrics) and consideration of other factors such as intestinal absorption.

[h] The increased requirement during pregnancy cannot be met by the iron content of habitual American diets nor by the existing iron stores of many women; therefore the use of 30–60 mg of supplemental iron is recommended. Iron needs during lactation are not substantially different from those of nonpregnant women, but continued supplementation of the mother for 2-3 months after parturition is advisable in order to replenish stores depleted by pregnancy.

Food and Nutrition Board. *Recommended Dietary Allowances, 9th Revised Edition.* Washington, D.C.: National Academy of Sciences, National Research Council, 1980.

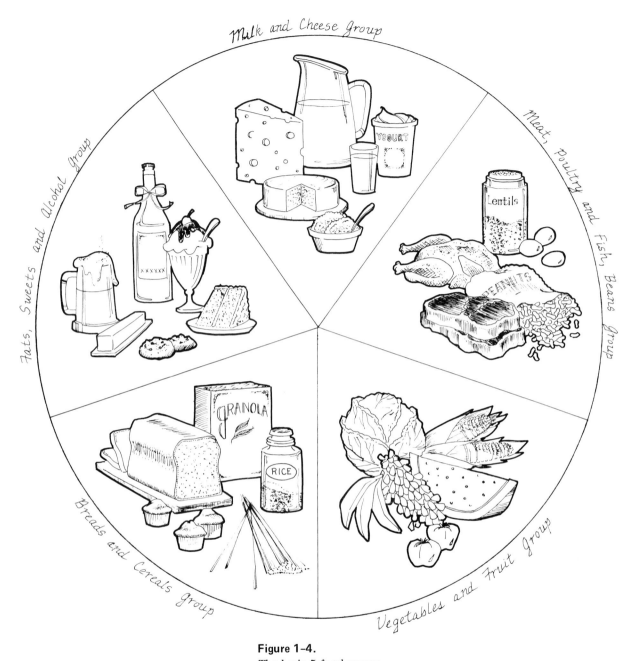

Figure 1-4.
The basic 5 food groups.

should be eaten each day. An average serving is one slice of bread; 1/2 to 3/4 cup of cooked cereal, cornmeal, grits, macaroni, noodles, rice, or spaghetti; or 1 ounce of ready-to-eat cereal. This group is an important contributor of the B vitamins, iron, and carbohydrate. Some protein is also added.

Fats-Sweets-Alcohol. Foods in this group include fats, such as butter or margarine, and foods high in fat content, such as mayonnaise and salad dressing; foods high in sugar content, such as candy, sugar, jams, jellies, and other sweets and sweet toppings; highly sugared beverages, such as soft drinks; and alcoholic beverages. There are no recommended servings for this food group. Some of the foods in this group are ingredients in food products, and other foods in the group, such as butter or margarine, are added to food at the table. With the exception of the foods, which are high in fat content, the nutrient level of these foods is minimal and their calorie content is high. Therefore, it is wise to concentrate any additional food intake on the first four food groups.

A daily eating plan following the Basic four food groups can vary widely in its calorie content, depending on the foods selected. The average diet from the Basic four food groups contains approximately 1,200 to 1,400 calories. Most individuals need additional food to provide the energy needed for activity.

Chemical Factors Affecting Food Preparation

Although this text is not designed to provide an in-depth study of the chemical changes that occur when food is prepared, it is important to understand some of changes that occur in food as it is prepared. These explanations will serve as a constant referral as food is studied.

Enzymes

An enzyme is a protein produced by a living substance that acts as a catalyst to allow certain chemical transformations to take place. The following examples provide some illustrations of how enzymes function in food preparation.

1. Enzymes are responsible for the breaking down of the disaccharide sucrose to glucose and fructose.
2. Enzymes are responsible for the ripening of fruit.
3. The enzyme, papain, found in the papaya fruit can be used to tenderize meat.
4. Fresh pineapple cannot be used in a gelled salad because the enzyme, bromelin, found in fresh pineapple hydrolyzes the protein in gelatin and prevents gelation.

Hydrolysis

Hydrolysis is a term used to describe the breakdown of a compound by the addition of water. Several examples of this in food preparation are noted.

1. The heating of a starch with an acid such as lemon juice breaks the starch into smaller polysaccharide units with the result having less thickening power. This is why the acid, lemon juice, for a lemon pie filling is added after the sauce has thickened.
2. When foods, which naturally contain water, are deep fried, the water causes the breakdown of the fat into glycerol and fatty acids. The free fatty acids cause the smoke point to lower.
3. When sugar is hydrolyzed, the resulting components are glucose and fructose.

pH

This term on a scale of 1 to 14 describes the acidity or alkalinity of a food with pH 7 being neutral. Water has a pH of 7. Foods high in acidity have a pH below 7 and foods high in alkalinity have a value above 7. Baking soda and baking powder are both alkaline in value; whereas, cream of tartar and vinegar are acidic in nature. The quality of many food products can be improved or made worse by the pH value.

1. Vegetables have a low acidic content and the addition of baking soda when cooking vegetables creates a mushy texture.
2. Baking soda is used in recipes calling for sour milk or molasses to decrease the amount of acid.

3. A baked product with a higher pH will have a browner crust and a finer texture.

Fermentation

Fermentation is the breakdown of a compound without the use of oxygen. Substances causing fermentation to take place include bacteria and yeast.

1. A yeast bread rises by the breakdown of the sugar by the yeast present. This causes carbon dioxide and alcohol to form.
2. Cheese is produced by the bacterial fermentation of milk.
3. Fermentation is the process by which cucumbers are transformed into pickles.

LEARNING ACTIVITIES

1. Survey a group of 20 people outside of class to find out their most popular convenience foods. Report your findings to the class.
2. If possible, compare the eating patterns of a traditional working family and a single individual to determine the differences in their eating patterns. Report your analysis to the class.
3. Interview a paid working mother or an active volunteer in the community to determine how she makes food selections to fit her family needs.
4. Interview an individual who is the sole support of a family unit to find out the difficulties encountered by that person in planning nutritious and creative meals for family members.
5. Interview a senior citizen who is living as a single person to find out what his or her life-style of eating is.
6. Make an analysis of the discoveries in number 3, 4, and 5 and report to the class.
7. Conduct a survey in class to discover what psychological meanings each student attaches to food. Make a chart noting similarities and differences.
8. Have a group of 10 people make a list of their 10 most-liked foods and 10 most-disliked foods; see if they can trace the reasons for their choices. Report your findings to the class.
9. For 1 week keep track of the foods you eat in a social setting. Note if there were any reasons why eating made the occasion a more sociable situation.
10. Make a list of foods that you like because they are associated with your cultural heritage. Share with class members 1 recipe that reflects your cultural background.
11. Keep a chart for 1 week of the number of times you eat snack foods, and deter-

---

mine the nutrient content of these foods.

12. Make a survey of the fast-food outlets in your community and determine the cost for one meal at each of them. Figure the cost for feeding a family dinner at one of these outlets, and decide what nutrients might be lacking because of this type of meal.

13. For 3 days, survey the food advertising on television and determine whether what is being advertised is a healthful addition to your knowledge. Make a list of the advantages and disadvantages of television food advertising from what you have learned.

14. Make a list of the different types of grocery stores found in your locality. Compare the prices of three food items in each of these stores and analyze the results.

15. Compare the unit pricing of three products and decide whether this would be beneficial in making a decision of what to purchase.

16. If possible, compare the food costs of a family with two preschool children and one with two teenagers.

17. Read the suggestions for preparing a shopping list in this chapter; add other helpful ideas after doing additional reading and interviews.

18. Design a menu for 1 day for an 8-year-old child that is responsible for feeding him or herself; be sure that the menu meets the nutrient needs of the Basic 4 food groups.

19. Make a survey of 18- to 21-year-olds to determine their food intake for 3 days; analyze this information to determine if the daily intakes provides the necessary nutrients.

20. Compare the diets of two male and two female teenagers to determine if these individuals could be lacking in calcium, iron, and ascorbic acid from what they had consumed. Make a list of foods that could be added to their diets to improve them.

21. Compare the diets of two individuals, one who eats breakfast and one who does not, to note if there is any difference in the daily nutrient intake of these individuals.

22. Investigate 10 school-age children to find out when they eat snacks and what their favorite snacks are. Determine if these snacks contribute to a healthful diet.

23. Contact a local governmental agency to find out what government food programs are available in your local area and how many people these programs assist.

24. Do a research paper on the advantages and disadvantages of the Food Stamp Program and share your findings with the class.

25. Visit a day-care center for preschool children to find out what type of eating program is planned for the children. Find out what guidelines are used for planning menus and what the average cost is for serving each child.

REVIEW QUESTIONS

1. What are five factors that influence how food is selected and eaten?

2. What is the approximate percentage of take-home pay spent on food?

3. What are two good points and two poor points that advertising can influence on food purchasing?
4. What are the characteristics of the five basic types of food stores? Which types are the best for most major food purchasing?
5. How is unit pricing used?
6. How is the cost per serving determined when purchasing food?
7. What are five items that should be considered prior to shopping?
8. What are the six major nutrients?
9. What is meant by the term *nutrition*?
10. Why should some nutrition literature be carefully evaluated?
11. What are carbohydrates? From what food sources do they come?
12. What are the three classes of carbohydrates?
13. Why is carbohydrate called a protein-sparer?
14. What is the value of cellulose in the diet?
15. Why are carbohydrates a better source of energy than protein?
16. What is the recommended calorie portion of fats in the diet?
17. What are five functions of fat in the diet?
18. What are three major sources of saturated and unsaturated fats in the diet?
19. What is the major function of protein in the diet?
20. How can incomplete protein foods be made more complete?
21. How do vitamins contribute to a healthy individual?
22. Name one major function for thiamine, riboflavin, niacin, and vitamins A, D, E, and K.
23. Why should a deep-green or yellow vegetable be eaten every other day?
24. What is a major source of vitamin D in the United States?
25. What is the purpose of iron in a dietary plan?
26. Why should an individual purchase and use iodized salt?
27. Why is calcium important to good health besides promoting growth and maintenance of bones?
28. How much liquid should an individual consume each day?
29. What is a calorie?
30. What two nutrients must be carefully consumed during pregnancy?
31. How many additional calories may be needed during the last part of pregnancy in an average diet?
32. Why do nursing mothers need increased protein?
33. What are the characteristics of the eating patterns of preschoolers?
34. Why is breakfast an important meal for school-age children?
35. What are the major nutrients in which the diets of teenagers may be deficient?
36. What nutrients do adults need? What nutrients may be neglected?
37. Define an enzyme.
38. What happens during hydrolysis?

Equipment and Measurements for Cooking

Successful food preparation partly depends on the proper selection, use, and care of kitchen equipment, a vast amount of which is available on today's market. Although the individual's life-style and amount of available income will determine which items will be selected, some are essential for food preparation, whereas other kinds are nice to have if storage space is available. Because certain kinds of equipment are great time- and energy-savers when they are used efficiently, the instruction and care booklets that come with them should be carefully read and stored where they can be easily located.

The key to quality food products is dependent upon the use of standard measuring equipment and the following of specified procedures for measuring foods. As with the use of equipment, kitchen safety is vital to the prevention of accidents; this chapter contains a short section pertaining to this subject.

The selection and use of large appliances such as the stove, refrigerator, and automatic dishwasher are not discussed, but the care of these major equipment items is covered in the chapter on Food Safety.

Types of Cookware

Cookware includes all the saucepans, fry pans, bakeware, portable electrical appliances, and other nonclassifiable items that are used for mixing and cooking food. This section describes the basic cookware used in cooking foods, the advantages and disadvantages of the construction of cookware, and its proper care.

Saucepans and Fry Pans

A pan that has deep sides and a lid with either one long handle or two short handles is called a

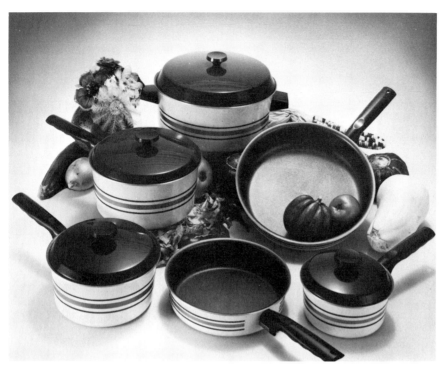

Figure 2-1.
Saucepans and frying pans are available in a variety of sizes and many have attractive decorative finishes. (The West Bend Co.)

saucepan. It is used for simmering or boiling foods. A fry pan, sometimes called a skillet, has low sides and is used for cooking foods that require a high temperature for browning or for foods that cook quickly. Although many saucepans and skillets can be used in the oven, most are considered as top-of-the-range cookware.

Size. Most cooking can be done with three or four saucepans and one or two fry pans, but this varies with need and the kinds of portable electric appliances that are available. The 1-quart saucepan is used to reheat or cook small portions of food and the 2- or 3-quart saucepan is necessary for cooking foods to serve four to six people. A 6-quart or larger saucepan is essential for foods that require a large amount of water for cooking, such as boiling less tender cuts of meat or various macaroni products.

Another type of saucepan is the double boiler, which consists of two pans one of which fits inside the other. The bottom part of the double boiler is used for holding water at a simmering or boiling temperature while food that would tend to scorch or burn when cooked over direct heat warms or cooks in the upper pan. The bottom section of the double boiler can also serve as a regular saucepan.

Fry pans are available in varying widths; the two widths that are most essential for cooking are the 6- to 8-inch for preparing various sauces, cooking individual eggs, and frying small amounts of food; and the 10- to 12-inch for such cooking as frying several pieces of meat, stir-frying vegetables, or cooking pancakes. Several sizes of saucepans and fry pans are shown in Figure 2-1.

A pan that is called a Dutch oven or roaster is a heavy saucepan with deep sides and a lid that is used for frying and cooking foods with liquid. It is used for cooking foods that require a long cooking time and may be used in the oven or on top of the range.

Material Construction. Saucepans and fry pans can be constructed of many different types of materials or combinations of materials; each has its advantages and disadvantages for use in cooking.

1. The lightweight metal, aluminum, is the best conductor of heat. It is a good choice for foods that cook quickly over high heat, but not as good a choice for foods that are to be cooked for longer periods of time, because if the food is not watched, there is danger of its scorching. Because aluminum is a soft metal, it is easily dented and it may pit if salty foods or hard tap water are allowed to stand in the pan. Also, alkaline foods and strong detergents such as those used in automatic dishwashers may cause the surface of the pan to become a dull gray; acid foods, such as tomatoes, may have a metallic taste if cooked in aluminum ware. However, these characteristics are not harmful to an individual's health, and aluminum cookware is the most inexpensive to purchase.

2. Stainless steel is a strong, dent-resistant metal whose surface is unaffected by a food's chemical composition. However, contrary to aluminum, stainless steel is not a good heat conductor and foods tend to cook unevenly, stick, or scorch if they are not watched. Thus, stainless-steel fry pans are not a wise choice, but stainless-steel saucepans that use liquid as a cooking medium are satisfactory.

3. Some cookware is made of stainless steel and another metal to increase the heat conductivity of the steel. These pans either have a bonded coating of copper or aluminum, or a part of the inner core of the pan is constructed of another metal. These pans are stain-resistant and have more even cooking.

4. Cast-iron cookware has been popular for hundreds of years. It resists stains, distributes the heat slowly but evenly, retains the heat, and is of moderate cost. Its advantages make it a particularly good choice for fry pans. The disadvantage of cast-iron cookware is that it is heavy and rusts easily.

5. Porcelain enamelware is a glasslike finish that is applied to cast iron or plain steel. Coated cast-iron ware has more even heating than coated steelware, but the durability of either is dependent upon the thickness of the enamel. Thin-coated enamelware chips easily.

6. Glass cookware for top-of-the-range cooking allows clear inspection of the food being cooked, but is susceptible to chipping and breakage. A metal trivet must be placed between the direct heat source and the pan. Some top-of-the-range glassware has been developed for use with the glass ceramic-type stove and does not require this special care.

7. Some cookware has a nonstick finish applied to the cooking surface that prevents food from sticking and eliminates, if desired, the necessity of additional cooking fat. Teflon is a registered trademark for this type of finish.

8. Copper cookware is an ideal type for fast cooking because of the metal's rapid heat conductivity. However, it is very expensive and copper requires continuous polishing to keep it attractive. Copper pans used for cooking are lined with another metal, such as tin or stainless steel, because the toxicity of copper can contaminate the food.

Care. All saucepans and fry pans are best cleaned by washing in hot, soapy water, and then rinsing and drying the pans. Stainless and porcelain enamelware, steel, glass, and pans with a nonstick finish can all be washed in an automatic dishwasher. If food particles adhere to the pan, they are best removed with a plastic scouring pad. Steel wool pads can be used on aluminum ware. Another method for removing sticky substances from the pan is to boil water in the pan for 5 minutes. Stained pans can be cleaned by boiling 2 tablespoons of baking soda with 1 quart of water in the pan for 5 minutes. Stains in pans with a nonstick finish are removed by boiling for 5 minutes a mixture of 1 cup of water, 1/2 cup of household bleach, and 2 tablespoons of baking soda.

Both cast-iron pans and pans with a nonstick finish should be seasoned before they are first used. Pans with a nonstick finish are seasoned by wiping the surface with a small amount of vegetable oil, washing, rinsing, and drying. Cast-iron pans are seasoned by washing, rinsing, drying, and coating the cooking surface with a small amount of vegetable oil. The pan is then placed in a moderate oven at a temperature of 350° F (175° C) for 1 hour. After repeated use, this seasoning process may need to be repeated; for nonstick surfaces the process should be repeated if the pan has been cleaned to remove stains. Cast-iron cookware should never be washed in a dishwasher because the oily surface will be lost and the pans will rust.

Cooking Equipment for Baking

Bakeware

Bakeware includes the pans and dishes used for cooking foods like cakes, cookies, pies, breads, casseroles, and meats in the oven. There are many sizes, kinds, and shapes of bakeware, which may be constructed of many different materials. A few basic pieces are essential for food preparation, whereas a collection of other pieces is determined by available storage space and need.

Certain features are important to all bakeware to make it easier to handle, to remove food from it, and to care for it. A hot pan is easier to remove from the oven if the handles are built-in; food is easier to remove from baking pans and the pans are easier to clean if they have rounded corners and seamless construction. Angel food cakes and cheese cakes are easier to remove if the pan has a loose bottom, and foods such as muffins are easier to remove if the pan surface has a nonstick finish. An array of bakeware items is shown in Figure 2–2.

Size. To achieve the best cooking results, it is very important to use the pan size called for in a recipe. Pan sizes for bakeware are standardized, and most manufacturers imprint the pan size on the bottom of the pan. The size of a rectangular baking pan is stated in inches as length $\times$ width $\times$ depth. An example would be a $13 \times 9 \times 2$-inch pan. Dimensions for a round pan are given as diameter $\times$ depth; an example for a 9-inch cake pan would be 9×1–$1/2$ inches.

Bakeware should be chosen that will fit the oven. To allow heat to circulate evenly there should be 1 inch of space between the pan and the oven walls and 1 inch of space between 2 or more pans in the oven at the same time. Table 2–1 lists the recommended sizes and number of bakeware that a kitchen should have for food preparation. However, more or less of bakeware items may be needed to fit individual needs.

Some bakeware has a variety of uses, whereas other pieces may have only 1 or 2 uses. Shallow metal or glass pans can be used for baking such foods as cakes, casseroles, and some breads, whereas a muffin pan, bundt pan, or pizza pan has limited use. A jelly roll pan, having a 1-inch edge on all four sides, is used

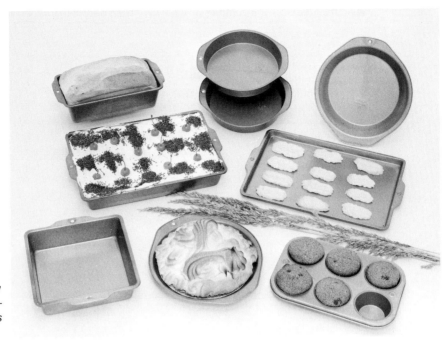

Figure 2-2.
Bakeware is available in many sizes and shapes to fit cooking needs. (Ecko Housewares Company)

for making cake rolls or it may be used for baking foods such as cookies or biscuits. A loaf pan is used for baking breads, some cakes, and meat loaves, and may be used for molded salads. A soufflé dish is a round dish with straight sides that may double as a serving or casserole dish. A broiler pan is a shallow pan with a rack used for broiling foods; the pan section may be used for roasting meats.

Material. The material from which bakeware is constructed can make a difference in the specified oven temperature of a recipe. If glass, anodized aluminum, or glass ceramic bakeware is used, the temperature is reduced by 25° F (10° C). For example, if a cake recipe calls for a temperature 350° F (175° C), and a glass baking pan is used, the temperature is reduced to 325° F (165° C).

The baking surface will affect the finished baked product. Shiny pans, which reflect heat, yield a product that has a light, tender crust and should be used for baking cakes, cookies, muffins, and quick breads. Dull, finished pans absorb heat and should be used for baking foods such as breads and piecrusts where a browner crust is more desirable. The materials used for bakeware construction are the same as those used for saucepans and fry pans, but the reasons for selecting specific kinds of material construction are different.

1. Aluminum bakeware is an excellent choice because the heat is spread quickly and evenly to all areas of the pan. There are two kinds of finish applied to aluminum pans: a shiny finish and a dull, frosty-looking finish called anodized aluminum. Heavy aluminum pieces are cast (poured into a mold) and this is desirable for ware such as roasters that are used for long periods of cooking. Other bakeware is stamped or formed from sheets of aluminum such as cookie sheets and pie pans.

Table 2-1

Recommended Size and Number of Bakeware for Food Preparation

Item	Size	Recommended Number
Cake pans, round	8 × 1-1/2	2, or
Cake pans, round	9 × 1-1/2	2
Cake pan, oblong	13 × 9 × 2	1
Tube cake pan	10 × 4	1
Jelly roll pan	15-1/2 × 10-1/2 × 1	1
Casserole dish	1 quart	1
Casserole dish	2 quart	1
Casserole dish	3 quart	1
Cookie Sheet	15-1/2 × 12	1
Loaf pan	8-1/2 × 4-1/2 × 2-1/2	2
Pie pan	8 × 1-1/4	1
Pie pan	9 × 1-1/4	1
Soufflé dish	1-1/2 quart	1
Springform pan	9 × 3	1
Muffin pan	2-1/2 × 1-1/4	2/6-cup or 1/12-cup
Broiler pan and rack	Optional size	1

2. Because heat conductivity is not as important in baking, stainless steel bakeware is satisfactory. It may be tin-plated or enameled.

3. Specialty pans, such as corn stick pans and pans for making foods like *ebelskiver*, a Danish dessert, are made of cast iron. Cast-iron casserole-type dishes are made with a Teflon coating on the inside and a porcelain coating on the outside.

4. Some copper bakeware is sold for casserole-type dishes and baking pans. It is always lined in stainless steel or tin for cooking and is expensive.

5. Heat-resistant glass is a popular bakeware that comes in many different sizes and shapes for cooking casseroles, pies, cakes, and many other food dishes.

6. Glass-ceramic ware can be used in the oven, on top of the range, and under the broiler, and comes in varying sizes and shapes.

7. Some types of china and earthenware can also be used for oven cooking, but it is best to check the manufacturer's instructions.

Care. The directions for care of bakeware are the same as those discussed in the section on saucepans and fry pans in this chapter.

Microwave Oven Cookware

Any ovenproof glass, glass ceramic bakeware, strong plastic, or paper is suitable for use in a microwave oven. However, metal or any type of cookware that has a metal trim and some types of glass ceramic dinnerware cannot be used in a microwave oven. Strong plastics can be used for very short cooking periods, but longer times may cause the plastic to melt. Paper products should be used only for those foods that require no longer than 3 to 4 minutes of cooking.

A simple test to check a nonmetal's usability in a microwave oven is to place the container and 1 cup of water in the oven and heat for 1 minute. If the water becomes hot and the dish does not, then the dish can be used. Dishes that get hot must not be used in a microwave oven.

Small Electrical Appliances

Small electrical appliances, sometimes called portable appliances, are a convenience and time-saver when they are properly used. If they are used in place of the range, they may also be an energy saver. Most homes have at least 1 small electrical appliance, whereas other homes may have as many as 30 small appliances to use in food preparation. The list of available portable appliances continues to grow each year, but only those that fit an individual's need and life-style should be purchased. The instruction and care booklet for each appliance must be carefully read so that the appliance is used to its fullest advantage.

These appliances should be stored in an easy-to-reach place and, if possible, at the site of first use. Appliances are seldom used if they have to be taken from the back of a cupboard or from a high shelf. This section discusses a few of the most commonly used small electrical appliances, their special features, and how they can be used in food preparation.

Fry Pans. The electric fry pan is a very versatile appliance that can be used to fry, roast, bake, and simmer foods. It can also serve as an additional cooking element when preparing a meal, or it may be used in place of the range for preparing many foods, thus saving energy. The portability of the fry pan allows it to be used as a cooking element in many different areas of the home. For example, quick cooking foods such as pancakes can be prepared at the table if an electrical outlet is close by, thus allowing the host or hostess to enjoy mealtime conversation while the food is being cooked. A fry pan may also be used to keep foods like sauces and dips warm when entertaining in another area of the home.

Electric fry pans come with many different features and are constructed of either aluminum or stainless steel. Aluminum fry pans are the least expensive and those made of stainless steel are very durable. Teflon-lined pans require a minimum of care and offer the same advantages as other types of cookware lined in Teflon. Fry pans are designed with one or two handles, some having deep sides, and this style may be safely used for deep frying. Other fry pans may have a high-domed lid that is an advantage for cooking foods such as a roast, and some have a broiling element in the lid.

All electric fry pans have thermostatically controlled heat that assures even cooking. Most heat control units can be removed so that the pan may be submerged in water for cleaning. The heat unit is never put in water but may be cleaned with a damp cloth. Before cleaning the pan should first be cooled to room temperature to ensure the life of the appliance.

Blenders. The blender is a time saving appliance that mixes, chops, grinds, liquefies, and blends foods. Foods are either prepared for eating in the blender or they may require further preparation, but in both situations, the blender simplifies food preparation and saves time. Examples of some tasks that can be done with a blender include reconstituting dried milk and frozen juices, preparing instant puddings, pureeing foods for babies and those on special diets, and whipping cream. Other jobs that can be performed by the blender include chopping nuts, mixing salad dressings, making dips and spreads, and preparing cake mixes.

Blenders come with two speeds or a multiple of speeds. The appliances are easier to clean if they have blades that can be removed. Some blenders feature a lid with a section that can be removed for adding other food while the blade is activating, and some feature a handle and pouring lip.

Food Processor. The food processor is relatively new on the small appliance market. Its work action is so quick that it is revolutionizing many food preparation jobs that have been considered time consuming when performed by traditional work methods. The basic parts of the food processor include the motor base, the work bowl, the cover with feed tube, and the pusher. The major tools of the food processor include the metal blade, the plastic blade, the shredding disk, and the serrated slicing disk.

Using the major tools, the food processor chops, pulverizes, slices, shreds and combines food ingredients. It can be used for kneading, making pie crusts, and sauces. Most food processors will hold up to 2-1/2 cups of a watery product. However, this will vary with individual manufacturers.

Mixers. The electric mixer was one of the first small electrical appliances to be used in the home. It is used to mix many ingredients by blending, beating, creaming, stirring, and whipping and has eliminated the need for performing many of these manipulations by hand.

Mixers are available either with or without a stand. Stand mixers are the most powerful, and the stand has a lever that allows the user to adjust both the small and large bowl that comes with the mixer. Mixers without a stand are lighter in weight and should not be used for heavy mixing jobs, such as beating candy, as the motor will burn out if it is overworked. It is important always to have a nonslip pad under the bowl when using a portable mixer so that the bowl does not slide on the counter.

Slow Cookers. The slow cooker is a low-wattage appliance that has been introduced in the home in recent years. The principal advantage of the slow cooker is that various food ingredients can all be added at once without prior preparation, and the food being cooked does not need further attention until it is ready to be served because the heat setting is so low that moisture is retained within the pot and there is no danger of foods scorching or burning. Foods that require 1 to 2 hours of cooking on top of the range require 4 to 8 hours in the slow cooker. Foods that are best suited for slow cookers include the tougher cuts of meat like pot roasts or stew meat, chicken, and raw vegetables. Seafoods will break apart with extended cooking but may be added during the last part of cooking time, as can milk and milk products and frozen vegetables. Pastas and rice are best if precooked or added during the last hour of cooking.

The main difference between models of slow cookers is the method of heat distribution. One type features heating coils wrapped around the sides or bottom of the pot, and another features a separate heating base upon which the pot rests. Some brands have an inner pot that can be removed. The heating temperature may be adjusted by a "low" or "high" setting on some brands, whereas others feature a variable heat setting. The size capacity ranges from 2- to 6-quart models. Various models have different interior and exterior finishes, examples of which are shown in Figure 2-3.

Figure 2-3.
Many sizes of slow cookers are available with differing interior and exterior finishes. (The West Bend Co.)

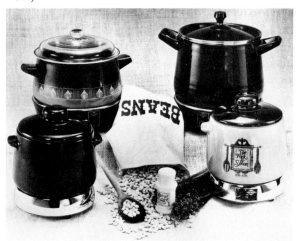

Microwave Ovens. The countertop microwave oven is considered a small electrical appliance because it receives its electrical energy from a 110-volt outlet, just as other small appliances do. However, the heating of food in a microwave oven operates on a different principle from that of conventional cooking. In conventional cooking, food is cooked either by heating the surface of a pan, which transfers this heat to the food, or by heating the air of the oven, which is then transferred to the food. In a microwave oven, a magnetron tube converts the electrical energy to electromagnetic energy; this, in turn, produces short energy waves, called microwaves, that are sent into the oven.

Microwaves bounce off the metal of the oven walls but pass through the cookware and are absorbed by the food. When the microwaves are absorbed by the food, they cause the molecules of food to vibrate and rub together, which causes friction; the heat produced from this friction is what cooks and heats the food. Foods cook very quickly by this action. Most foods can be cooked in the microwave oven. Each chapter of this book dealing with food includes a section on microwave cooking.

Other Cookware

Three other pieces of cookware are commonly used in food preparation and deserve special consideration.

Pressure Cookers. A pressure cooker is a specially designed pan that seals in steam under pressure when a liquid is heated in the pan. Foods cook more quickly in a pressure cooker because the temperatures reached are higher than the boiling point of water. The pressure cooker is a great time-saver for cooking less tender cuts of meat, and most other foods can be satisfactorily cooked in this pan. Because foods cook so quickly, the cooking times listed in the instruction booklet must be carefully followed so that the food is not overcooked.

Wok. The wok is a bowl-shaped Chinese cooking utensil that has become a popular pan in this country for stir-frying meats and vegetables. Woks that are used on top of the range have metal rings upon which they sit; other woks are electric.

Fondue Pots. A fondue pot is a ceramic or metal pot used to keep foods warm or to cook foods. The fuel source, depending on the design of the pot, is either an alcohol burner, a butane-gas burner, or canned fuel such as Sterno. Some fondue pots are electric, and these maintain a more even heat and are safer to use. Electric fondue pots are used for any type of fondue cooking.

The ceramic fondue pot is used for cooking foods that require a low temperature, such as cheeses and chocolate. Metal fondue pots are used for cooking foods that require a higher temperature, such as meats, but may also be used to make cheese fondues. A nonelectric fondue pot should have a sturdy base because of the danger of tipping over.

Types of Tools

Kitchen tools are the utensils used to mix, cut, measure, and further prepare foods for eating. Some are essential to food preparation, some are luxury items that may prove to be great time-savers, and others are often called gadgets because they are seldom used.

Mixing Tools

Mixing tools are used to blend, stir, and beat foods. The most essential mixing tool is the spoon. Most individuals prefer wooden spoons for mixing, but sturdy metal spoons may also be used. Another utensil used for mixing is the loop-wired whisk which is particularly convenient for eliminating lumps in sauces. The rubber spatula is mainly used for scraping the sides of bowls, folding ingredients together, and measuring fats. In addition to the electric mixer, the rotary or hand beater is convenient for small beating jobs.

Cutting Tools

One or two good cutting knives are most important to food preparation; the best knife has a blade made from high-carbon steel and has a comfortable handle. The small paring knife has a triangular-shaped blade that tapers to a point and varies from 2-1/2 to 4 inches. It is used for peeling, cutting, and doing other small jobs such as removing stems and roots and cutting out food blemishes.

The second important knife is called the French chef's knife; it has a heavier, thicker, and longer triangular-shaped blade. Blade sizes of the French chef's knife range from 8 to 14 inches. For most cutting jobs the 10- to 12-inch blade is easiest to operate. It is designed primarily for chopping and dicing but may be used for carving meats and slicing other foods. Another knife that is convenient to have has a long, slender blade with a serrated edge and is used for slicing foods like breads, cheese, and meat.

Kitchen shears are useful for finely mincing vegetables such as parsley; if they have a serrated edge, shears can be used for boning poultry and meats. A tool called a parer or peeler removes a thin layer of skin from such foods as potatoes and apples.

Measuring Tools

For success in food preparation, three kinds of measuring tools are essential. They are available in both standard and metric units, and include a set of dry measuring cups, a liquid measure, and a set of measuring spoons. These measuring tools are not the same as the ware used for eating because they are standardized to hold specific amounts of ingredients.

A set of standard dry measuring cups includes 1/4, 1/3, 1/2, and 1 cup measures, and some sets include a 2/3 cup measure. These are sometimes referred to as Mary Ann measures. Dry metric measuring devices are usually sold as units of 60, 75, 125, and 250 milliliters. Dry measures are important for accurate measurement of all dry ingredients, such as flour and sugar.

Standard liquid measures for home food preparation are the 1-cup, 1-pint, and 1-quart measures. Liquid metric measures are available in 250, 500, and 1,000 milliliters. Liquid measures are made from glass or a plastic and have decreasing measures imprinted on the container. Some sizes of liquid standard and metric measures are shown in Figure 2-4. Dry ingredients cannot be accurately measured in liquid measures because of the lip at the edge. A standard measuring spoon set includes 1/4, 1/2, 1 teaspoon, and 1 tablespoon. Similar metric measures are 1, 2, 5, 7, 15, and 25 milliliters.

Other Tools

Several sizes of mixing bowls are needed. A sifter is necessary for sifting dry ingredients, a rolling pin for rolling dough, a strainer or sieve for letting foods drain, and a grater to shred food. A wire rack is necessary to allow certain baked foods such as cookies and cakes to cool.

A metal slotted spoon is helpful to remove food from liquid, and a metal fork and metal spatula are needed for turning foods as they are cooking. Various tools needed for food preparation are shown in Figure 2-5.

Measurements

Until recent years most household measuring of weight (mass), volume, and length has been done by the English or Standard system of measurement, and temperature has been re-

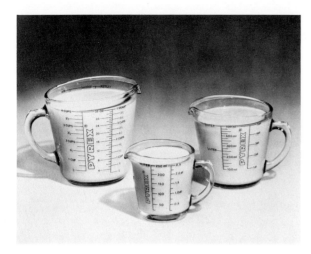

Figure 2-4.

Liquid measuring cups are in cup, pint, and quart standard measure and are also available in metric measure. (Corning Glass Works)

corded in degrees Fahrenheit. However, since 1960 and the passage of the U.S. Metric Act in 1975, there has been an increasing voluntary usage of the metric system in the United States. The metric system is commonly referred to as the International System of Units (SI). The metric system is simple to understand and the easiest way to master it is to learn the terms, practice using the measurements, and "think metric." In food preparation this means to cook metric.

The most common metric terms that will be used in the American household to measure volume and weight (mass) for food preparation are the *liter*, which equals slightly more than 1 quart, and the *milliliter*, which is 1,000th of a liter. The milliliter measure is similar to the spoon and cup in standard measure. One cup is slightly less than 250 milliliters, 1 tablespoon

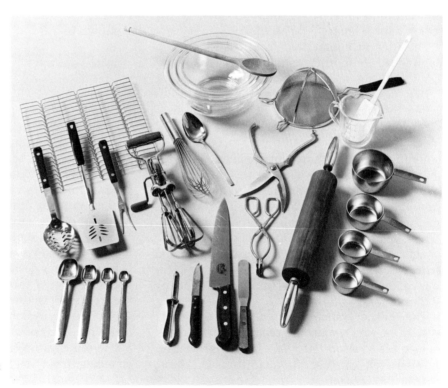

Figure 2-5.

These basic food preparation tools make cooking easier.

Table 2-2

Terms, Abbreviations, and Equivalents for Commonly Used Standard and
Metric Measuring Units

Term	Abbreviation	Equivalent
Teaspoon	tsp., or t.	5 milliliters
Tablespoon	Tbsp., or T.	3 tsp., 15 mL or 1/2 fl. oz.
Cup	c.	16 Tbsp., 250 mL, 8 fl. oz.
Pint	pt.	2 cups
Quart	qt.	2 pt., 1,000 mL
Gallon	gal.	4 qt.
Ounce	oz.	28.35 gms
Fluid ounce	fl. oz.	2 Tbsp.
Pound	lb.	16 oz., 453.59 gm
Few grains	f. g.	few grains
Milliliter	mL	0.001 L
Liter	L	1.06 qts., 1,000 mL
Gram	g	0.035 oz.
Kilogram	kg	2.21 pounds

equals approximately 15 milliliters, and 1 teaspoon approximates 5 milliliters.

The liter in abbreviated form is written as a capitalized *L* to differentiate from the number *1*, and the milliliter is written as *mL*.

Dry measure may also be done very accurately by using the *gram* or *kilogram*. To measure foods in kilograms or grams, a set of metric scales is used. Although the gram is a common unit for measuring ingredients in many countries and is used in this country for quantity food measurements, the average household in the United States will not use this method because the scales are not available. When scales are used for measurement, the weight of the container used must be deducted from the total weight. The kilogram replaces ounces and pounds, with 1 kilogram equaling 2.2. pounds.

The metric system is based upon a decimal system in which units are related to each other in simple factors of 10. The abbreviation symbols tell whether the quantity is in 10ths, 100ths, 1,000ths, or in lesser or greater amounts as shown in the following.

deci equals 0.1	deka equals 10
centi equals 0.01	hecto equals 100
milli equals 0.001	kilo equals 1,000

Conversion of metric units is simply done by moving the decimal point the appropriate number of spaces to the left or right.

With the standard system, food for home preparation is measured by teaspoons, tablespoons, cups or fractions thereof, pints, quarts, gallons, pounds, and ounces.

Most measurement terminology used in recipes is abbreviated (as shown) in Table 2-2. It is sometimes desirable to increase or decrease the quantity of food ingredients to meet serving needs: it is therefore important to understand the equivalency or quantity of various measurements, as is also shown in Table 2-2.

The temperature measurement system is also changing from degrees Fahrenheit to degrees

Celsius. The following shows a comparison of temperature terminology that is commonly used in food preparation.

	Fahrenheit	Celsius
Water freezes	32° F	0° C
Water boils	212° F	100° C
Slow oven	300° F	150° C
Moderate oven	350° F	175° C
Hot oven	425° F	220° C
Very hot oven	450° F	230° C

Although it is easier just to use the metric system for measurements, some favorite recipes may need to be converted to the metric system; Table 2–3 and Table 2–4 demonstrate the method for conversion. Because metric measurements are slightly greater than standard measurements, converted recipes, particularly those for baked products, need to be tested and the measurements may need to be adjusted to achieve the same quality results.

Whether the metric system or the standard system of measurement is used, certain techniques for various food measurements need to be followed.

Dry Ingredients

Dry ingredients include flours, sugars, leavening agents, salt, spices, and herbs. Other dry ingredients include the various pasta products and rice.

Flour. All-purpose flour, except for instant blending and cake flour, need to be sifted before measuring. To do this the approximate amount of required flour is put into the flour sifter and sifted onto waxed paper. The flour is then lightly spooned into a cup and leveled off even with the edge of the cup, using the straight edge of a knife. The flour is then either resifted with other dry ingredients or put into the mixing bowl, depending on the recipe. If a sifter is not available, a sieve may be used.

Some flours are labeled "presifted" but these still tend to pack down when they are spooned into a cup. A relatively accurate adjustment to sifted flour can be made by removing 2 tablespoons of the presifted flour from the cup.

Instant-blending flour is an all-purpose flour that, as the name implies, does not need to be sifted before measuring. The granular texture of instant blending flour allows it to be easily mixed with cold water and it does not pack down. With the sifting step eliminated, it is a time-saver. However, the cost of instant-blending flour over other types of flour may make it an expensive major ingredient in baked goods.

Other flours like whole wheat or rye are not sifted. They are stirred, spooned lightly into the cup and leveled, and then stirred into other dry ingredients to thoroughly mix.

Table 2–3
Conversion of Standard Measurements to Metric

To Change Standard	To Metric	Multiply by
teaspoons	milliliter	5
tablespoon	milliliter	15
cup	liter	0.24
pint	liter	0.47
quart	liter	0.95
gallon	liter	3.8
ounce	gram	28.35
fluid ounce	milliliter	29.575
pound	kilogram	0.45

Table 2–4
Conversion of Metric Measurements to Standard

To Change Metric	To Standard	Multiply by
milliliters	fluid ounces	0.03
liters	pints	2.1
grams	ounces	0.035
kilograms	pounds	2.2
milliliters	tablespoons	0.068
milliliters	cups	0.0042

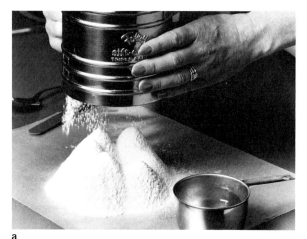

a

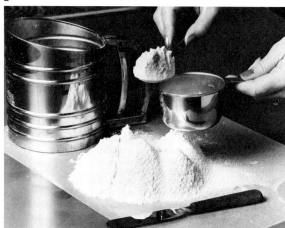

b

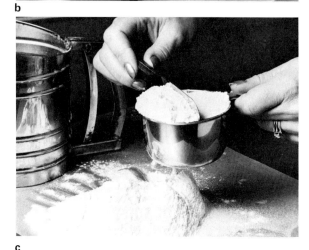

c

Sugar. Granulated and brown sugar are not sifted before measuring, but lumps must be crushed before measurement. After sugar is measured, it may be sifted or thoroughly stirred into other dry ingredients, or used as directed in the recipe.

Brown sugar is packed into a cup so that it molds to the cup without air spaces. Powdered sugar is sifted before measuring because it, like flour, packs down during storage. Figure 2-6 demonstrates the method for measuring flour.

Leavening Agents, Salt, and Spices. The leavening agents, soda and baking powder, as well as salt and spices are usually measured in fractions of teaspoons. The spoon is put into the container and the ingredients are leveled off as with flour. These ingredients are never leveled off over other foods.

Other Foods. The measurement for pasta and rice products is discussed in the chapter on cereals. Other foods, such as nuts, raisins, fruits, vegetables, and chopped or ground meats, are lightly spooned into the cup for proper measurement.

Fats

Solid and semisolid fats, such as hydrogenated shortening, lard, butter, or margarine, are either measured in a dry measuring cup or as cubes or sticks; 1 cube equals 1/2 cup. The best way to measure hydrogenated shortening and lard is to pack the fat into a dry measuring cup with a rubber spatula and level off to the rim as shown in Figure 2-7. Care must be taken that all of the fat is removed from the measuring cup when it is scooped out.

Figure 2-6.
(a) The proper way to measure flour is to first sift the flour onto waxed paper. (b) Spoon the sifted flour into the measuring cup. (c) Level the flour to the edge of the cup with a straight edge.

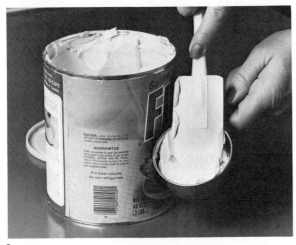

a

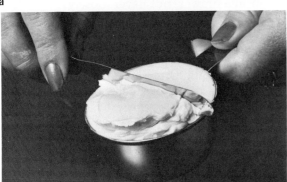

b

Figure 2-7.

(a) Fat is measured by packing it into a dry measuring cup. (b) Then it is made level to top of the cup by use of a straight edge.

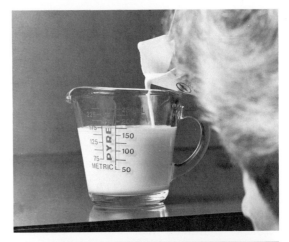

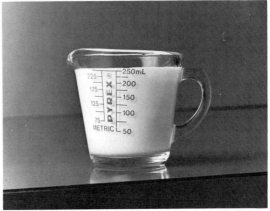

Figure 2-8.

Liquid measures are set on a flat surface and checked at eye level for accuracy.

Liquid fats or vegetable oils are measured in a liquid measuring cup. Some recipes indicate 1/4 cup butter, melted. This means that the butter is measured and then melted. If a recipe indicates 1/4 cup melted butter, the butter is melted and then measured.

All liquid ingredients are measured in a liquid measuring cup that is placed on a level surface. The liquid is filled to the desired mark on the cup and then checked for accuracy by looking at eye level with the container remaining on the surface. This method is shown in Figure 2-8. Sticky liquid substances, such as honey or corn syrup, must be thoroughly removed from the measuring container to assure accuracy of ingredients. This is best done by cleaning out the container with a rubber spatula.

Kitchen Safety

Many needless accidents occur in the kitchen because of individuals' failing to follow basic safety procedures in the handling of foods, equipment, and kitchen furnishing. The following basic list of safety instructions will hopefully create an increased awareness of safety and help to eliminate accidents.

1. All electrical cords should be kept neatly bound on the counter; a plastic tie facilitates this. Dangling cords can be easily caught when walking by, and they create a sense of curiosity in young children.

2. For the same reasons as listed in number 1, all pan handles must be turned toward the center of the stove.

3. Long hair, for both sanitary and safety reasons, must be either covered or tied back. Synthetic hair wigs are extremely flammable and should not be worn when cooking, particularly when the oven is in use.

4. Harmful cleaning substances, including detergents, must be stored on a high shelf, not under the sink, when young children are in the household.

5. Gas appliances that must be ignited to start the flame should be lit immediately after the gas is turned on. Otherwise too much gas will accumulate and an individual is likely to be burned.

6. Electrical cords should always be pulled from the outlet, not the appliance. If it is left plugged into the outlet, the cord can be a source of shock to an individual or a cause of fire.

7. Sharp tools such as knives should be placed in dishwater only when they are ready to be washed. If placed in a pan prior to washing, the tools may not be seen when the hands are placed in the water.

8. Hot fat should never be left unattended. If a grease fire does start on the stove, a heavy dosage of salt will put it out. The pan should never be carried to the sink flaming, nor should water be thrown on it because this will cause the flames to flare higher.

9. Glass dishes that have chipped edges and cracks should be discarded. Chipped dishes have the potential of cutting the user and are also a source for bacterial growth.

10. Knives should be stored in racks on a wall or in a drawer, but never loosely.

11. Beaters for electric mixers should never be inserted when the mixer is plugged into the outlet.

12. Proper equipment should be used for performing specific household tasks. For example, a can opener not a knife, should be used to open cans.

13. Pot holders of a heavy thickness, not towels, should be used for lifting and moving hot equipment.

14. Spills on the floor must be immediately wiped, and rugs should have a nonskid backing to prevent falls.

15. Kitchen drawers and cupboards should be closed when not in use to avoid bumps and bruises.

16. All hot liquids and foods must be handled with care to eliminate spillage and burns to the individual.

LEARNING ACTIVITIES

1. Make a list of the cookware and bakeware that would be most essential for a single individual and a family of four.

2. Take a field trip to a local department store and price the cost of equipment listed in number 1.

3. Make a list of kitchen equipment that you have that is seldom used. Decide if

this is because of the storage location or lack of usability of this equipment.

4. Make a list of the small electrical appliances that you consider most essential to your life-style. Select one or two of these items and investigate the cost, different features, and material construction of the appliances. Decide which appliance would be the best purchase and where it should be stored for greatest usability.

5. Examine the equipment that is available in a foods laboratory and determine if you know the specific use for each piece.

6. Plan a menu in which all foods could be prepared in an electric fry pan.

7. Convert a favorite recipe with standard measurements to the metric system.

8. Cut the measurements of a recipe that will serve four to six people in half.

9. Triple the measurements of a recipe that will serve four to six people.

10. Write the standard abbreviations commonly used in recipes for the following terms: teaspoon, tablespoon, cup, pint, quart, ounce, liter, and milliliter.

11. Make a list of the kitchen tools you consider essential for a kitchen to have.

12. Investigate the kinds of metric measuring tools that are now for sale in your area.

13. Do an investigation and present to the class a report on the reasons for and against the United States converting to the metric system.

14. Demonstrate to the class the proper way to measure dry, fat, and liquid ingredients.

15. Investigate and report to the class the features of five different brands of microwave ovens.

REVIEW QUESTIONS

1. What is the difference between a saucepan and a fry pan in design construction?

2. What three sizes of saucepans should most kitchens have?

3. What two sizes of fry pans should most kitchens have?

4. Which metal used in cookware construction is the best conductor of heat?

5. What are three disadvantages of the metal named in number 4?

6. Why is a stainless steel fry pan not satisfactory?

7. What is the advantage of stainless steel saucepans that are coated with copper or aluminum?

8. What is one disadvantage and one advantage of fry pans made of cast iron?

9. What is porcelain enamelware?

10. What is the advantage of a nonstick finish when it is applied to cookware?

11. What are two methods for removing stuck-on food substances from pans?

12. What are two methods for removing stains from cookware?

13. How are cast iron pans seasoned?

14. What are three important features to look for when buying bakeware?

15. What should be remembered about bakeware and oven size?

16. What three materials that bakeware is made from require a reduction of 25° F (10° C) in the specified oven temperature?

17. What kinds of baked products should be cooked in pans with a shiny surface? Why?
18. What foods are best baked in pans with a dull finish? Why?
19. What is the best metal for bakeware?
20. What types of cookware may be used in the microwave oven?
21. What kinds of cookware cannot be used in the microwave oven?
22. What is a test for checking the suitability of cookware for microwave oven use?
23. Why is the electric fry pan such a versatile small appliance?
24. How should an electric fry pan with a separate heat unit be cared for?
25. What are five different jobs that a blender can perform?
26. What kinds of food are best cooked in the slow cooker?
27. What are the two different kinds of heat distribution in slow cookers?
28. How are foods cooked with microwaves?
29. Why are foods so quickly cooked in a pressure cooker?
30. What two kinds of knives are essential to food preparation?
31. What are three kinds of measuring tools that every kitchen should have?
32. What is the proper method for measuring all-purpose or cake flour?
33. How is brown sugar measured?
34. How is powdered sugar measured?
35. How is fat measured?
36. What type of measuring cup would be used for measuring milk?
37. Name 10 safety factors that must be remembered when working in the kitchen.

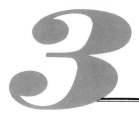

Food Safety

Protecting our food supply and keeping food safe to eat is a major job of the food industry and the governmental protection agencies. As technological advances have increased, so has farm production, and this has led to improved food processing and packaging while research and education have made great advances in protecting food from the ravages of insects, pests, and disease. Many laws and regulations help to protect the safety and quality of food as it travels the chain from farm, processor, packager, wholesaler, and supermarket to the home.

Despite the safeguards employed, food contamination continues to occur. Today, unsafe food is most commonly found in the home and in the public eating establishment. Unsafe food is caused by the presence of harmful yeast, bacteria, and molds called *microorganisms*, toxins produced by microorganisms, parasites from infected animals, or certain chemicals coming in contact with food.

Since the American public generally assumes that food is safe until it reaches the individual who prepares and serves the food, each individual is responsible for learning the causes of unsafe food and developing a knowledge of the principles involved in food safety.

Foodborne Illness

There are two common causes of foodborne illness in the United States: (1) eating food that has become unsafe by a toxin-producing bacteria present in the food, and (2) eating food that has acted as a carrier for harmful bacteria. General symptoms of a foodborne illness are vomiting, diarrhea, abdominal cramps, chills, and fever. Indications are that cases of *salmonella* infection that are commonly diagnosed as the flu may be the direct result of bacterially contaminated food.

43

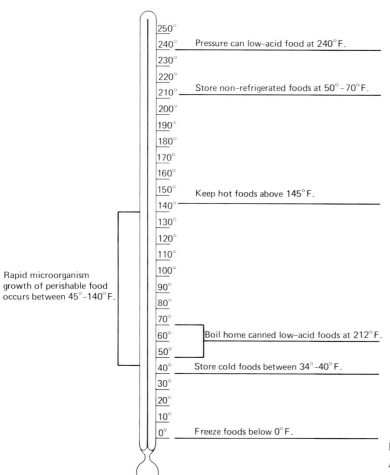

Figure 3-1.
Keep food safe by cooking and storing at the proper temperature.

Labels on the thermometer figure:
- Pressure can low-acid food at 240°F.
- Store non-refrigerated foods at 50° - 70°F.
- Keep hot foods above 145°F.
- Boil home canned low-acid foods at 212°F.
- Store cold foods between 34° - 40°F.
- Freeze foods below 0°F.
- Rapid microorganism growth of perishable food occurs between 45° - 140°F.

Unsafe Food

Unsafe food may be spoiled, deteriorated, or chemically contaminated; it may contain mircoorganisms or toxins harmful to man; or it may be in itself poisonous to man. Certain bacteria, yeasts, and molds are microorganisms that cause food to become unsafe. For micro-organism growth to occur the conditions for growth must be right. Most bacteria multiply rapidly where moisture and warmth are present, as in high-protein foods that have a high moisture content. Some bacteria grow at extremely low temperatures and some bacteria require oxygen for growth whereas others do not. Bacteria my be present in dry food, such as crackers or cereal, but will not multiply in sufficient quantity to cause illness. Figure 3-1 shows the range of temperature at which bacteria will grow.

Yeasts grow best when both sugar and mois-ture are present, and undesirable yeast growth may be found in fruit juices and other products with a high sugar concentration such as jams and jellies. Molds grow on the surfaces of food and appear first as grayish-white matter; then they change in color to blue, green, brown, or black substances. Mold on the surface of food such as jelly can be removed and the food is safe to eat. Not all microorganisms are harmful and many are used as ingredients in the making of certain foods, such as yeast in bread making and molds in the making of cheese.

Enzymes occur naturally within food. An enzyme is a protein substance that causes certain changes to take place without entering into the reaction itself. Fruits ripen as a result of enzymatic activity; if fruits are not used at the ripened stage, enzymatic activity continues and the fruit ripens to the point of spoilage. Oxidation of food also causes spoilage and deterioration as with the surfaces of fruits such as peaches or bananas turning brown when they are exposed to air. Fats, oils, and foods containing a high proportion of fat, such as meats, oxidize when exposed to air and become rancid.

Some foods are directly harmful because of their composition. For example, certain varieties of mushrooms are poisonous to human beings. Rhubarb and tomato leaves are toxic to human beings, but the rhubarb stalk and the tomato are safe.

Signs of spoilage or deterioration in food can sometimes be detected by the smell or appearance of cooked and raw food, as is explained later. Microorganism growth and parasitic infestation are difficult to detect in food. Parasitic infestation in food is caused by eating food that contains another harmful living organism which produces an infection in the human body. *Trichinosis* is a disease caused by eating pork that has been infected with the parasite, *trichinella spiralis;* it is usually caused by feeding hogs with infected, uncooked garbage. The cooking of pork to a proper internal temperature will kill the parasite as discussed in Chapter 14 Meats. A knowledge of the types of raw and cooked food that are most susceptible to microorganism growth and parasitic infestation can help prevent the occurrence of foodborne illness.

Raw Food

Checking the appearance of food before it is prepared will provide several clues to its safety. For example, raw beef that is gray-greenish in color and has a slimy appearance and a pungent odor is spoiled as is fish with unfirm flesh, an odor similar to that of ammonia, and a change in its normal color. Fruits and vegetables that show a change in texture and have bruised areas and mold developing on the surface may also not be safe to eat.

Frozen foods that are not immediately used after thawing are quickly susceptible to organism growth because of the breakdown in tissue caused by the freezing process.

Eggs, raw meat, poultry, and dairy products are susceptible to the infectious bacteria *salmonella*, which enter through cracks in the egg shell. Eggs with cracked shells should thus not be purchased and eggs should be checked for cracks prior to purchase. Other foods susceptible to *salmonella* growth include processed meats such as lunch meats and hot dogs that are not properly wrapped and stored; foods that are browned on the outside but not thoroughly cooked inside, such as croquettes; and the brown bag lunch that sits in a warm room for several hours before being eaten.

Salmonella growth can occur in poultry stuffing cooked in the bird cavity that does not reach an internal temperature of 165° F (74° C) during the cooking time. Dressing left in the bird after cooking also may develop bacteria growth.

Meat, poultry, eggs, and dairy foods that are prepared by an individual who has a *streptococcus* infection are potentially unsafe foods because these bacteria are easily transmitted by the individual's talking, sneezing, or coughing over the food.

Fruits and vegetables that are not washed before they are used may be carriers of harmful bacteria from soil contamination and human handling. Even thick-skinned fruits such as oranges and grapefruit should be rinsed before they are peeled for eating.

Milk that has not been pasteurized is susceptible to *brucella*, an organism that causes undulant fever. Bovine tuberculosis affects human beings via the consumption of infected milk and milk products, but standards developed by the U.S. Public Health Service and followed by most state and local agencies help to keep a check on this disease.

Cooked Food

Moist, high-protein foods such as poultry, beef, egg dishes, custards, and cream-filled pies are susceptible to the toxin-producing bacteria, *staphylococcus*. Other foods susceptible to *staphylococcus* include those that are rehandled after initial preparation, such as a potato or meat salad, and food which is handled many times during preparation, such as ground meat. *Staphylococcus* bacteria are found in cuts, pimples, and skin infections and grow best in a warm temperature. Individuals who carry a *staphylococcus* infection and prepare food can quickly transmit these bacteria to the food.

Meats and meat dishes such as stews, broths, and gravies are susceptible to a second toxin-producing bacteria, *clostridium perfringens*. This bacteria is commonly found in the soil, and foods that have been grown in the soil can be carriers.

Inadequate processing of home-canned meats and low-acid foods such as string beans, beets, and corn produces a growth medium for the third toxin-producing bacteria, *clostridium botulinum*, the most deadly bacterial growth

that can occur in food. *Clostridium botulinum* grows without oxygen. A pressure canner always must be used for processing these foods, and before home-processed vegetables are tasted the food must be brought to a rolling boil, covered, and boiled for at least 10 minutes. Meats, spinach, and corn should be boiled for 20 minutes.

Bulging ends and leaks along the seams of cans indicate that the food is unsafe. If the interior of the can is rusty or darkened, the contents may be spoiled. Food contents of any can that has an off-odor or a foam or milkiness in the juice should be discarded and not tasted.

Leftovers need to be checked for discoloration, off-odor, and mold. Any leftovers held for more than 24 hours are potentially unsafe foods. Leftovers that are not completely heated are dangerous foods.

The picnic and the potluck dinner are two meals in which many of these conditions for causing unsafe food can occur. Cold foods need to be kept cold and hot foods hot, and food should not be left out for long periods of time. Rules for personal sanitation need to be closely followed.

Other Causes of Unsafe Food

Rodents, flies, and other insects are all bacteria carriers that can transmit harmful bacteria to food upon contact. Proper storage of food, the use of garbage containers with covers, and the use of screens on windows help to eliminate these pests.

Certain chemicals react with food and make it unsafe to eat. Utensils that should not be used for food preparation include chipped enameled pans, pans with a copper interior, galvanized iron containers, homemade pottery, or foreign-made pottery purchased in the United States before 1974 because the chemicals in these utensils may penetrate the food.

Quality food control and modern food packaging provide a high assurance that food purchased today is safe to eat. After the food is purchased, each individual has to learn and practice the safety rules involved in storing and preparing food, caring for and using kitchen equipment, and following good habits of personal sanitation.

Food Storage

Proper food storage is most important in maintaining the safety, quality, and nutritional value of food. Many foods keep best when they are stored at low temperatures, with a minimum exposure to moisture, air, and light. A vast amount of food is wasted each day as a result of improper storage or in storing foods for too long a period of time before they are used. Only the amount of perishable food that can be used in a short period of time should be purchased.

Refrigerator Storage. All perishable foods, such as eggs, dairy products, most vegetables, meats, lard, potato and macaroni salads, and leftovers, must be refrigerated to prevent food spoilage. Even though food has been cooked it is not safe to leave it sitting out. A temperature of 40° F (5° C) or less will keep food cold. A meat that has been cooked should be served and then promptly refrigerated. Meat should not be allowed to cool to room temperature before being refrigerated.

Foods that are wrapped in heavy paper should be unwrapped and loosely covered before they are refrigerated. Heavy paper keeps the heat in and the cold out. Prepackaged meats can be stored in their original wrappings if the meats are used in 1 to 2 days after purchase. If the meat is to be stored for a longer period, the meat should be unwrapped and covered lightly with waxed paper, which allows the surface of the meat to dry out; bacteria do not grow well on dry surfaces.

The refrigerator should not be overloaded because air cannot circulate freely in a crowded refrigerator. Cooked foods must be stored in the refrigerator to eliminate the possibility of bacteria entering the cooked foods, and prepared foods should be covered with a tight-fitting lid, foil, or plastic wrap.

Once foods are put in the refrigerator they need to cool rapidly to prevent the start of microorganism growth. Foods should be stored in small portions and to a depth of not more than 4 inches. Large quantities of food can be spread in a shallow pan for quick cooling and then stored in a different container if this is necessary. Large portions of food, such as a cooked turkey, should be cut into smaller sections for adequate cooling during refrigeration.

The kind of food and the conditions under which it is stored in the refrigerator determine the length of storage time. Table 3–1 lists the recommended refrigeration storage time for certain groups of food.

Freezer Storage. Frozen foods need a temperature of 0° F (–10° C) or less to maintain food quality. To preserve the quality of frozen food and to prevent its deterioration, it is important to use the proper wrappings or containers for frozen food and to have an airtight seal. Proper wrapping materials include freezer foil, plastic wrap, and paper that is wax or plastic coated on one side. Waxed paper, bread paper, paper bags, or regular cellophane should not be used as these wrappings are not moisture-or vapor-proof. Proper freezer containers include plastic freezer containers, glass dishes or jars with a wide opening, metal cookware, and heavy-duty plastic bags. Figure 3–2 illustrates one method for wrapping freezer packages and achieving an airtight seal.

It is better from the safety perspective to

Table 3-1
Recommended Refrigeration Storage Time

Food	Maximum Storage Time
Meat, Fish, and Poultry	
Ground meat	2 days
Fresh sausage	2 days
Roasts, chops, and steaks	5 days
Luncheon meats	5 days
Processed meats	7 days
Poultry	2 days
Fish and shellfish	1 day
Dairy Products	
Hard cheese (well-wrapped)	1 month
Ricotta and cottage cheese	5 days
Cheese spreads	2 weeks
Butter or margarine	2 weeks
Milk, liquid forms	1 week
Fresh Fruits and Vegetables	
Ripened soft fruits	5 days
Firm fruits	1 month
Leafy greens	1 week
Soft-skinned vegetables	1 week
Root vegetables	2 weeks
Cooked and Opened Canned Foods	
Leftovers	2 days
Egg and cream dishes	2 days
Salads (other than fresh green)	2 days

reheat frozen, cooked main dishes without thawing. If the food is to be completely thawed before reheating, the food should be left in the refrigerator and heated immediately after thawing is completed. Partially thawed frozen foods can be refrozen only if many ice crystals still remain in the food. Foods should not be eaten or refrozen after they have reached a temperature of 50° F (10° C). Bacterial growth can begin after 2 hours when frozen food stands at room temperature.

Some refrigerators, which have a freezing section that is not a separate compartment, do not have a low enough temperature to hold frozen foods for more than a few days. It is important to put no more food in the freezer or refrigerator-freezer compartment than will freeze in a 24-hour period. Table 3-2 shows the recommended storage time for frozen foods.

Other Food Storage. Dried, canned, and bottled foods should be stored in a cool, dry place. Packages and cartons should be securely closed to prevent microorganisms or insects from entering. It is best to store dry food items such as crackers and cereals in their original package unless the food is in a plastic bag and the food is being stored under humid climatic conditions. Then it is best to store the food in a container with a tight-fitting lid. Flour and sugar are best stored in a glass or plastic container with a tight-fitting lid to prevent insects from entering.

Canned goods and other nonperishable items should be shelf-rotated as new items are purchased because this eliminates older items from remaining on the shelf over a long period of time. Table 3-3 lists the recommended storage time for nonperishable foods.

Potatoes and dry onions need not be refrigerated but must be stored in a cool, dry place. Citrus fruits, bananas, and melons keep best at a room temperature of between 60° F (15° C) and 70° F (21° C). Bread will keep for several days at room temperature but in warm, humid weather it is best to freeze bread to prevent mold growth.

Hydrogenated fats and salad oils need to be stored in a cool, dry place and rancidity is prevented by avoiding overexposure of fats and oils to light and air. Nuts contain a high

Figure 3–2.

Packages must be wrapped air tight for freezer storage. (a) The freezer paper is brought up to even edges and folded under in a 1-inch crease. (b) The paper is continuously folded down in 1-inch creases. (c) until it is even with the container. (d) The center seam is taped securely; the ends folded as illustrated and brought up to the center seam and taped. The package is lastly marked with freezing date, contents, number of servings, and any special cooking instructions.

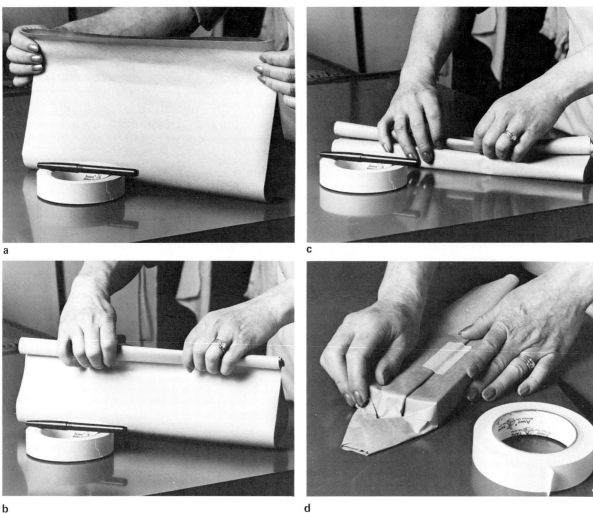

a

c

b

d

Table 3-2

Recommended Storage Time for Frozen Food

Food	Maximum Storage Time
Meat, Poultry, and Fish	
Ground beef	3 months
Steaks and roasts	12 months
Pork	6 months
Poultry	6 months
Fish and shellfish	4 months
Dairy Products	
Butter or margarine	4 months
Cheese	4 months
Ice cream	1 months
Milk	4 months
Fruits and Vegetables	
Fruits (sugar-packed)	12 months
Vegetables	12 months
Baked Food	
Yeast bread and rolls	8 months
Quick breads	3 months
Prepared food, stews, and soups	3 months
Sandwiches	1 month
Cakes	4 months
Pies, unbaked	4 months
Pork and chicken, cooked	3 months
Beef, cooked	6 months

Table 3-3

Recommended Storage Time for Nonperishable Foods

Food	Maximum Storage Time
Bread	3 days
Canned foods	1 year
Crackers, unopened	3 months
Dried fruit	6 months
Mixes	
Cake	1 year
Casserole	18 months
Hot-roll	18 months
Pancake	6 months
Piecrust	6 months
Pudding	1 year
Sauce and gravy	6 months
Nonfat dry milk	6 months
Herbs and spices	1 year
Salad oils	3 months
Peanut butter, opened	2 months
Jams and jellies	1 year

proportion of fats and are best stored in a cool, dry place or they can be refrigerated or frozen.

Food Preparation

Harmful bacteria thrive best in moist, high-protein foods at a temperature between 45° F (7° C) and 140° F (60° C). Therefore, high-protein foods such as eggs, meats, and dairy products need to reach an internal temperature of at least 145° F (63° C) during cooking. Therefore, it is advisable to use a meat thermometer to check the internal temperature of meat and other food dishes, and it is important to allow ample cooking time for these dishes.

Pork needs to reach an internal temperature of 150° F (65° C) to kill the parasite *trichinella spiralis*. This parasite is undetectable in meat inspection and is commonly found in home-cured hams, undercooked sausages, and pork. The disease from *trichinella spiralis* is called trichinosis. The label on purchased pork must be checked to see if the meat is uncooked or cooked. Some food scientists believe that all pork products should be heated to assure food safety. Canned hams should be heated to an internal temperature of 140° F (60° C).

Foods prepared with egg and/or dairy products need prompt refrigeration after cooking and should not be held at room temperature for even a short time.

Kitchen Equipment and Dishes

Work surfaces, utensils, appliances, and dishes that are used in food preparation and serving can transmit harmful bacteria to food if they are not clean. Unclean work areas attract rodents, flies, and other insects more quickly than clean areas do. During food preparation countertops should be continuously wiped clean with a clean cloth and sinks need to be scoured daily.

Utensils and cutting surfaces become micro-organism carriers between uses for different foods. For example, both the knife and the cutting board used to cut raw meat need to be thoroughly cleaned with soap and water before vegetables are chopped on the same surface with the same knife. Food that is allowed to harden on utensils is a breeding ground for bacteria and care must be taken to remove all food particles from hard-to-clean areas of such utensils and appliances as rotary beaters, can openers, food grinders, meat slicers, and cookie presses.

The cooking surface and the exterior of small appliances should be thoroughly cleaned after each use. The manufacturer's instructions for special care directions should be followed.

The exterior and interior surfaces of the major kitchen appliances are in constant contact with both the hands and food. The stove surface area should be cleaned after each use and the oven should be frequently cleaned. Spilled and baked-on food particles are removed more easily if they are not allowed to remain on the cooking surfaces. The manufacturer's directions for special cleaning hints should be read. For both efficiency of operation and sanitation the microwave oven interior should be wiped clean often.

The outside surface of the refrigerator should be cleaned frequently. The interior parts of the refrigerator should be washed weekly and the interior walls cleaned. Some refrigerators require manual defrosting; after the ice has been removed, the defrosted section needs to be thoroughly washed. The manufacturer's directions will suggest the proper cleaning agents to use. The exterior of the freezer should be wiped clean frequently and the freezer interior should be defrosted and cleaned a minimum of once a year.

Many homes have automatic dishwashers. The exterior of the dishwasher should be cleaned and the manufacturer's directions followed for the care of the interior. Whether dishes are washed by hand or in the automatic dishwasher, they must first be scraped and rinsed to remove excess food particles. Dishes and utensils with baked-on food may need to be soaked before being washed. The directions of the manufacturer for loading the automatic dishwasher should be followed and only automatic dishwashing detergent should be used.

For hand dishwashing it is important to have the proper cleaning equipment. Suggested cleaning equipment includes a dishpan, a draining rack, a dish cloth or cellulose sponge, a plastic and steel wool abrasive pad, and clean dish towels. The choice of which abrasive pad to use depends upon what is to be cleaned. Utensils with special nonstick finishes such as Teflon and plastic ware are best cleaned with a plastic pad, whereas hard surfaces such as metal and glass can be cleaned with either a plastic pad or steel wool.

A recommended sequence for washing dishes is first glasses, then silver, dishware, utensils, and pans. All dishes should be rinsed with water to remove excess food particles before they are washed. Some dishes are easier to clean if they are soaked first to help remove encrusted food. A detergent and water that is as hot as the hands can stand is essential to cleaning dishes, and the water should be changed as it becomes greasy. After washing, dishes are placed in a draining rack and rinsed with water that has been heated on a surface burner until it is boiling (212° F) (100° C). If it is impossible to have very hot water for washing dishes, 1/4 ounce of laundry bleach per gallon of hot water should be used as the final rinse. The procedure is to wash the dishes with hot water and detergent, and then to rinse the dishes in hot water and then in the sanitizer solution. Dishes should air dry and then be stored. Air-drying helps to prevent bacterial contamination.

The one exception to air drying is items that tend to rust when water remains on the surface. For example, cast-iron utensils should be dried immediately after being washed and rinsed. Wooden ware may be washed in soapy water, and air dried. However, to prevent wooden ware from cracking and to maintain the finish, some prefer to only wipe thoroughly with a clean, wet cloth.

The garbage can must be cleaned after disposing of refuse, relined, and kept covered. The garbage can should never be situated near food.

Personal Sanitation

The cleanliness of the person handling, preparing, and serving food is of utmost importance. Clean clothing, clean hair, clean hands, and clean nails help to prevent the transmission of germs to food. Hands are always washed before beginning food preparation, between the handling of different kinds of food, and always after going to the toilet.

Coughing and sneezing over food that is being prepared must be avoided, and if cuts, pimples, or boils are present, food should not be handled. While working with food, the hands must be kept away from the mouth, nose, and hair. If hair is long, it is advisable to keep it tied back or to wear a hair covering.

In food preparation and serving, tools should be used for lifting and mixing food and the food-hand contact should be kept to a minimum. To sample food, a tasting spoon is used and the spoon is not returned to the food after the spoon has been in the mouth. Another clean spoon should be used to taste the next sample.

Government Protection Agencies

Laws, standards, and guidelines have been established by both private industry and governmental agencies to provide that the food purchased is wholesome, of high quality, and safe to eat. Private industry has made great progress in developing safe processing, storage, and transportation methods for food. Private industry safeguards on food vary with the specific functions of individual plants and are not discussed here. Federal, state, and local governmental agencies cooperate with the food industry in developing quality-controlled safe food.

Federal Agencies

Five federal agencies are directly concerned with protecting our food supply. Each agency covers a major aspect of food safety.

Food and Drug Administration. Operating under the Department of Health, Education and Welfare, the FDA is responsible for a large segment of laws that regulate food safety. The FDA's work began in 1906 with the passage of the original Pure Food and Drugs Act, which prohibited interstate transportation of adulterated food and drugs and the shipment of misbranded drinks in interstate commerce.

The Federal Food, Drug and Cosmetic Act was passed in 1938. Items of the act that directly relate to food safety include (1) authorized standards of identity, quality, and fill of container for foods; (2) authorization of factory inspections; (3) provisions for truth-in-labeling. The act covers both imported and exported food.

Standards of identity define the ingredients a food should contain when it is purchased; more than 200 food items have established standards of identity and the ingredients need not be listed on the container. For example, the ingredients for mayonnaise are not listed on the label if they meet the standard specifications as registered with the FDA, but if the mayonnaise does not meet the specifications, then the label must indicate this.

The act provides for minimum standards of quality for certain canned fruits and vegetables. A standard of quality is judged by a food's freedom from defects, color, and tenderness.

Standards of fill have been established for seafoods, tomato products, and certain canned fruits and vegetables. This segment of the law states how full the container must be when the food item is purchased. The act also provides for the FDA to regulate the use of the term *enrichment* to guarantee uniformity among products so labeled.

In 1954, the Miller Pesticides Amendment set safety limits for pesticide residues left on raw agricultural products. Once a safe tolerance level is established by the user of the pesticide, the legal residue level must be equal to, or exceed, the standard set by the FDA.

The 1958 Food Additives Amendment established requirements for proof of safety before an additive may be used in food. Because many food additives are common household foods, such as salt and sugar, the GRAS (Generally Recommended as Safe) list was established. The GRAS list, which includes over 600 items, eliminates the testing of commonly used household foods. As a part of the 1958 amendment, the Delaney Clause states that any additives shown to induce cancer in human beings or animal are prohibited from use in food.

In 1960, the Color Additive Amendment was passed. The 1938 act required only that synthetic colors be tested and certified for use by the FDA and there was no limit as to the quantity of the coloring material that could be used. The 1960 amendment brings all colors under the law and provides for all colors to be reevaluated for safety, especially regarding cancer-inducing properties. In addition, the law provides for the amount of color that can be used and states that no coloring agent can be used that will deceive the consumer.

Enacted in 1966, the Fair Packaging and Labeling Act requires that consumer products sold in interstate commerce be honestly and informatively labeled. Although the 1938 act states that foods must be honestly and informatively labeled and packaged, the 1966 act requires more complete information to enable the consumer to make more adequate value comparisons between products.

Information required by law on the food label includes (1) the food's identity and any variations in form, such as sliced, diced, or whole; (2) the quantity of food contents by weight or liquid measure; (3) the name and address of the manufacturer, packer, or distributor; (4) the listing of the ingredients in decreasing order if the food does not have a Standard of Identity; and (5) the listing of any artificial flavoring or chemical preservatives.

Nutrition-labeling regulations were established by the FDA in 1975. Providing nutrition information on the label is voluntary on the part of the manufacturer except when the food contains added nutrients or makes additional nutritional claims. Any nutritional information included on the label must include in terms of the stated serving or portion (1) calorie content to the nearest 5-calories increment; (2) the number of grams of protein, fat, and available carbohydrate to the nearest gram; (3) the amount of vitamins and minerals expressed in 10 per cent increments of the US RDA; and (4) the listing of vitamin A, vitamin C, thiamine, riboflavin, niacin, calcium, and iron in percentages of the US RDA. Informative nutritional labeling is illustrated in Figure 3–3.

U.S. Department of Agriculture. The USDA is responsible for both mandatory and voluntary food inspection programs, and for establishing grading standards of quality for specific foods. Both grading and inspection programs are under the auspices of the Consumer and Marketing Service of the USDA.

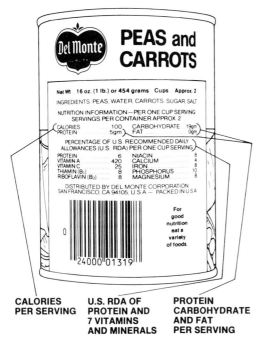

CALORIES PER SERVING   U.S. RDA OF PROTEIN AND 7 VITAMINS AND MINERALS   PROTEIN CARBOHYDRATE AND FAT PER SERVING

Figure 3–3.

Informative nutritional labeling can be a helpful guide to the consumer. (Del Monte)

Grading offers to both the food industry and the consumer an avenue of quality food control with the establishment of definite standards of size, color, shape, maturity, lack of defects, and gradation of the food's value and usability. Quality-grading standards have been established by the USDA for fruits, vegetables, and nuts. Although the U.S. grade may not be printed on the label, it is probably used by the wholesaler in purchasing lots of food. Grading is not required by law but is available upon request to the USDA for a fee. Figure 3-4 shows the USDA shield and grade mark used for eggs.

Meat grades have been established by the USDA on the basis of conformation, finish, and quality, but it is not mandatory that these grades be used. Carcass meat that is quality graded by the USDA must also be yield graded.

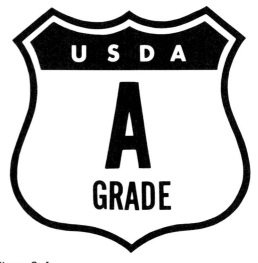

Figure 3–4.

Official USDA grade mark used on egg cartons when the egg size is designated on the carton.

See Chapter 14 for a more complete discussion on meat grading.

Except for meat and poultry inspection and egg inspection, upon request and for a fee, voluntary food inspection is provided by the USDA. Inspection assures the consumer that the food meets the minimum standards required, that the food is wholesome, and that the statements on the label are true. Food-processing plants that most often use this service include canned and frozen fruits and vegetable plants, dairy product plants, and processors of fresh eggs. Mandatory food inspection by federal or federally trained state inspectors is now being required for meat, poultry, and egg products. Figure 3-5 shows the USDA inspection shield.

In 1906, federal meat inspections began with the requirement that all meat-packing plants involved in the slaughter or manufacture of meat food products sold in interstate or foreign commerce be federally inspected. The Wholesome Meat Act of 1967 required the inspection of all meat that is entered in commerce

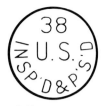

Figure 3–5.
This is the USDA inspection shield for meat.

and capable of being used as human food. The act requires that each state provide an inspection program "equal to" the federal standards of inspection for products prepared and sold in that state (intrastate commerce) or be designated as one requiring federal inspection for that state. The USDA monitors the state programs at least quarterly to assure compliance with that law.

The Wholesome Poultry Products Act of 1968 provides for the federal or state inspection following federal guidelines of all poultry and poultry products sold in the United States. Specifically, inspectors check for processing under sanitary conditions, product wholesomeness, and truthful labeling.

The Egg Products Inspection Act of 1970 provides for the inspection of plants where egg products are manufactured and sets specifications for the labeling of such products. The act regulates the type of eggs used in egg products and established control over imported egg products and imported fresh eggs.

U.S. Department of Commerce. Inspection and grading of fish and shellfish is performed by inspectors from the U.S. Department of Commerce. The voluntary inspection is paid for by the seafood company requesting the service.

U.S. Public Health Service. The primary function of this agency is to guard the public against food hazards. The Center for Disease Control of the U.S. Public Health Service investigates the occurrence and the cause of food poisoning outbreaks throughout the country. The Grade A Pasteurized Milk Ordinance, developed by the Public Health Service, is a set of standards for protecting the nation's milk supply. In state and local areas that have adopted the ordinance, this agency advises in its administration.

Federal Trade Commission. The FTC helps to protect the safety of food by investigating and taking action against false and misleading advertising, deceptive packaging, and unfair price fixing.

State Agencies

Some states have departments of health, or agriculture, and/or consumer protection that along with special state boards and commissions help to regulate food safety within the state's boundaries. State departments of agriculture are mainly responsible for the inspection and grading of raw foods, the proper use of food additives and pesticides, and the sanitation of food handling establishments. State and federal inspectors work together to enforce the mandatory inspection of meat and poultry. Most often state regulations regarding food and drinking establishments are handled by the state departments of health. State consumer protection departments are most responsible for investigation of food mishandling and the education of the public.

Many state departments have laboratories to analyze food products for contamination and to develop better methods for quality food control.

Local Agencies

Local food safety controls vary with the needs of the area. The main responsibility is normally undertaken by city and county health departments.

1. Contact the director or public information offices of a city or county health department to determine the agency's role in maintaining food safety in the community.
2. Contact the director or public information offices of the state department of health and the state department of agriculture to determine the specific functions of these agencies in your state in maintaining food safety.
3. Set up a display picturing foods that are susceptible to harmful bacterial growth.
4. Contact the manager of a major restaurant and fast-food outlet in your area to discover how each deals with food sanitation.
5. Make a chart of poisonous plants specific to your locale and plan a way for disseminating this information to mothers of preschool children.
6. Make a study of the food sanitation procedures followed in your home and note important changes, if any, that need to be made.
7. Check the local grocery store to determine which foods carry the USDA shield.
8. If a food-packing plant is in your area, learn the specific rules and regulations that the plant enforces to ensure food safety.
9. Collect a group of labels with nutrition information and determine the effectiveness of these labels in educating the consumer.

1. What are the two major causes of foodborne illness?
2. Name the five causes of unsafe food.
3. Which foods are highly susceptible to bacterial growth?
4. What foods are susceptible to spoilage and deterioration because of oxidation?
5. What signs in the appearance of food may suggest that the food is unsafe?
6. What foods are susceptible to *salmonella* growth?
7. Why should one purchase only pasteurized milk?
8. What personal health situations determine whether or not one should handle food?
9. Give three examples of moist, high-protein foods. What kinds of bacteria grow in moist, high-protein foods?
10. Why should home-processed foods not be tasted before being heated?
11. What are three factors that would warn you that canned food is spoiled?
12. What is the proper care for refrigerated leftovers?
13. Why can the family picnic become a dangerous meal?
14. Name four rules to remember when storing refrigerated foods.
15. What is the reason for shelf-rotation of canned foods?
16. What disease can be contracted from eating improperly cooked pork? How can this disease be avoided?
17. How does one care for wooden cutting boards?
18. Why should one not use the same knife and cutting board without cleaning for

chopping vegetables and cutting raw meat?

19. List six important rules for personal sanitation when handling food.

20. What is the meaning of standard of identity as set forth in the 1938 Food, Drug and Cosmetic Act?

21. How do the Miller Pesticide Amendment and the Food Additives Amendment assure us that food is safe?

22. What information is required by law to be included on a food label?

23. What two groups of foods are now under mandatory federal inspection?

24. What is the difference between mandatory and voluntary inspection?

25. How does the grading of certain foods help the consumer?

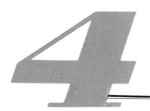

Cereals

Cereals are a group of foods derived from plants, which are called *grains*. Cereal grains such as wheat, oats, rye, and barley are seeds that are derived from dried grasses. Cereals are the main food for most of the world's population and are one of the least expensive foods available. In some parts of the world, more than 80 per cent of an individual's calorie intake is obtained from cereals.

Now and in the future, grains are expected to help solve much of the world's hunger problem because they can be grown under most soil and climatic conditions. Food researchers are working to develop grains with a higher nutritive quality and that give a higher yield per acre. For the weight-conscious American, the cereal group is often overlooked, and yet it is a needed and staple food, which is low in calories.

Nutritional Factors to Consider

Carbohydrate. Cereal grains are a major source of energy in the diet because they are high in carbohydrate. It is recommended that the individual consume four or more servings daily from the cereal group. One slice of bread, 1 ounce of ready-to-eat cereal, or 1/2 cup of cooked rice constitutes one serving, as shown in Figure 4-1.

Fat. The fat of cereal grain is located in the germ of the kernel. Whole-grain cereals which contain the germ provide fat in the diet, and vegetable oils derived from the germ and used in the diet. Figure 4-2 illustrates the structure of the grain kernel.

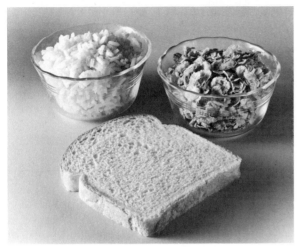

Figure 4-1.
One slice of bread, 1 ounce of ready-to-eat cereal or 1/2 cup of cooked rice constitutes one serving from the bread and cereal group.

Protein. Cereal proteins are incomplete proteins because they lack one or more of the essential amino acids, lysine, threonin, or tryptophan. However, many cereals are eaten with complete protein foods and this combination serves to make the food eaten a more complete source of protein. For example, cooked oats combined with milk is a good protein source.

Vitamins and Minerals. Whole-grain cereals are excellent sources of the B vitamins. When cereals are refined in processing, some of the nutrients are lost. Federal law has established standards for adding back the nutrients lost in processing and most cereals today are enriched with thiamine, riboflavin, niacin, and iron. Additional vitamins, minerals, and protein are added to some cereal products. Supplements to cereals must be stated on the container label and it is important to read the label of a cereal box to determine the ingredients and additions.

The minerals calcium, phosphorus, and iron are present in unrefined cereals. Iron is returned to cereals by the enrichment process, but other minerals may or may not be added.

Calories. Cereals and cereal products are not high in calories when they are consumed in the recommended amounts. One slice of enriched white bread contains 41 calories, 1 cup of cooked oatmeal contains 132 calories, and 1/2

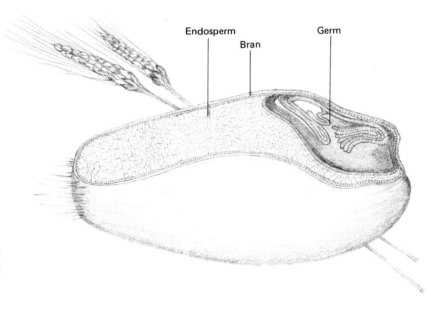

Endosperm   Bran   Germ

Figure 4-2.
The grain kernel is composed of the bran, endosperm and germ layers.

cup of cooked enriched rice contains approximately 112 calories.

Menu-Planning Points

Cereals and their products are important foods to include in all meals. They not only are important nutrient contributors, available at a relatively low cost, but they give a pleasing balance of flavor and texture. For example, a dry, crisp cereal adds textural quality to a breakfast and the flavor of a rye bread or a cornbread adds variety to many meals.

Cereal grains play an important role in the food of a culture. Corn is the principal food for the peoples of South America, and rice is the most important and most widely eaten food for the people of Asia. Wheat is the principal cereal grain eaten by people of the Western world.

Kinds of Cereal

Many different kinds of cereals and cereal products are available on the market. Some of these products are composed of a single grain and some are mixtures. One of the most popular ways to eat cereal is in the form of breakfast food. Breakfast cereals are sold either in a ready-to-eat form that has been cooked during processing or in a form that must be cooked prior to eating. Other products made from cereal grains include flours, meals, and starches.

The kernel is the part of the grain that is eaten. During harvesting the outer covering or hull of the grain is removed and the kernel is left. The kernel is composed of three different layers. The outer layer, known as the *bran*, is composed mainly of cellulose. The middle layer, the *endosperm*, is the main starch portion of the kernel. The third layer or portion of the kernel, the *germ*, is located at the lower end of the kernel. See Figure 4-2.

Cereal grains go through a process called *milling* to separate the various particles and to make various grain products. White or refined rice and white flour has had both the bran and germ removed. Unless the product is a whole grain, the germ is removed and sold separately, because it contains the fat of the kernel and tends to become rancid when it is exposed to air, thereby affecting the keeping quality of the product.

Cereal grains include barley, corn, oats, rice, rye, and wheat. Cereals are either consumed in grain form or are further processed and refined into many different food products. Flour, a refined cereal product with a high starch content, is the principal thickening agent in food preparation.

Barley. Barley is sold as pearl barley, from which the hull and bran have been removed in processing. This cereal is mainly used in making soups and some casserole-type dishes. Barley flour is used in baby foods and in some types of breakfast cereals.

Corn. Corn meal, corn grits, hominy, corn syrup, cornstarch, corn oil, and several types of breakfast cereals are the products of corn. Cornmeal is made either from the whole kernel or by removing the bran and germ and grinding the endosperm. Hominy, usually made from white corn, has both the hull and germ removed. Corn grits is made by breaking the endosperm. Corn oil is processed from the germ of the kernel. The popular breakfast cereal, corn flakes, is made by blending corn grits with other ingredients. When the whole kernel of corn is eaten, it is considered a vegetable.

Oats. Oats, sold as either rolled oats or oatmeal, are used mainly as breakfast foods. They

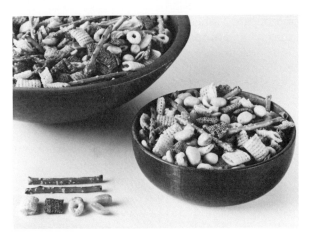

Figure 4–3.

A mixture of cereals and other ingredients heated with seasonings and small amount of fat makes a nutritious snack.

are made from the whole kernel including the bran and the germ portions. They may be combined with wheat, mainly in the form of flour, for making such baked products as cookies and bread. Figure 4–3 shows a combination of cereals served for a snack.

Rice. Rice is discussed in Chapter 10, rather than in this chapter. However, rice is considered a cereal grain.

Rye. Rye is made into flour and is principally used in the preparation of bread, most often in combination with wheat flour. Because of its chemical characteristics, rye flour produces a baked product that has a very compact texture.

Wheat. Wheat is classified as either hard or soft. Durum wheat is a hard wheat used in making pasta products. The major portion of wheat is milled into flour and sold as white, or "enriched white," sometimes referred to as "all-purpose," and whole wheat. These flours may be made from soft wheat or be a mixture of hard and soft wheat. Soft wheat is used in making cake flour. The uncooked wheat cereal, called farina, is made from the endosperm. Various forms of ready-to-eat breakfast cereals made from wheat are available.

Purchasing and Storing Cereals

Cereals are considered to be among our least expensive foods and therefore can be a great saving to the food budget. The more highly processed and refined cereal products are usually the most costly. For example, ready-to-eat breakfast cereals are more costly than those that must be cooked prior to eating, and sugar-coated cereals are not only more expensive but less nutritious. Instant-cooked cereals are more costly than those that require longer cooking. One exception at the present is that the less refined whole wheat flour and brown rice are more expensive than all-purpose flour and white rice.

Although most cereal products are enriched, it is advisable to check the label for added nutrients and the listing of ingredients, which are listed in decreasing order of quantity contained. A 1-ounce serving is considered an average serving and therefore cereals should be purchased by net weight, not by the package size. Cereal should be purchased in accordance with personal preference, the use intended, the time available for preparation, and the storage space allowance in the kitchen.

Cereals are best stored in a dry, well-ventilated area. Proper covering and storage of cereal grains are important to prevent insects from entering. Processed cereal grains, such as flour, are more conveniently stored in a container with a tight-fitting lid. Breakfast cereals are best stored in their original package that should be properly reclosed after each use. In humid climates, it is better to store plastic-packaged cereals in a metal or glass container.

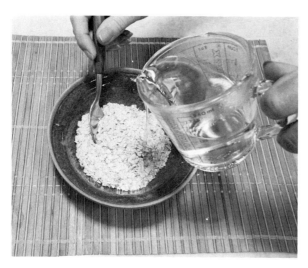

Figure 4–4.

Instant cereals can be quickly mixed and when served with milk make a complete protein food.

Cooking of Cereals

Uncooked cereals are either cooked by pouring them into boiling, salted water, or if finely ground, they are first mixed with cold water and then added to the boiling, salted water. Instant and precooked cereal grains have greatly shortened the length of time involved in meal preparation. Figure 4–4 shows instant cereal mixed with boiling water, which is ready-to-eat. The cooking time required for cereals is dependent upon whether they are cooked over direct heat or in a double boiler, and whether they are a precooked, instant, or a regular form. Precooked and instant cereals take from 1 to 5 minutes cooking time, whereas uncooked cereals take from 30 minutes to 2 hours to cook.

Cereal is cooked by stirring it into rapidly boiling water. If the cereal is finely ground, it may be mixed first with cold water to form a paste and then added to the boiling water. Cereal thickens by the release of starch from the grain. It should be stirred only at the start of cooking, since further stirring will yield a gummy and unpalatable mass. For a more in-depth discussion on the cooking of starch, refer to Chapter 6, "Sauces."

The amount of water used in cooking will determine the thickness of the cereal. The usual proportion is 1 cup of cereal to 2 cups of boiling water, but it is best to read the cooking directions on the package. Cooking instructions vary for the different types of cereal.

Cereals may also be cooked in a microwave oven. It is important to use a large enough glass dish so that the cereal will not boil over. In microwave cooking, the mass is stirred several times to keep the food evenly distributed. A single serving needs less stirring than a larger amount. Allowance must also be made for carry-over cooking, which is caused by heat remaining in the food even though it has been removed from the oven.

Other Uses of Cereals

Cereals are also used in the preparation of many food dishes to provide added nutrition, flavor, and texture. For example, oatmeal may be added to meat loaf or other dishes prepared from a ground meat, as shown in Figure 4–5, not only to increase the number of servings but also to reduce the amount of meat used. This helps to reduce the cost of the food. Cereal grains are nutritious additions to all kinds of baked products, including breads and cookies. Adding 1/2 to 1 cup of ready-to-eat cereal to cookie recipes and topping casserole dishes with a crushed ready-to-eat cereal adds flavor to the finished product.

Convenience Cereal Food Products

In addition to dry and ready-to-cook cereals that are available today, other convenience cereal food products continue to increase on the market. Particularly popular are snack foods such as crackers and chips. Although these are flavorful and popular with all age groups, care must be exercised that additional sodium and fat intake are not added to the daily dietary plan.

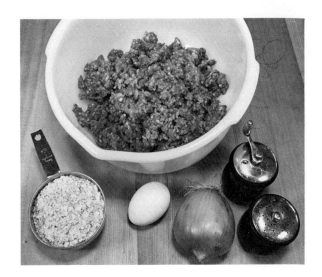

Figure 4-5.
When uncooked oatmeal is added to ground meat mixtures, the number of servings is increased and the nutrition, flavor, and texture of the food is improved.

RECIPES

——————— Cereal Snack ———————

	Standard	Metric
Butter or margarine	3/4 cup	180 mL
Worcestershire sauce	1 Tbsp.	15 mL
Seasoning salt	2 Tbsp.	50 mL
Wheat squares	2 cups	500 mL
Rice squares	2 cups	500 mL
Oat puffs (cereal circles)	1 cup	250 mL
Pretzel sticks	2 cups	500 mL
Peanuts	1 cup	250 mL

1. Preheat oven to 250° F (121° C).
2. Combine butter or margarine, Worcestershire sauce, and seasoning salt in a large shallow baking pan or in the bottom of a broiler pan and place in oven. Heat until the fat is melted.
3. Add cereals, pretzel sticks, and peanuts. Bake for 1 hour, stirring ingredients every 15 minutes.
4. Store in a tightly covered container in a dry area.

Yield: approximately 2 quarts

Variations
1. Measurements of cereal ingredients may be altered to suit personal taste. Mixed nuts may be substituted for peanuts.
2. The recipe may be prepared in a microwave oven. Melt butter or margarine, Worcestershire sauce, and seasoning salt in 2 C. glass measure. Use a large glass bowl for mixing and cooking and cook 20 minutes, stirring every 5 minutes.

——————— Fruity Granola ———————

	Standard	Metric
Quick or regular oats, uncooked	5 cups	1250 mL
Brown sugar, firmly packed	1/3 cup	75 mL
Wheat germ	1/2 cup	125 mL
Vegetable oil	1/3 cup	75 mL
Honey	1/4 cup	60 mL
Almond extract	1/4 tsp.	1 mL
Raisins	1 cup	250 mL
Dried chopped apricots	1 cup	250 mL

1. Preheat oven to 350° F (175° C).
2. Add oats to a 13 × 9 × 2 inch ungreased pan and bake in the oven for 10 minutes.

3. In a bowl combine oats, brown sugar, and wheat germ. Add oil, honey, and almond extract. Mix until the dry ingredients are well coated.
4. Bake in the same ungreased pan used in Step number 2 for 20 to 25 minutes. Stir every 5 minutes to ensure even browning. Cool.
5. Stir until crumbly; add raisins and apricots.
6. Refrigerate in a tightly covered container.

Yield: 8-1/2 cups

--- Hominy Grits ---

	Standard	Metric
Water	5 cups	1250 mL
Salt	1 tsp.	5 mL
Hominy grits	1 cup	250 mL

1. Heat water to boiling; add salt.
2. Slowly add the grits to the boiling water, stirring constantly; cover and cook for 25 to 30 minutes. Stir occasionally.
3. Serve with butter and sugar as a cereal or with butter or gravy as a meat accompaniment.

Yield: six servings

--- Cornmeal Mush ---

	Standard	Metric
Cornmeal	1/2 cup	125 mL
Water, cold	1/2 cup	125 mL
Salt	1/2 tsp.	2 mL
Water, boiling	2 cups	500 mL

1. Mix cornmeal with cold water.
2. Gradually add cornmeal mixture to boiling salted water, stirring until mixture comes to a boil. Cover and cook for 10 minutes, stirring occasionally.

Yield: 2 cups

--- Fried Cornmeal Mush ---

1. One recipe (4 servings or 2 cups) thick cornmeal mush.
2. Pour cooked cornmeal into a loaf pan. Chill until set.
3. Unmold and slice into 1/4-inch slices. Melt a small amount of fat in a heavy skillet. Fry the slices on each side until they are a light, golden brown.
4. Serve with syrup, honey, or jam.

Yield: four servings

--- Cornmeal Squares with Mushroom Sauce ---

	Standard	Metric
Milk	2 cups	500 mL
Cornmeal	1/2 cup	125 mL
Salt	3/4 tsp.	7 mL
Grated cheddar cheese	3/4 cup	175 mL
Minced green pepper	1 Tbsp.	15 mL
Dry mustard	1/4 tsp.	1 mL

1. Preheat oven to 350° F (175° C).
2. Scald 1-1/2 cups milk. Combine remaining 1/2 cup milk with cornmeal and stir gradually into scalded milk. Add salt.
3. Bring mixture to a boil, stirring constantly.
4. Cover; reduce heat to low; and cook for 30 minutes.
5. Remove from heat and add cheese, green pepper, and dry mustard. Stir until cheese has melted. Pour into greased loaf pan and cool.
6. Slice chilled mixture and place slices in greased 8-inch square baking pan and cover with mushroom sauce.

Mushroom Sauce
1. Mix 1 can cream of mushroom soup with 1/2 cup milk or prepare a medium thick white sauce and add 1/2 cup chopped mushrooms that have been sauteed in 2 Tbsp. butter or margarine. The basic proportions for a medium white sauce and method of preparation are given in Chapter 6, Sauces (page 80).

Yield: four servings

Cracked Wheat with Mushrooms

	Standard	Metric
Butter or margarine	1/4 cup	60 mL
Chopped onion	1/2 cup	125 mL
Sliced mushrooms	1/2 cup	125 mL
Cracked wheat	1 cup	250 mL
Chicken broth	3 cups	750 mL
Salt	1 tsp.	5 mL

1. Melt butter or margarine in a heavy saucepan and sauté onions and mushrooms until lightly browned.
2. Add cracked wheat and cook 5 minutes, stirring constantly.
3. Add chicken broth and salt; bring to a boil. Cover and reduce heat to low. Cook for 30 minutes.

Yield: 4 to 6 servings

Barley Casserole

	Standard	Metric
Butter or margarine	2 Tbsp.	30 mL
Pearl barley	1 cup	250 mL
Chopped celery	1/2 cup	125 mL
Dehydrated onion	1 tsp.	5 mL
Chopped parsley	1 Tbsp.	15 mL
Salt	1 tsp.	5 mL
Pepper	1/4 tsp.	1 mL
Chicken bouillon cubes	2	2
Water, boiling	2 cups	500 mL

1. Preheat oven to 350° F (175° C).
2. Melt butter or margarine in heavy fry pan and sauté barley lightly; do not let brown.
3. Combine barley, celery, onion, parsley, salt, and pepper in a casserole dish.
4. Dissolve bouillon cubes in boiling water and add to the barley mixture.
5. Bake for 1 hour.

Yield: 4 to 6 servings

Farina Pudding

	Standard	Metric
Milk, scalded	2 cups	500 mL
Butter	2 Tbsp.	30 mL
Grated lemon peel	1-1/2 tsp.	7 mL
Salt	1/4 tsp.	1 mL
Farina	1/3 cup	75 mL
Eggs, separated	4	4
Sugar	1/4 cup	60 mL

1. To the hot scalded milk add the butter, lemon peel, and salt and stir. For discussion on milk scalding, refer to Chapter 8, Milk.
2. Gradually add the farina, stirring constantly. Cook over low heat, stirring constantly, until thick.
3. Cool mixture to lukewarm.
4. Beat egg yolks until thick and lemon colored. Blend into farina mixture. For discussion of egg cookery, refer to Chapter 7, Eggs.
5. Beat egg whites until frothy and gradually add sugar, beating continuously.
6. Gently fold farina mixture into egg whites and spoon into a buttered 2-quart casserole.
7. Set casserole dish in a larger pan and pour boiling water to a depth of 1 inch on the sides of the pan.
8. Bake for 1 hour and 35 minutes or until a knife inserted near center comes out clean. Serve immediately.

Yield: 6 to 8 servings

Indian Pudding

	Standard	Metric
Yellow cornmeal	1/2 cup	125 mL
Sugar	1/4 cup	60 mL
Salt	1 tsp.	5 mL
Cinnamon	1 tsp.	5 mL
Ginger	1/2 tsp.	2 mL
Milk, scalded	3 cups	650 mL
Egg, well-beaten	1	1
Molasses	1/2 cup	125 mL
Butter or margarine	2 Tbsp.	30 mL
Milk, cold	1 cup	250 mL

1. Preheat oven to 300° F (150° C).
2. Mix together in a bowl the cornmeal, sugar, salt, cinnamon, and ginger.
3. Slowly stir cornmeal mixture into hot, scalded milk.
4. Mix together the egg and molasses.
5. Blend 2 tablespoons of the hot cornmeal mixture into the combined egg and molasses.
6. Stir the warmed egg and molasses into the cornmeal mixture and cook over boiling water for 10 minutes or until thick, stirring constantly. Stir in the butter.
7. Turn the mixture into a casserole and pour the 1 cup of milk over the top of the mixture.
8. Bake in oven for 2 hours or until the top is lightly browned.
9. Serve warm with whipped cream or ice cream.

Yield: 6 servings

Scottish Bread

	Standard	Metric
Barley flour, or 1 cup oatmeal and 1 cup cornmeal	2 cups	500 mL
Soda	1 tsp.	5 mL
Powdered ginger	1/2 tsp.	2 mL
Grated lemon rind	1 Tbsp.	15 mL
Butter or margarine	1 Tbsp.	15 mL
Buttermilk	1 cup	250 mL
Butter or margarine, melted	2 Tbsp.	30 mL
Honey	2 Tbsp.	30 mL

1. Preheat oven to 375° F (190° C).
2. Mix barley flour, soda, ginger, and lemon rind together in a mixing bowl.

3. Combine buttermilk, melted butter, and honey and add to dry ingredients. Stir to mix well.
4. Melt butter in a 12-inch heavy fry pan that is ovenproof.
5. Add bread mixture and cook on top of the stove for 10 minutes over a moderately low heat.
6. Bake in oven for 20 minutes. Serve hot.

Yield: 4 to 6 servings

Oatmeal Griddle Cakes

	Standard	Metric
Buttermilk	3 cups	750 mL
Rolled oats	1 cup	250 mL
Flour, sifted	1 cup	250 mL
Sugar	2 Tbsp.	30 mL
Baking soda	1 tsp.	5 mL
Salt	1 tsp.	5 mL
Eggs, beaten	2	2

1. Combine the buttermilk and oats; cover. Refrigerate 4 hours or overnight.
2. When ready to cook, sift the flour, sugar, baking soda, and salt together into a mixing bowl.
3. Combine the eggs and buttermilk mixture and add all at once to the sifted dry ingredients. Stir until the dry ingredients are just moistened. For a further discussion on mixing batter, refer to Chapter 17, Breads.
4. Add a small amount of fat to a griddle or heavy fry pan. Pour the batter from a pitcher onto the hot surface and cook over medium heat, turning once to lightly brown each side.

Yield: 1 to 1-1/2 dozen griddle cakes

LEARNING ACTIVITIES

1. Investigate the types of cereal grains that are available at a local market. Categorize them into regular, precooked, or instant. Read the label to determine what type of fortification or enrichment each type has. Make a price comparison between a grain that is available in more than one form.

2. Prepare an instant-cooking cereal and long-cooking cereal of the same grain. Analyze the time of preparation and the difference in flavor and texture. Determine which would be the best buy for the working individual who has limited time for food preparation.

3. Investigate the different kinds of flour available at the grocery store. Make a price comparison both between different brands of the same kinds of flour and between different kinds of flour, and report as to which would be the best buy for general food preparation.

4. Listen to the advertisements during a popular children's television or radio program and note the different cereals that are advertised. Go to the store and investigate to see whether there is any difference in price between the advertised cereals and those cereals that are not advertised. Note the ingredients of the advertised cereals.

5. Make a list of the ways advertisers try to sell food through children on the basis of what is learned in number 4.

6. Make a list of the different ways that cereals can be used in cooking in addition to being used as breakfast cereals.

7. Plan a complete breakfast menu around some type of cooked breakfast cereal. Analyze the meal for its nutrient contribution to the day. Determine which nutrient areas need more foods to complete one's daily requirements.

8. Plan a breakfast menu a family of four could prepare for themselves in the morning. Presume that the ages of the children are 6 and 12.

9. Make a list of toppings that could be used for cereal that would still be nutritious but could be used in place of milk. Determine how milk could still be a part of the menu.

10. Develop a recipe for a cereal granola using your own cereal variations. Analyze the recipe for carbohydrate and fat content.

11. Compare the cost of the recipe in number 10 with a commercially available granola.

12. Make a list of recipes containing a cereal grain as the main food ingredient that could be used as a satisfactory substitute for potatoes in a meal.

13. Make a list of foods containing a high-protein food that would be less expensive to prepare if extended with a cereal.

REVIEW QUESTIONS

1. Why is cereal such an important food to the world population?

2. Why is cereal a major source of energy in the diet?

3. Why is cereal not considered a good source of protein when eaten alone?

4. If a cereal grain is enriched, what nutrients are put back?

5. Which mineral is predominant in whole-grain and enriched cereals?

6. What are the three sections of a cereal kernel?

7. From which section of the kernel is flour milled?

8. What is the name of the uncooked wheat cereal?

9. Which cereal is the most expensive and which is the least expensive?
10. Why is it important to read the label on a cereal container?
11. What are three important things to remember about storing cereal grains and cereal products?
12. What are the two ways to cook a cereal? What determines the thickness of the cooked product?

5

Fats

Fat is present in both plants and animals. Its importance in food preparation can be evaluated from the high proportion (40%) of the daily food consumption of the average American. In food preparation fat contributes flavor and texture, and serves as a medium in which foods are cooked.

Fat may be solid, semisolid, or liquid at room temperature. The term *oil* is used when referring to a liquid fat. Fat is either unsaturated, saturated, or polyunsaturated. For a further discussion of the latter, refer to Chapter 1.

Nutritional Factors to Consider

Fat is a major energy source in the diet, providing almost 2-1/4 times as many calories per gram as either protein or carbohydrate. Table 5-1 shows the high energy content of some food products. Foods that are high in fat content are good sources of the fat-soluble vitamins, A, D, E, and K. Whole milk and butter are good sources of vitamin A and other dairy products may be enriched with both vitamin A and/or vitamin D. Margarine, which is made from vegetable oils, is usually fortified with vitamin A. Vegetable oils are also a good source of vitamin E.

Kinds of Fat

Butter. Butter is made from the fat of milk and by federal law must contain no less than 80 per cent milkfat. Butter contributes an appreciable flavor to many foods, and is used chiefly as a spread and as the fat ingredient in some baked products and sauces.

Margarine. Margarine is a mixture of skim milk and other ingredients, mainly vegetable oils.

Table 5-1
Energy Content of Some Food Products

	Food Energy (Calories)	Fat (gms)
Apple pie, 3-1/2 inch sector arc	302	13
Bacon, 2 slices, broiled or fried, drained	86	8
Butter, 1 Tbsp.	2	12
Ground Beef Patty, 3 oz. 21 per cent fat	235	17
Margarine, 1 Tbsp.	102	12
Mayonnaise, 1 Tbsp.	101	11
Peanut butter, 1 Tbsp.	94	8
Whole milk, 1 cup	159	9

Nutritive Value of American Foods. Agriculture Handbook #456. USDA. 1975.

By federal law, margarine must contain no less than 80 per cent fat. Most margarines are fortified with vitamin A and vitamin D. Margarine and butter are often used interchangeably as a fat ingredient. Those margarines that are labeled "imitation" contain about 40 per cent fat, and whipped margarines contain about 55 per cent fat. These margarines are more expensive and cannot be used interchangeably with butter in a recipe but are satisfactory to use as a spread.

Lard. Lard is processed from pork fat. When used in making a piecrust, lard makes a tender and flaky product. Some baked products for which lard is used as the fat ingredient may have a heavier texture because it does not hold air well. Lard contributes a definite flavor to any cooked product. If lard is exposed to air, it becomes rancid and thus needs to be kept continuously under refrigeration. Some lard products now on the market have been fortified with an antioxidant to prevent rancidity and are more acceptable for food preparation.

Vegetable Oils. Vegetable oils are processed from various seeds, legumes, and other foods. The most common vegetable oils are made from corn, olives, peanuts, safflowers, and soybeans. These oils are often combined to make a fat product. A highly nutritious butter is made from peanuts and is used as a spread or as an additional ingredient in various kinds of food preparation. This food is further discussed in Chapter 10 on Meat Alternates.

Hydrogenated Fat. A hydrogenated fat is a vegetable oil or a combination of vegetable oil and animal fats to which hydrogen has been added to create a semisolid fat. This fat is more plastic or moldable than fats such as butter or margarine. A hydrogenated fat is a highly desirable form of fat to use in many areas of food preparation because it is easily combined with other ingredients. A hydrogenated fat is commonly called a *shortening.*

Purchasing and Storing Fat and Oil

In general, fats and oils are purchased according to the individual's taste and flavor preference. Other factors in selecting a fat or oil include special dietary needs, the intended use for the fat or oil, and the price. Reading the label of a fat or oil product helps the consumer decide if the product will meet his or her specific needs. Ingredients of fats and oils are always listed in order of the percentage contained. As of January 1978, the labels of all fats and oils must also provide the common name of the fat used, such as coconut oil or lard, rather than just vegetable or animal fat.

The most expensive fat is butter. The prices of other fats will vary with the kinds of fats or oils used and the type of processing; oils are usually more costly than hydrogenated fats. Lard is available in most large markets and in specialty stores.

Animal fats need to be refrigerated because

they tend to oxidize and become rancid when exposed to air. For extended storage, butter should be frozen. Hydrogenated fats and vegetable oils can be stored at room temperature or they can be refrigerated. Vegetable oils go through a special process called winterizing to prevent a cloudy appearance when the oil is chilled. The cloudy appearance of vegetable oils is caused by some of the fat solidifying. Refrigerated hydrogenated fat will be easier to handle if brought to room temperature before use. All fats should be kept well covered because they can pick up flavors and odors of other foods.

Functions in Food Preparation

Emulsion Ingredient. Fat is a major ingredient of oil-in-liquid emulsions, in which the fat is dispersed in droplet form in another liquid such as water. Examples of foods in which fat is a major ingredient in emulsion formation are whole milk, various salad dressings, and ice cream.

Flavoring Agent. The type of fat used can greatly enhance the flavor of the food. Butter has a highly desirable flavor when it is added to certain foods such as cooked vegetables. Many baked products require the rather bland flavor of hydrogenated shortenings or vegetable oils. Olive oil has a distinctive flavor that may or may not be desirable in food. It is usually used in some ethnic dishes and in some salad dressings, and as a frying medium for certain meats. Lard and bacon fat have distinctive flavors that may or may not be appealing to the taste.

Tenderization Agent. Fat is a tenderizing agent in most baked products. Gluten is the protein portion of flour that develops elasticity when it is mixed with water. Because fat is insoluble in water it is able to encompass the gluten strands of the flour and prevent them from becoming

as strong, thereby producing a more tender product. This process is sometimes referred to as the "shortening" power of the fat. Butter and margarine do not have as much "shortening" power as hydrogenated fats.

Leavening Agent. Fat acts as a leavening agent for mixtures in which the fat is creamed and the mixture is beaten, because the fat holds in the air which has been incorporated.

Frying Medium. Fat helps to prevent food from sticking to the pan and serves as a medium for the transferring of heat to the food. Vegetable oils and hydrogenated shortening are the best fats for frying because they have a higher smoke point than butter, margarine, and most forms of lard.

All fats have a smoke point, the temperature at which a fat begins to decompose. At this stage smoke rises from the surface of the fat. The decomposition of fat is not only irritating to the nose and throat but is likely to give an off-flavor to foods being cooked in such fat. Fats vary at the temperature at which they melt and solidify.

Foods are either pan-fried or deep-fried. In pan frying the food is cooked in a small amount of fat until it reaches the desired stage of doneness. Foods that are deep-fried are submerged in hot fat and cooked.

Deep frying is done in a deep-fat fryer or in a deep heavy metal pan with straight sides and a small surface area. For pans that do not have a thermostatically controlled temperature unit, it is important to use a thermometer, which can be attached to the side of the pan to assure a proper temperature of the fat. A basket is helpful for lowering small foods into a pan and for removing them upon completion of cooking. A slotted spoon and tongs are also helpful. Proper deep-frying equipment is shown in Figure 5-1.

The fat to be used for deep frying must have a high smoke point; these include vegetable

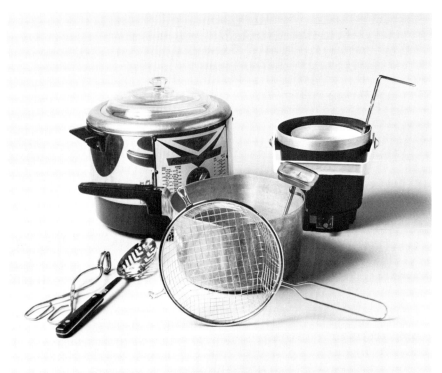

Figure 5-1.

Proper equipment for deep-fat frying includes a fryer or heavy saucepan, thermometer, basket, slotted spoon, and tongs. The smaller deep-fat fryer is suitable for frying small quantities of food.

oils, except olive oil, and hydrogenated fat. Olive oil, butter, and margarine are not suitable for use in deep frying; lard can be used but has a varying smoke point. The cooking container should not be more than half full of fat.

Fat can be reused for deep frying if it is clarified after each use. The fat is cooled to a warm temperature and ladled into a strainer lined with cheesecloth that has been set in another container as illustrated in Figure 5-2. If strongly flavored foods have been cooked, several thick slices of raw peeled potato can be put in the hot fat. The heat is turned off and, as the fat cools, the potato is discarded and the fat is strained after this process. Fat clarified in this manner can be used several times, but upon repeated use, it will deteriorate. This condition is noted by excessive foaming, the inability of the fat to brown foods properly and a strong odor. The fat should be discarded at this point.

Figure 5-2.

The safe and correct way to clarify fat after it has been used for deep-fat is to strain it through cheesecloth, placed in a sieve and store it in a tightly covered container.

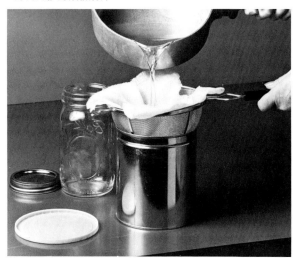

Vegetables should be free of moisture when cooked in deep fat, since moisture can cause the fat to spatter. With the exception of potatoes, most vegetables, meat, fish, and poultry are coated for deep frying. Coating develops a crisp outer brown crust and keeps the interior of the food moist. Suitable coatings include bread crumbs, cracker crumbs, cereal crumbs, a mixture of crumbs, a mixture of half cornmeal and half flour, flour, and egg mixed with water. The food is first dipped into the flour, then the egg mixture, and then the crumbs. The coating will adhere to the foods better if the coated food is allowed to chill before cooking. Some foods are also dipped into a batter composed of flour, egg, and milk and are then deep-fried. A deep-fried food mixture of chopped foods and a sauce is called a *croquette*.

In deep frying food, only a few pieces at a time should be cooked. Large quantities of food do not cook evenly and will lower the temperature of the fat. After the food is cooked, it should be drained on paper toweling to remove excess fat. Deep-fried foods should be served immediately.

Cooking in deep fat is dangerous and all safety precautions should be followed. Hot fat spatters when it comes in contact with a hot surface and it will flame; hot fat spatters when it is in contact with moisture.

The cord of an electric deep fryer should be in a place where it will not cause the pan to tip over, and the handles of pans used for deep frying on the top of the stove should be turned away from the edge. Hot fat must be constantly watched or removed from the heat, or the electric unit of an appliance must be turned off when the fat is not being used.

RECIPES

French Fried Potatoes

	Standard	Metric
Potatoes	4	4

1. Wash potatoes and peel.
2. Cut into narrow lengthwise strips and soak in ice water for 1 hour.
3. Drain potatoes and dry thoroughly between towels.
4. Fry potatoes in hot fat at 370° F (190° C) until desired brownness and crispness are reached. Drain on paper toweling.
5. Sprinkle with salt and serve.
6. If the cooked potatoes need to be held for a time, they may be recrisped in hot fat at 390° F (201° C).

Chicken Croquettes

	Standard	Metric
Ground cooked chicken	1-3/4 c.	430 mL
Celery salt	1/4 tsp.	1 mL
Lemon juice	1 tsp.	5 mL
Chopped parsley	1 tsp.	5 mL
Thick white sauce (see page 80)	1 cup	250 mL
Fine crumbs	1 cup	250 mL
Egg, beaten	1	1

1. In a bowl mix together the chicken, celery salt, lemon juice, chopped parsley, and thick white sauce.
2. Chill until the mixture is firm enough to shape into balls.
3. Shape into balls 1-1/2 inch to 2 inches in diameter. Mixture may also be shaped into cones or pyramids.

4. Roll in crumbs, dip into egg, and into crumbs again.

5. Fry in hot deep fat at 375° F (190° C) for 2 to 5 minutes or until golden brown.

6. Drain on paper toweling and serve.

Yield: 4 servings

--------- Corn Dogs ---------

	Standard	Metric
Flour	1 cup	250 mL
Sugar	2 Tbsp.	30 mL
Baking powder	1-1/2 tsp.	7 mL
Yellow cornmeal	2/3 cup	150 mL
Salt	1 tsp.	5 mL
Shortening	2 Tbsp.	30 mL
Egg, beaten	1	1
Milk	3/4 cup	180 mL
Frankfurters	1 pound	454 gm
Wooden skewers		

1. Sift flour and measure; sift again with sugar, baking powder, and salt into a bowl. Stir in cornmeal until thoroughly mixed.

2. Cut shortening into flour mixture until it resembles fine crumbs.

3. Combine egg and milk and add to dry ingredients; mix well.

4. Insert wooden skewers into the end of the frankfurters.

5. To a skillet with deep sides add oil to a depth of 1 inch. Heat the oil to a temperature of 375° F (190° C).

6. Dip the frankfurter into batter and fry, rotating the frankfurters to assure even cooking.

--------- Fish Fritters ---------

	Standard	Metric
Fish fillets	1 pound	454 gms
Water	1/4 cup	60 mL
Eggs, separated	3	3
Flour	3 Tbsp.	45 mL
Salt	1/2 tsp.	2 mL
Pepper	1/8 tsp.	1/2 mL
Minced garlic	1/8 tsp.	1/2 mL
Chopped parsley	1/8 tsp.	1/2 mL

1. Cook fish in 1/4 cup water until it flakes. Drain the water and mash the fish.

2. Beat egg yolks until light and thick.

3. Add flour, salt, pepper, garlic, fish, and parsley to egg yolks.

4. Beat egg white until stiff peaks form and fold into fish mixture.

5. Drop tablespoons of the mixture into hot deep fat at 370° F (190° C) and fry until golden brown. Note: For discussion on beating egg yolks and egg whites refer to Chapter 7 on Eggs.

--------- Thick Fritter Batter ---------

	Standard	Metric
Flour	1 cup	250 mL
Baking powder	1 tsp.	5 mL
Salt	1 tsp.	5 mL
Eggs	2	2
Milk	1/2 cup	125 mL
Melted fat or oil	1 tsp.	5 mL

This batter is used to coat small pieces of meat, fish, or poultry for deep frying, or 1-1/2 cups of drained, cooked vegetables may be folded into the batter and dropped by tablespoonsful into the hot fat for cooking.

1. Sift flour and measure; sift flour, baking powder, and salt into a bowl.

2. Beat eggs slightly and mix together with milk and melted fat or oil.

3. Dip food into batter and fry at 375° F (190° C) until golden brown.

--------- Thin Fritter Batter ---------

	Standard	Metric
Flour	1 cup	250 mL
Baking powder	1 tsp.	5 mL

Salt	1/2 tsp.	2 mL
Egg	1	1
Milk	1/2 cup	125 mL
Melted fat or oil	1 tsp.	5 mL

The thin batter is used to deep-fry small pices of food such as shrimp, onion rings, or thin slices of apples.

The batter will aid in retaining the shape of the food.

1. Sift flour and measure; sift flour, baking powder, and salt into a bowl.
2. Beat eggs slightly and mix with milk and melted fat or oil.
3. Dip pieces of food into the batter and fry at 375° F (190° C) until golden brown.

LEARNING ACTIVITIES

1. At the market compare the different prices of fats and oils. Determine which would be the best buy for your cooking needs.
2. Compare the difference in taste between a butter, margarine, whipped margarine, and "imitation" margarine. From the information gathered in number 1 determine if flavor will have any impact on your decision.
3. Prepare a baked product such as muffins in three different batches, using a vegetable oil, hydrogenated shortening, and lard as the differing fat ingredients.

Analyze the difference in flavor and texture of the three batches. Write your conclusions and present them to the class. Refer to Chapter 17, Bread, for the method of preparing muffins.
4. Evaluate the calorie content of a food prepared by deep frying and the same food prepared in another way.
5. Plan a menu and time schedule for preparing a meal for which the main entrée is a deep-fried food.
6. Investigate the cost of different types of equipment that are needed for deep frying and report to the class.

REVIEW QUESTIONS

1. What does the term *oil* mean when referring to a fat?
2. What is the difference between margarine and "imitation" margarine?
3. What are the characteristics of baked products that use lard as the fat ingredient?
4. What is a hydrogenated fat?
5. For what reason should animal fat be refrigerated?
6. Why is olive oil not suitable for all cooking?
7. Why are antioxidants added to fat products?
8. How does fat act as a tenderizing agent in baked products?
9. What is the "smoke point" of a fat?
10. What fats and oils are not suitable for deep frying?
11. How is fat clarified?
12. Why should only a few pieces of food at a time be deep fried?
13. What are three safety rules to remember when deep frying?

Sauces

Sauces are various combinations of ingredients mixed together, usually cooked, and in some stage of liquidity. Sauces are either combined with foods or served as an accompaniment to various food dishes. Sauces are used to enhance the flavor of food dishes and to hold ingredients together while a food dish is being cooked. Gravy is served with meat, cheese sauce may be served as a topping for a vegetable, or a sauce may be used to hold food ingredients in more compact form, as in the popular dish macaroni and cheese.

A cooked sauce is a combination of a fat, thickener, and liquid. The degree of thickness of the sauce will vary with the proportions of the ingredients, the gelling characteristics of the thickener, and the length of cooking time. The most commonly used sauce is the white sauce, which is usually composed of butter or margarine as the fat, flour as the thickener, and milk as the liquid.

Nutritional Factors to Consider

Sauces can add additional nutrients to a meal in the form of more protein, carbohydrate, fat, vitamins, and minerals. However, care must be exercised in using sauces to avoid adding unnecessary calories. Skim milk could be substituted for whole milk or cream, and the amount of sauce served can be a lesser amount and still add interest to the food.

Ingredients

Fat. The fat used in a sauce may be butter, margarine, bacon fat, or meat drippings. The choice depends upon ingredient availability and the flavor desired. Butter or margarine is used for sauces requiring a delicate flavor.

Liquid. Liquids used in cooked sauces include

76

milk, cream, meat stock, vegetable, or fruit juices, and wine. The richer the cream, the more satiny appearance of the sauce.

Thickener. A thickener is a food ingredient made from a grain product that, because of its gelling qualities, changes a liquid mixture into a more solid form. Milk in the presence of acid and egg, which are protein foods, coagulate when they are subjected to heat. The thickening properties of milk and eggs are discussed in more detail in Chapter 7, "Eggs," and Chapter 8, "Milk." Foods that are thickened in preparation include gravies, puddings, pie fillings, sauces, and some soups. The thickening power of a food is based on its starch content or its coagulation of protein, as with eggs and milk.

Cereal grains and tuber and root vegetables all have a high starch content. The grains that are most commonly used for thickening are corn in the form of cornstarch and wheat in the form of flour. Tapioca made from the root of the cassava is used mainly as a thickener in pudding and pie fillings, and the starch from the potato is used in some parts of the world as a thickening agent.

A starch is composed of minute grains, called *granules*. When water is added to the starch and the mixture is subjected to heat, the water penetrates the granules. This causes the granules to swell, soften, absorb liquid and a thickened paste is formed. This process is called *gelatinization*.

Starches vary in their thickening power. Wheat flour has one half the thickening power of cornstarch. Therefore, if a recipe calls for 1/4 cup of flour, and cornstarch is substituted, 2 tablespoons of cornstarch would be used. The flour may be all-purpose or browned all-purpose. Flour is browned by heating a small portion in a heavy fry pan over direct heat or in a shallow pan in the oven at 350° F (175° C). While browning, the flour should be occasionally stirred. Because the starch molecules are further broken down in browned flour,

more browned flour is needed for thickening. Browned flour is used in the making of gravies to give additional color and may be prepared in advance and stored in a tightly covered container.

Foods that are thickened with different agents look different. Wheat flour tends to look cloudy when cooked; cornstarch cooks to a more clear and translucent appearance.

Cooking with Thickeners

Basic Factors

When using starch as a thickener for other food ingredients, certain basic factors need to be understood about the cooking of starches in order to achieve a flavorful, smooth-appearing product of the proper consistency.

Lumping. Because some starch granules swell before others when a liquid is added and the mixture is heated, lumping may occur. Depending on what is being prepared, three methods of mixing the starch are available to prevent lumping. Lumping can be prevented by mixing the starch first with cold or lukewarm water and adding this mixture to a hot liquid, while stirring continuously. This method can be used when cooking some cereals and in the making of some gravies. A second process is to mix the starch first with a greater proportion of sugar, as in the making of puddings and pie fillings. The third way, which is commonly used in making sauces, is to melt the fat, add the flour, and then stir to coat the granules. This mixture should be cooked over moderate heat to decrease the starchy taste after which the liquid is added.

Effect of Heat. When heat is applied to the starch mixture, the granules swell and the mixture becomes thick. Starch mixtures may be heated in a heavy saucepan or in the top of a double boiler. Cooking the mixture over direct heat will cause rapid thickening, whereas cook-

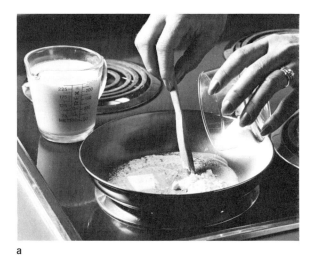

a

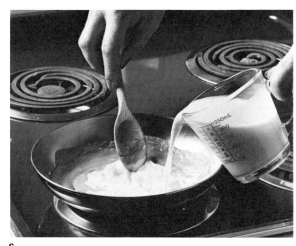

c

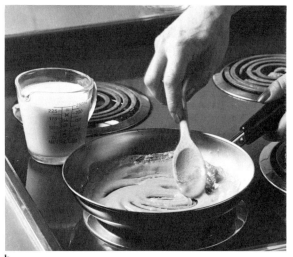

b

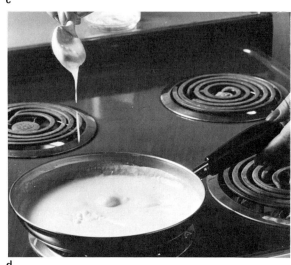

d

Figure 6-1.

(a) The basic sauce is made by melting the fat (usually butter or margarine) and adding the flour. (b) The butter-flour mixture is then cooked for 1 minute. (c) The liquid is added and the mixture is stirred until it thickens. (d) A thick white sauce has approximately this consistency.

ing in a double boiler is slower and yields a product that is of thinner consistency. Constant stirring of the mixture while it is heating helps to keep the granules separated and the mixture from scorching. Mixtures cooked in a double boiler require less stirring.

Once a starch mixture has thickened, it is cooked at the simmering stage for 3 to 5 minutes to improve the flavor and to assure maximum thickening. At this stage, only occasional stirring is necessary. Figure 6-1 shows the stages of sauce preparation.

When a starch is mixed with a fat, the liquid has to be added before the starch-fat mixture becomes too hot. If a liquid is not added, the heat causes the starch to break down and lose some of its thickening power. Once a starch mixture has thickened, too much stirring can also cause lesser thickening.

Effect of Other Ingredients. Too much sugar in proportion to the amount of starch can cause a decrease in the swelling or thickening power of the starch granules. If a recipe for a food such as a pie filling calls for an extremely high amount of sugar, a small portion of the sugar may be mixed with the starch at the beginning of cooking and the remaining amount added after the mixture has thickened.

Acids such as lemon juice or vinegar tend to decrease the thickening power of a starch. To prevent this the acid is usually added after the mixture is thickened.

The kind of liquid used in the starch mixture has little effect on the thickening action. Liquids are chosen on the basis of the food being prepared. Milk is usually used in preparing puddings, pie fillings, and most sauces. Water, meat stocks, the juice from cooked vegetables, or milk may be used in making gravies. Fruit juices are also used as the liquid in some thickened food dishes.

Effect of Cooling. As a starch-thickened mixture cools, it continues to thicken. Starch mixtures that are not immediately served must be refrigerated to prevent bacterial growth. Gravies, sauces, and other starch-thickened mixtures should not be left out for any extended period of time. To further protect the foods both from bacterial growth and the development of off-flavors, they need to be covered.

Equipment

A heavy, flat shallow pan or a double boiler is suitable for sauce preparation. A fork or a wire whisk helps to keep the starch granules apart. A liquid measuring cup is necessary to measure the liquid.

Microwave Cooking

Sauces can be readily made in the microwave oven. For making 1 cup of a sauce, a 2-cup glass measuring cup is best. Sauces need to be stirred every 30 seconds until they thicken.

Sauce Uses

A thin sauce is used as the base for making creamed soups or gravies.

A medium sauce is used for serving vegetables or in preparing creamed meats, poultry, fish, and eggs.

A thick sauce is used for filling crepes. A very thick sauce is used in preparing soufflés and croquettes.

Sauce Variations

Cheese Sauce. Add 1-1/2 cups of grated cheese to a medium-thick sauce.

Vegetable Flavoring. Sauté or cook lightly for 5 minutes 1/4 cup chopped onion, celery, green pepper, or mushroom in the fat before adding the flour and liquid.

Seasonings. Add 1/4 tsp. salt, 1/8 tsp. pepper, or 1/4 tsp. of such seasonings as basil, dill weed, or tarragon to 1 cup of sauce.

Convenience Sauce Food Products

Many instant-to-prepare sauces are available on the market. These instant sauces are particularly an aid in preparing various meat dishes of a cultural origin when time is short. Some canned sauces such as Hollandaise sauce can also be purchased. Instant sauces can be of particular value when stored on the emergency shelf of a kitchen.

————— Basic Sauces —————

	Standard	Metric
Thin sauce	1 Tbsp. fat	15 mL
	1 Tbsp. flour	15 mL
	1 cup liquid	250 mL
Medium	2 Tbsp. fat	30 mL
	2 Tbsp. flour	30 mL
	1 cup liquid	250 mL
Thick	3 Tbsp. fat	45 mL
	3 Tbsp. flour	45 mL
	1 cup liquid	250 mL
Very thick	4 Tbsp. fat	60 mL
	4 Tbsp. flour	60 mL
	1 cup liquid	250 mL

1. Melt the fat.
2. Stir in the flour and cook 1 minute, stirring constantly.
3. Add the liquid gradually and continue to stir until the mixture thickens. Cook an additional 1 or 2 minutes.
4. If using egg yolk, beat the egg slightly. Remove the sauce from the pan and stir 1/4 cup of the sauce into the egg yolk. Add the warmed egg to the sauce and cook another minute, stirring constantly. One egg yolk may be substituted for 1 tablespoon flour or 1 egg may be substituted for 2 egg yolks or an egg yolk may be added for flavor and color.
5. Serve immediately or chill.

Yield: 1 cup of liquid yields 1 cup of sauce

————— Lemon Sauce —————

	Standard	Metric
Cornstarch	1 Tbsp.	15 mL
Sugar	1/2 cup	125 mL
Salt	1/8 tsp.	0.5 mL
Water	1 cup	250 mL
Lemon juice	2 Tbsp.	30 mL
Grated lemon rind	1 tsp.	5 mL
Egg yolk, slightly beaten	1	1
Butter	1 Tbsp.	15 mL

1. Thoroughly mix cornstarch, sugar, and salt in a pan. Add water. Heat to boiling, stirring constantly.
2. Stir a small amount of the hot mixture into the beaten egg yolk. Return the egg mixture to the mixture in the pan and cook 1 minute. For further discussion on egg cookery, refer to Chapter 7, Eggs.
3. Add lemon juice and rind.
4. Add butter.

Yield: 1-1/4 cups

————— Orange Tapioca Cream —————

	Standard	Metric
Quick-cooking tapioca	2 Tbsp.	30 mL
Salt	1/8 tsp.	0.5 mL
Sugar	1/3 cup	75 mL
Milk, scalded	2 cups	500 mL
Egg yolk, slightly beaten	1	1
Egg white, beaten to form soft peaks	1	1
Grated orange rind	1-1/4 tsp.	6 mL
Diced oranges	1 cup	250 mL

1. Mix together in a saucepan the tapioca, salt, and 3 Tbsp. of the sugar. Add the milk and cook over moderate heat, stirring frequently until the mixture is clear.
2. Combine egg yolk and remaining sugar.
3. Stir a small amount of the hot mixture into the egg yolk and stir back into mixture in the saucepan. Continue cooking about 5 minutes, stirring constantly.
4. Fold in beaten egg white. Cool. Add orange rind and diced orange and chill.

Yield: 4 servings

Note: Refer to Chapter 7, "Eggs," for further knowledge in preparing this recipe.

1. Prepare six basic white sauces using a vegetable juice, a fruit juice, and milk as the liquid. Prepare three sauces using flour as the thickener and three sauces using cornstarch as the thickener. Compare the difference in texture, flavor, and appearance.
2. Prepare a sauce for a cooked vegetable. Add a flavoring ingredient that would enhance the vegetable's flavor. Refer to Chapter 12 on vegetables for methods of cooking these foods.
3. Prepare three sauces that use milk as the liquid but vary the fat by using shortening, butter, and bacon fat. Evaluate the sauces for flavor, texture, and appearance. Decide when each sauce might be suitable to use in food preparation.
4. Prepare a sauce for a dessert and analyze the additional calories added to the dish.
5. Note what happens to the consistency of a sauce after it has been removed from the heat and refrigerated for 20 to 30 minutes. What is the cause of the change in the sauce's characteristics?

REVIEW QUESTIONS

1. What are the two ways that a sauce is used?
2. What are the main ingredients of a cooked sauce?
3. What fats are used in cooked sauces?
4. What are the three thickening agents used in cooking?
5. What proportion of cornstarch is used in substituting cornstarch for flour?
6. What happens when heat is applied to a starch mixture?
7. How can lumping be prevented in cooking a mixture that is high in starch content?
8. What effect does a large amount of sugar have on the thickening power of a starch? How can this be avoided?
9. When should acids be added to a starch-thickened mixture?
10. How should cooked starch mixtures be stored?
11. What are the basic proportions for a thin white sauce yielding 1 cup? How are the ingredients increased to make a thick white sauce yielding 1 cup?

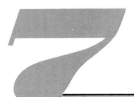

Eggs

The egg is one of the most versatile and valuable foods available. It is economical, nutritious, and simple to prepare. Cooked and served in the shell or without the shell, the egg can be the entrée for breakfast, lunch, or dinner, or it can be a snack food. The whole egg, the yolk, or the white may be combined with other ingredients to prepare baked products, casserole dishes, puddings, salads, sandwiches, and sauces.

Technological progress in handling, storing, and transporting eggs from the farm to the retail store allows the consumer to have fresh eggs within 2 days after they leave the farm. Mass-scanning equipment checks the interior quality of eggs and helps to assure the consumer of their soundness and wholesomeness.

Nutritional Factors to Consider

Carbohydrate and Fat

Eggs are not a contributing source of carbohydrate in the diet. An egg contains less than 1 per cent carbohydrate.

The fat of the egg is found mainly in the yolk, in the form of saturated fatty acids, and the related lipid, cholesterol. The egg white contains only a trace of fat.

Protein

Eggs are an excellent source of complete protein. Because of the quantity and quality of egg protein, the egg is an excellent meat substitute.

Table 7-1
Nutrient Value of One Egg

Per Cent Water	Food Energy Calories	Protein gm	Fat gm	Carbohydrate gm	Calcium gm	Iron mg	Vitamin A I.U.	Thiamine mg	Riboflavin mg	Niacin mg
74	82	6	6	Trace	27	1.2	590	0.05	0.15	Trace

Nutritive Value of American Foods, Agriculture Handbook No. 456, USDA, 1975.

The protein quality of food dishes prepared from cereal grains and legumes is improved with the addition of egg.

Vitamins and Minerals

Although the vitamin content of the egg may vary slightly with the type of food the hen consumes and the season of the year, eggs are considered a good source of vitamin A, thiamine, and riboflavin, and a fair source of vitamin D. The minerals found in eggs include iron, calcium, phosphorus, and sulfur. Each of these vitamins and minerals is essential for growth and body maintenance.

Calories

One raw egg contains 75 calories. However, the addition of other ingredients in egg preparation can increase the calorie content of an egg dish. For example, frying an egg in 1 tablespoon of fat increases the calories of the egg dish to 175. Table 7-1 shows the nutrient value of an egg.

Menu-Planning Points

Inherent Factors

Color. The whole egg or the egg yolk adds color to sauces, breads, other baked products, and puddings. However, when the egg is the featured attraction of a meal, it is important to add foods of contrasting color to prevent a monotone appearance. For example,

a luncheon of creamed eggs on toast points can be balanced in color with a crisp, green lettuce and tomato salad.

Texture and Flavor. Since eggs are soft in texture, the accompanying foods need to be crisp and firm to create a balance in the meal. A meal featuring a French cheese omelet served with stir-fried green beans and almonds gives a balance between soft and firmer textured foods.

Eggs are rather bland in taste and combine well with more flavorful foods. The addition of various cheeses, sauces, vegetables, spices, and herbs to egg dishes creates many interesting taste combinations.

Shape. The egg can be sliced, diced, cut in halves, or left whole to add a variety of pleasing shapes to a meal. A hard-cooked egg yolk can be crumbled and used as a colorful garnish topping for a salad or casserole, or a hard-cooked egg may be cut in half, the yolk mixed with a salad dressing, mayonnaise or sour cream; the yolk put back in the white and be served as part of the meal.

External Factors

Age and Culture. Eggs are an acceptable food in most cultures of the world and their year-round availability makes them a main food in many meals. The egg's low calorie content makes it a suitable food for the weight-watcher.

Economics. In nutrients provided per serving portion, eggs are considered one of the least expensive protein foods. For example, if a dozen eggs cost $.72 and two eggs are consumed, the cost of the dish would be $.12.

There is no difference in the quality of eggs relative to the color of the shell, and there is no advantage to buying fertile eggs over non-fertile eggs. When purchasing eggs, it is important to open the carton to inspect for tiny openings or cracks in the shells. Eggs with defective shells should not be purchased, since salmonella bacteria may have been able to penetrate the shell. A small blood spot in an egg broken out of the shell is not harmful and the spot can easily be removed.

Time Scheduling. When preparing a time schedule for meal preparation, it must be remembered that with the exception of hard-cooked eggs, most other egg dishes are served immediately upon the completion of cooking. Some egg dishes are quick and easy to prepare and are an asset to last-minute meal preparation. Examples of quick-to-prepare egg dishes are the fried, poached, scrambled, and soft-cooked egg and the French omelet. Preparation time for egg dishes that include other ingredients vary.

Equipment. Egg cookery will be more successful when kitchen tools such as a wire whisk with flexible wires, a rotary beater, an electric beater, egg separator, and an egg slicer are used. Egg cookery is improved when the proper pans are used. Special pans for making omelets and poaching eggs are available on the market. An ovenproof dish with straight sides is preferably used to bake soufflés to achieve maximum volume. Eight-ounce custard cups are suitable containers for baking and serving individual baked custards. For the proper beating of egg whites, a deep bowl with rounded sides is important to achieve the best volume. See Chapter 2 for a more complete discussion on equipment.

Grading

Eggs sold to the consumer are graded for quality on the basis of the thickness of the white, the firmness and height of the yolk, and the condition and appearance of the shell. These standards have been set by the USDA and appear on the egg carton as Grade AA, Grade A, and Grade B. All grades are suitable for most egg cookery, but Grade AA and Grade A give a better product when preparing fried or poached eggs. There is no difference nutritionally between the three grades. Grade A is the most common grade found in the retail store.

The terms *Jumbo*, *Extra Large*, *Large*, *Medium*, *Small*, and *Peewee*, which refer to the size and weight of the egg, have been established by the USDA. Each egg in the carton does not need to meet the specified weight for the size designated on the carton; the combined weight for that size egg must be met and in most instances is stated on the carton as minimum weight. Unit pricing also allows the consumer to determine the cost per ounce.

Refer to Chapter 3, "Food Safety," for additional information on egg grading and inspection.

Purchasing

Eggs are available 12 months of the year but their price will be slightly lower during the late spring and summer months because of the increased production during these months. In general, if the price difference between two sizes of eggs is $.07 or less per dozen, the better buy is the larger size.

Most recipes are based on the use of large-sized eggs. If using another size, an increase or a decrease in the amount of egg used in the recipe must be made.

Storage

Fresh Eggs

Eggs deteriorate rapidly when they are stored at room temperature, and it is important to note the method of egg storage at the place of their purchase. Only the number of eggs that will be used in a 1- to 2-week period should be purchased, and these must be refrigerated immediately after they are purchased. They may be stored either in the covered carton or in the rack provided in some refrigerators. Eggs are stored with the large end of the egg facing up to prevent the air cell located at the large end from rupturing, the membrane from stretching, and the yolk from moving. The longer the egg is stored, the more fragile the yolk membrane becomes, and the greater is the chance of the yolk breaking when the egg is separated from the shell.

Both egg yolks and egg whites can be refrigerated out of the shell for 1 to 2 days. Egg yolks tend to develop a thick outer surface and will keep best if covered with a thin layer of water. Both egg yolks and egg whites should be tightly covered for storage. They will stay fresher and will have less tendency to pick up other food odors and bacteria.

Frozen Eggs

The whole raw egg, the yolk, and the white can be frozen. Cooked egg white becomes rubbery when frozen, but cooked egg yolk freezes satisfactorily. To prevent whole raw eggs and the raw yolks from solidifying, 2 tablespoons sugar or light corn syrup or 1/2 teaspoon salt are added to 1 cup eggs or about 12 egg yolks. The kind of food preparation for which the egg is to be used after freezing is the determining factor in whether to use either salt or sugar. Whole eggs and egg yolks are stirred but not beaten before being frozen. Egg whites require no additional ingredients for freezing nor are they stirred or beaten. It is important that no particle of the yolk be present in an egg white that is to be beaten as the egg white will not beat properly.

An ice-cube tray makes an ideal freezing container to freeze individual amounts of egg. After the egg cubes are frozen, they can be removed from the tray and stored in a container with a tight-fitting lid or sealed in a heavy plastic bag. The amount of egg frozen should be labeled.

Dried Eggs

Dried eggs are used in many commercial mixes by the food industry and are available only on a limited basis to the home consumer. If purchased, dried eggs need to be stored in a tightly covered container in the refrigerator to prevent bacterial growth.

Functions in Food Preparation

Thickening Agent

Eggs are used as thickening agents in the preparation of food products such as cream pies, cooked salad dressings, custards, and sauces. As the whole egg, the yolk, or the white is heated, the egg protein coagulates or thickens. The temperature at which an egg coagulates depends upon the amount of egg present and the other ingredients used.

The addition of sugar to a mixture increases the temperature at which the egg coagulates, whereas the addition of salt decreases the temperature of coagulation. The more diluted the egg is, the higher is the temperature needed for coagulation. Mixtures containing acid ingredients tend to coagulate at a lower temperature.

In the preparation of sauces, cream pie fillings, and cooked salad dressing, both a starch such as flour or cornstarch and the egg are used as the thickening agents. The egg is added after the starch-sugar-liquid solution has reached the thickening point. To prevent rapid coagulation, a small amount of the starch mixture is stirred quickly into the egg to warm it. The egg mixture is then rapidly stirred into the remaining starch solution and cooked until the mixture has completely reheated. Before the egg is added, the cooking temperature must be lowered.

Mixtures containing egg as a thickening agent tend to curdle if they are cooked too rapidly at a high temperature. Best results are attained when the mixture is slowly heated and stirred constantly. If a mixture should curdle, it can be beaten with a rotary beater to improve both the texture and appearance. Chapter 6, "Sauces," contains more information on sauces.

Coating Agent

The whole egg, lightly beaten, and sometimes diluted with a small portion of milk or water is used to coat foods that are to be cooked by baking, deep-fat frying, or pan frying. The egg coating is usually supplemented with an additional layer of flour, cereal, bread, or cracker crumbs. The egg coating helps to hold the other layer in place during cooking. In the case of baked products, such as bread, the egg coating is brushed on before baking to provide a crust that develops into a rich, brown color.

Binding and Emulsifying Agent

As a binding agent, the egg helps to hold food masses together in a desired shape while they cook. For example, a meat loaf or a croquette will have a better shape when an egg is used as the binding agent.

As an emulsifying agent, the egg coats the oil droplets in a mixture and prevents them from separating out from the other substance.

Examples of food products in which the egg acts as the emulsifying agent include mayonnaise and some ice creams.

Leavening Agent

As an egg white is beaten to a foamy consistency, air is incorporated into the mixture. During cooking, air expands and the egg white becomes rigid. Examples of food products that use the trapped air in the foam as a leavening agent include omelets, souffles, cake rolls, and meringues.

Basic Cookery

A low-to-moderate temperature and proper timing result in tender and evenly cooked eggs. High-protein foods such as eggs shrink and lose moisture when they are overcooked and become tough, rubbery, and unpalatable. Eggs that have been diluted with a liquid such as milk in the preparation of a custard have a tendency to curdle when the mixture is heated at too high a temperature.

Baked Eggs

Eggs may be baked in individual custard cups. The egg is broken into the buttered custard cup, covered with 1 tablespoon cream or tomato juice, and baked at 325° F (165° C) for 20 minutes or until set. In the last 5 minutes of cooking time, the egg should be checked to make sure it does not overcook.

Fried Eggs

There are several acceptable methods for frying an egg, with personal preference being the deciding factor. All frying methods use a small amount of fat in the fry pan, or the egg may be fried in a special pan with a nonstick surface. A tender fried egg is cooked over low heat and the length of cooking time varies with the desired result. Some people like a thin white coating over the yolk and a firm white; others prefer an egg "sunny-side up" with a more runny yolk. Still others prefer the egg to be turned over and cooked yolk-side down until the yolk reaches a desired degree of firmness. A better-shaped fried egg is achieved by breaking the egg first into a saucer, and then sliding it off the saucer into the fry pan.

One method of frying an egg is to heat a small amount of fat until it is hot but not bubbly in a fry pan. The egg is added and cooked until the desired doneness is reached. Another method is the same as the first except that after adding the egg to the fry pan, 1 tablespoon of water per egg is added, the fry pan is covered, and the egg is cooked by steam. A third method is to cook the egg in fat and spoon the fat over the yolk until the desired coagulation of the yolk and white is reached. A fried egg is served immediately.

Scrambled Eggs

To prepare scrambled eggs, the eggs are beaten with milk, cream, or water and seasonings. The use of milk or cream increases the nutrient content and makes a creamier product, whereas the use of water makes a fluffier product. One tablespoon of liquid per egg is used. As in frying eggs and in making omelets, fat is heated in a heavy fry pan until it is hot but not bubbly. The eggs are gently stirred during the cooking time. Eggs may also be scrambled in a double boiler. This is advantageous if the eggs need to be held for a short period of time before they are served. For variation, seasonings and other foods such as cheese, small pieces of vegetables, or meats can be added to scrambled eggs.

Poached Eggs

Eggs poach best in a shallow pan or skillet with enough water in the pan to cover the egg by 1 inch. A specially made pan for egg poaching may also be used. The water is heated to just below the boiling point. The egg is broken onto a saucer, then slipped into the water and cooked over low heat. Eggs will poach in 3 to 5 minutes. Fresh eggs with thick whites are best for poaching as the egg will not spread out. Eggs may be poached in other liquids, such as milk or tomato juice.

Soft- and Hard-Cooked Eggs

The length of time the egg cooks determine whether an egg is soft-cooked or hard-cooked. Soft-cooked eggs are cooked for 2 to 5 minutes, depending on personal preference and the size of the egg. Hard-cooked eggs are cooked for 10 to 15 minutes, depending on the size and the number of eggs being cooked. Regardless of the length of cooking time, eggs should be at room temperature prior to cooking.

To soft or hard cook an egg, the egg is submersed in cold water in a covered pan and allowed to simmer. After cooking, the egg is submerged in cold water to prevent further cooking and to facilitate peeling. If the egg is to be sliced or deviled, a firmer white is more desirable. To achieve this, the egg is cooked in simmering water for 20 to 25 minutes. Soft-cooked eggs are served immediately but hard-cooked eggs may not be. If this is the case, the egg should be refrigerated and held for not longer than 2 days.

The green discoloration appearing around the yolk of some hard-cooked eggs is harmless, but it does make them less appetizing. It is the result of the iron and sulphur present in the egg combining to form ferrous sulfide, which is the result of overcooking. Proper cooking and cooling will eliminate this discoloration.

Omelets

There are two kinds of omelets, the plain omelet, which is similar to scrambled eggs, and the fluffy omelet, in which the egg yolks and the whites are beaten separately and folded together. The fluffy omelet resembles the soufflé. Both kinds of omelets need a heavy fry pan with hot melted fat.

To prepare a plain, two-egg omelet, the eggs are beaten with 4 teaspoons of water. Beating with a wire whisk makes a lighter omelet but a rotary beater may also be used. A small amount of fat is heated in a heavy 6- or 8-inch fry pan and the egg mixture is added. The burner is turned to low heat and the fry pan is gently shaken across the burner until the bottom of the mixture begins to set. With a spatula, the sides of the egg mixture are lifted to allow the remaining mixture to flow to the bottom. When the omelet has set, grated cheese, sautéed mushrooms, chopped onions, cooked bacon or meat pieces, or numerous other foods may be added before rolling or folding the omelet in half. A sauce is often served with the omelet. Although plain omelets may be prepared to serve more than one person, best results are attained from single-serving omelets. Figures 7-1 (a) through (e) illustrate the steps in making a plain omelet.

Figure 7-1.

Making an omelet. (American Egg Board)

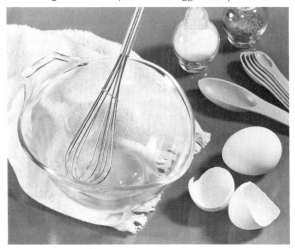

(a) mix eggs with water.

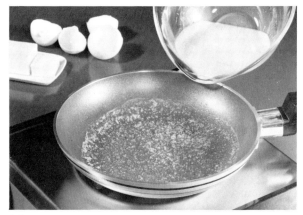

(b) Add eggs to melted fat.

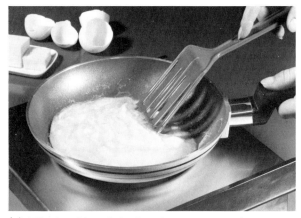

(c) Lift the sides of the forming omelet to allow the remaining mixture to flow to the bottom.

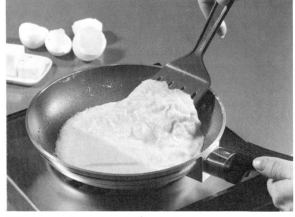

(d) The omelet is then folded in half.

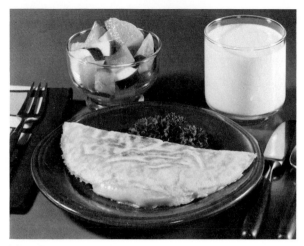

(e) A finished cheese omelet.

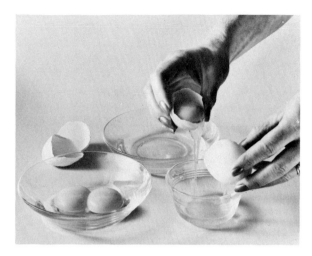

Figure 7-2.
(a) A yolk is separated from the white.

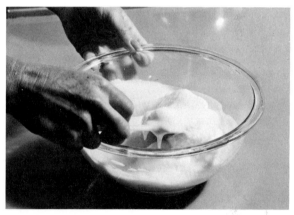

(b) Egg yolks or a sauce are gently folded into beaten egg whites. A rubber spatula is the best tool to use for this process.

A fluffy omelet is prepared by separating the egg yolk from the egg white and then beating each separately. To separate the egg yolk from the egg white, (See Figure 7-2(a)) the egg shell is cracked, opened, and the yolk is poured back and forth between the two shell halves as the egg white drips into a bowl or an egg separator may be used. An egg white is always separated in another bowl before it is added to other egg whites or ingredients because egg whites will not foam properly if any of the yolk is present in the white. The proper way to separate an egg is illustrated in Figure 7-2 (a). The section on egg white foams in this chapter should be studied before preparing a fluffy omelet.

A fluffy omelet can be prepared to serve more than one or two people. To prepare a four-egg fluffy omelet, the egg whites are beaten until frothy, 1/4 teaspoon salt is added, and beating continues until moist and shiny stiff peaks form. The egg yolks are beaten until they are thick and lemon-colored and then poured over the surface of the beaten egg whites. The egg whites are lifted and folded over the egg yolks with a rubber spatula until the yolks and whites are blended. Figure 7-2(b) illustrates the proper method of folding egg yolks or a sauce into beaten egg whites. The mixture is then put into a fry pan in which fat has been heated until hot. A fluffy omelet should be cooked over moderate heat until the bottom of the omelet is a light brown. Then the mixture is put in a 325° F (163° C) oven and cooked until set, which takes only 8 to 10 minutes. A fluffy omelet may be served with a sauce, such as a cheese or mushroom sauce.

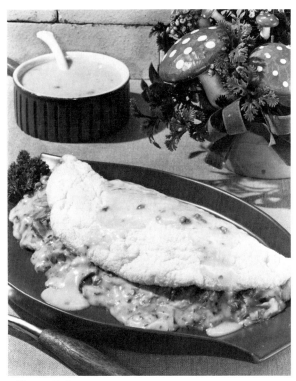

Figure 7-3.

A fluffy omelet is filled with a mushroom sauce. (American Egg Board)

Both fluffy and plain omelets can be served as the entrée for breakfast, lunch, or dinner. Serving an omelet immediately upon the completion of cooking time is important to preserve the taste and texture of the omelet. Figure 7-3 shows a fluffy omelet served with a cheese sauce.

Soufflés

A soufflé is a light and airy, baked or steamed pudding served either as the main course or as the dessert portion of the meal. It is composed of egg yolks, egg whites, a thick white sauce, and a main flavoring ingredient such as cheese, a vegetable pulp, a pureed fruit, or a ground meat. Dessert soufflés may include other ingredients such as sugar, chocolate or a liqueur.

A variation of the classic soufflé is a baked fondue, which uses bread crumbs or thin bread slices in place of the white sauce, and is less likely to shrink immediately after cooking. A fondue is normally baked in a shallow baking dish.

A baking dish with straight sides is used to make the classic soufflé. A grease-free bowl must be used to beat the egg whites as the whites will not foam properly when fat is present. Glass or metal bowls are recommended, rather than plastic.

Prior to mixing the ingredients for a soufflé, the oven is turned on to preheat. Most soufflés are baked at a moderate temperature of between 350° F (175° C) and 375° F (190° C). The rack is placed in the lower third of the oven to permit even cooking of the soufflé from the bottom and the top. The eggs should be at room temperature before they are beaten.

The white sauce is prepared following the basic directions given in Chapter 6. The egg yolks are beaten until they are light and lemon-colored, and are then added to the white sauce. Some of the warm white sauce is blended into the yolks before all of the egg is added to the white sauce to prevent the yolks from curdling; additional ingredients and seasonings are then added. The section in this chapter on egg white foams should be studied before beginning soufflé preparation.

The egg whites are beaten until they are stiff but still moist and shiny. The sauce is gently folded into the beaten egg whites with a rubber spatula by lifting the egg whites up and over the sauce mixture. The bowl should be rotated while blending the mixture until the yolks and whites are evenly distributed. The mixture is spooned into a soufflé dish to lose as little air as possible. Before baking the soufflé, a circle, 1-inch deep, is cut around the inner two thirds of the soufflé with a kitchen table knife. This produces the "top hat" of the soufflé, as is illustrated in Figure 7-4.

Soufflés baked in the oven will cook more

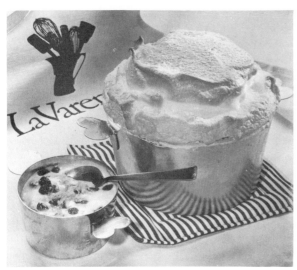

Figure 7-4.
Dessert soufflé with a top hat. (California Raisin Advisory Board)

evenly if the soufflé dish is placed in a pan of hot water that comes up to 1 inch on the dish.

To test the soufflé for doneness a metal kitchen knife is inserted into the side of the soufflé, or a wire cake tester or long trussing needle is inserted into the center. If any of the mixture clings to the tester, the soufflé is not sufficiently cooked. Soufflés are best served immediately. When a soufflé is removed from the oven, it begins to lose the air that was incorporated into the mixture during the beating process and some shrinkage will take place. An insufficiently cooked soufflé will shrink rapidly.

Custards

Custards are of two types, the stirred custard and the baked custard. The stirred custard is cooked on top of the range in a double boiler and the finished product is of a liquid consistency. The water in the boiler is kept at a simmer. The custard is continuously stirred and it is done when the mixture lightly coats a spoon as illustrated in Figure 7-5. In contrast to the rapid heating of a starch mixture, custards are cooked slowly at an approximate temperature of 160° F (70° C). Custards may be cooked over direct heat in a pan with a heavy bottom, but care must be taken with this method so that the mixture does not reach a high enough temperature to cause curdling.

The cooking of a baked custard is similar to that of a soufflé in that it is not stirred during cooking. The baking container for the custard is placed in another pan of water for cooking in the oven, and the point of a sharp knife is inserted halfway between the center and the outside of the custard to check for doneness. When the knife comes out clean, the custard is done.

The major ingredients of a custard are eggs, milk, sugar, and flavoring with the proportions being one egg to 2 tablespoons sugar per 1 cup of milk. Some recipes call for scalded milk but this process does not produce a better quality product; scalded milk shortens the cooking time since the mixture is heated before cooking.

Figure 7-5.
A soft custard is cooked when it lightly coats the spoon.

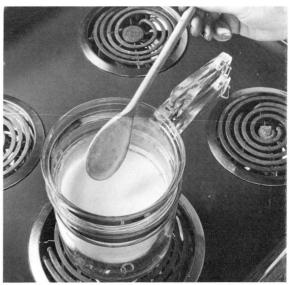

Stirred custards are normally served as the dessert portion of a meal. Baked custards are cooked alone or in a pie shell and are usually served as a dessert. Unsweetened custards that use cheese as a main ingredient are served as entrées.

Microwave Cooking

Eggs can be fried, scrambled, or poached successfully in a microwave oven. Eggs cannot be cooked in the shell because they will explode as a result of the rise in the internal temperature of the egg as it is heated in a microwave oven. Other egg dishes that can be prepared in a microwave oven include custards, fondues, and casseroles having eggs as an ingredient.

Cooking time for eggs must be carefully watched. Eggs cook quickly and it is easy to have a tough and rubbery product. Eggs should thus be removed just before they are done; the carry-over heat will complete the cooking. Cooking eggs on a defrost or slow-cook setting will lengthen the cooking time but will lessen the danger of overcooking.

When poaching or frying an egg in a microwave oven, the yolk should be pricked with a fork just prior to cooking. The yolk has a thin membrane covering and the pricking allows the air to circulate and prevents the egg from exploding. Eggs that are to be poached or fried should be covered with plastic wrap or waxed paper before cooking. Eggs to be fried are cooked in a 10 oz. glass dish. Eggs to be poached will cook more evenly if the water is heated in the dish prior to adding the egg.

Egg-White Foams

As an egg white is beaten, air is incorporated, and the egg white changes to a foamy mass. The foam's stability is dependent upon the degree of beating and the addition of other ingredients. The addition of an acid, such as cream of tartar, and sugar increases an egg white foam's stability, whereas the addition of salt decreases it.

Foams of egg whites develop in varying degrees. In the initial beating stage bubbles form on the surface, but the egg white mass is still in a semiliquid state. This is called the "foamy stage" and it is the point at which acid, salt, and other flavorings are added. Further beating of the foamy mass changes it to a nonfluid mass of tiny bubbles which will temporarily hold soft peaks. At the beginning of this stage sugar is gradually added. As beating continues, the mixture becomes shiny and opaque, and when the beaters are removed, the soft peaks retain their shape. This is the desired stage of foam development for a recipe which calls for stiffly beaten egg whites. Egg whites that are beaten beyond this stage become dry, break apart in chunks, and do not hold nicely shaped peaks. The varying stages for beaten egg whites are illustrated in Figure 7-6(a) to (d).

The type of beater used and the shape of the bowl in which the egg whites are beaten will affect the development of a satisfactory egg-white foam. Electric beaters will develop a better foam than a rotary beater. A bowl with rounded sloping sides is better than a straight-sided bowl.

Egg-white foams are used to prepare fluffy they are at room temperature prior to beating. The presence of egg yolk or fat on the beater, in the egg white, or on any utensil in contact with the egg white will retard foam formation.

Egg-white foams are used to prepare fluffy omelets, soufflés, hard and soft meringues, angel and sponge cakes, and some frozen desserts.

Meringues

A meringue, which is an egg-white foam containing sugar, is of two types, the soft meringue and the hard meringue.

Soft Meringues. Soft meringues are used as toppings for puddings and pie fillings. The

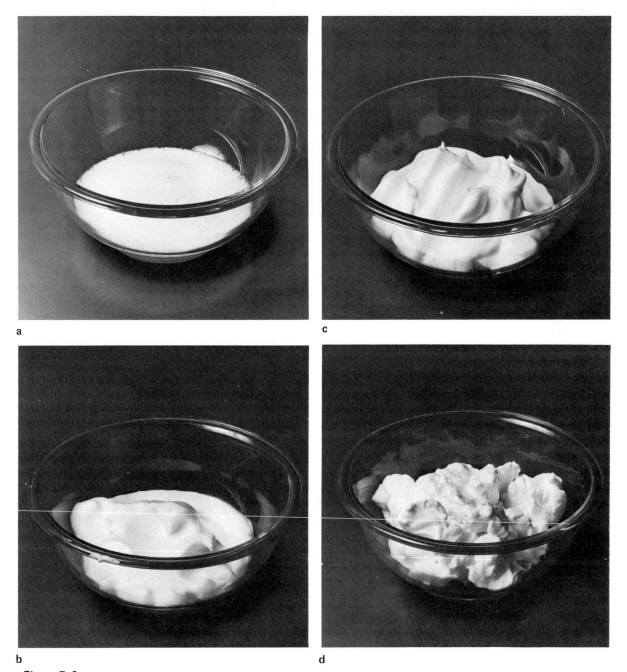

Figure 7–6.

(a) Egg whites beaten to the foamy stage; (b) to the soft-peak stage; (c) to the stiff-peak stage; (d) to the over-beaten stage, where they have a lumpy, dry-grained appearance.

basic proportion for a soft meringue is 2 tablespoons of sugar per egg white and 1/8 teaspoon cream of tartar. After the egg white is beaten to the frothy stage, the cream of tartar is added. As beating continues and the egg white foam develops, the sugar is added gradually. The egg whites are continuously beaten until the meringue holds soft peaks and all of the sugar is dissolved in the mass. For a pie, the meringue is placed on top of the baked hot pie filling and sealed to the edges. Meringues are baked at a temperature of 350° F (175° C) for 12 to 15 minutes.

Hard Meringues. A hard meringue is a combination of egg white, sugar in the proportion of 4 tablespoons per egg white, and 1/8 teaspoon cream of tartar per egg white. Hard meringues are used as an elegant crust for various cooked pie fillings and as a base for ice creams and fruits. The cream of tartar is added to a frothy beaten egg white. As beating continues and the soft peak foam stage is reached, the sugar is added gradually until the peaks become stiff.

Figure 7-7.

Individual hard meringues are molded with the back of a spoon, or the mixture can be put through a cookie press onto a cookie sheet lined with heavy paper.

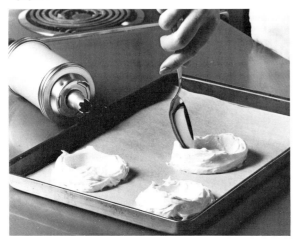

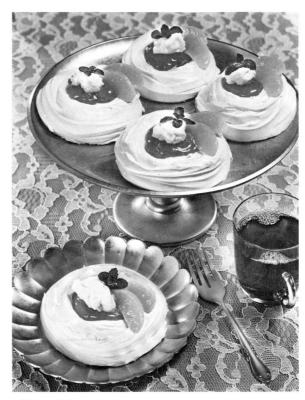

Figure 7-8.

Meringue shells are tasty dessert dishes. (Sunkist Growers, Inc.)

Hard meringues are best baked on a sheet of heavy brown paper placed on a baking sheet. The mixture should be stiff enough to mold into the desired form with the back of a spoon as illustrated in Figure 7-7. After the meringue is baked, the oven is turned off and the meringue is left in the oven for several hours or overnight. Long, slow baking and a drying-out period result in a meringue that is dry, crisp, tender, and delicately browned. A hard meringue with a gummy interior has not been allowed to dry out properly. Hard meringues can be stored in a tightly covered container for a short period of time or tightly wrapped and frozen for a period of 1 month. Figure 7-8 depicts a hard meringue as a shell for pudding and fruit.

Convenience Egg Products

Several egg products are available on the market that require a minimum of preparation including egg custard, soufflés, eggnog, egg rolls, and a complete breakfast with eggs. In addition, eggs are used in many ready prepared mixes, as well as in bakery and pasta products.

RECIPES

Fluffy Omelet

	Standard	Metric
Eggs, separated	4	4
Water, milk, or tomato juice	1/4 cup	60 mL
Salt	3/4 tsp.	4 mL
Butter or margarine	1 Tbsp.	15 mL

1. Beat the egg yolks with the liquid and salt.
2. Rinse the egg beater with cold water, wash, and dry.
3. Beat the egg whites until they are stiff but not dry.
4. Fold the egg yolk mixture gently into the beaten egg whites until evenly distributed.
5. Melt the butter or margarine in a heavy 10-inch fry pan until hot.
6. Pour the omelet mixture into the skillet and spread evenly with a rubber spatula.
7. Turn the heat to low and cook approximately 8 minutes or until the bottom turns a light golden brown.
8. Place in a moderate oven, 325° F (165° C) for approximately 10 minutes or until the top has dried out or a knife inserted in the center comes out clean.
9. Loosen the sides of the omelet with a metal spatula.
10. Make a slight crease in the center of the omelet; fold over and slide on to a platter.
11. The omelet may be served with a sauce.

Yield: 2 to 3 servings

Creamed Eggs

	Standard	Metric
Fat	2 Tbsp.	30 mL
Flour	2 Tbsp.	30 mL
Milk	2 cups	500 mL
Salt	1/4 tsp.	1 mL
Hard-cooked eggs, chopped	4	4

1. Melt fat in a heavy saucepan or in the top of a double boiler.
2. Stir in flour. Cook 1 minute.
3. Add milk and stir constantly over a low heat until thick. Add salt.
4. Add eggs to the sauce and heat through.
5. Serve creamed eggs over toast points, biscuit halves, in popover shells, or in tart shells.

Yield: 2 to 3 servings

Deviled Eggs

	Standard	Metric
Hard-cooked eggs, halved	4	4
Mayonnaise	2 Tbsp.	30 mL
Vinegar	1/2 tsp.	2 mL
Salt	1/2 tsp.	2 mL
Prepared mustard	1/2 tsp.	2 mL
Paprika	To garnish	To garnish

1. Remove yolks from egg white and mash in a bowl.
2. Mix mashed egg yolk with mayonnaise, vinegar, salt, and prepared mustard.
3. Fill egg white halves with egg yolk mixture. Sprinkle tops of stuffed eggs lightly with paprika.

4. Serve as part of a salad, as a garnish, or as an appetizer.

Stirred Custard

	Standard	Metric
Egg	1	1
Milk	1 cup	250 mL
Sugar	2 Tbsp.	30 mL
Vanilla extract	1/4 tsp.	1 mL

1. Blend together the egg, milk, and sugar.
2. Cook in a double boiler over low heat, stirring constantly until the mixture thinly coats a spoon.
3. Add the vanilla.
4. Immediately pour the stirred custard into a chilled bowl or immerse the pan holding the custard into a container of cold water to stop the cooking.
5. Serve plain or as a sauce over fruit or cake.

Yield: 1 to 2 servings

Baked Custard

	Standard	Metric
Egg	1	1
Milk, scalded or not	1 cup	250 mL
Sugar	2 Tbsp.	30 mL
Vanilla extract	1/4 tsp.	1 mL

1. Preheat oven to 350° F (175° C).
2. Blend together the egg, milk, and sugar. Add the vanilla extract.
3. Pour the mixture into two 4-ounce custard cups and set in a pan of water that comes up 1 inch on the side of the custard cups.
4. Bake for approximately 45 minutes or until a table knife inserted in the center comes out clean.

Yield: 2 servings

Quiche Lorraine

	Standard	Metric
Egg, slightly beaten	4	4
Milk	2 cups	500 mL
Salt	1/2 tsp.	2 mL
Dry mustard	1/4 tsp.	1 mL
White pepper	1/8 tsp.	0.5 mL
Shredded Swiss cheese	2 cups	500 mL
Bacon slices, cooked and crumbled	6	6
Chopped green onion	2 Tbsp.	30 mL
Baked pie shell, 9-inch	1	1
Grated Parmesan cheese	2 Tbsp.	30 mL

1. Preheat oven to 375° F (190° C).
2. In a bowl combine eggs, milk, salt, dry mustard, and white pepper.
3. Mix together cheese, crumbled bacon, and onion. Spread evenly in the pie shell.
4. Pour over milk mixture. Sprinkle with Parmesan cheese.
5. Bake for 35 to 40 minutes or until a knife inserted in the center comes out clean. Allow to stand 10 minutes before serving.

Yield: 6 servings

Eggs Benedict

	Standard	Metric
English muffin halves, toasted	4	4
Ham, thin slices, sautéed	4	4
Eggs, poached	4	4
Hollandaise sauce	1 cup	250 mL

1. Place the ham on top of the toasted English muffin and the poached egg on top of the ham. Pour the hollandaise sauce over the tops.

Yield: 2 to 4 servings

Hollandaise Sauce

	Standard	Metric
Butter or margarine	1/2 cup	125 mL
Egg yolks, well beaten	3	3
Lemon juice	1 Tbsp.	15 mL
Salt	1/2 tsp.	2 mL

1. Melt butter in the upper portion of a double boiler. The water in the lower portion of the double boiler should be simmering. Do not let the water boil.
2. Add the beaten egg yolks to the melted butter, stirring constantly until thickened.
3. Remove from the heat and stir in the lemon juice and salt.

Yield: 3/4 cup

Cheese Soufflé

	Standard	Metric
Butter or margarine	1/4 cup	60 mL
Flour	1/4 cup	60 mL
Salt	1/2 tsp.	2 mL
Dry mustard	1/2 tsp.	2 mL
Minced onion	1/2 tsp.	2 mL
Milk	1 cup	250 mL
Grated cheddar cheese	1–1/2 cup	375 mL
Eggs, separated	4	4
Cream of tartar	1/2 tsp.	2 mL

1. Preheat oven to 350° F (175° C).
2. Melt butter or margarine in saucepan.
3. Stir flour, salt, and dry mustard into melted butter or margarine. Add the onion.
4. Gradually add milk and cook until thick, stirring constantly.
5. Add grated cheese and allow to just melt.
6. Beat the egg yolks. Stir a small amount of the hot sauce into the egg yolks and then quickly stir the egg yolk mixture into the sauce in the pan. Remove from heat.
7. Beat the egg whites until frothy; add the cream of tartar and beat until stiff but still moist and shiny.
8. Fold the sauce gently into the egg whites.
9. Spoon the soufflé mixture into an ungreased 1-1/2 quart soufflé dish.
10. Place in a pan on a shelf in the lower third of oven. Add hot water to cover 1 inch of the soufflé dish.
11. Bake for 50 to 60 minutes. To check for doneness, insert a table knife near the center. If the knife comes out clean, the soufflé is done. Serve immediately.

Yield: 4 servings

Baked Fondue

	Standard	Metric
Butter or margarine	2 Tbsp.	30 mL
Hot milk	2 cups	500 mL
Shredded mild or sharp cheddar cheese	2 cups	500 mL
Soft bread crumbs	2 cups	500 mL
Salt	1/4 tsp.	1 mL
Egg yolks, beaten	6	6
Egg whites, stiffly beaten	6	6

1. Preheat oven to 350° F (175° C).
2. Melt butter or margarine in a heavy saucepan. Combine the milk, cheese, bread crumbs, and salt and add to the fat. Stir constantly until thickened.
3. Stir a little of the hot mixture into the beaten egg yolks. Then stir the egg yolks into the rest of the hot mixture.
4. Gently fold the sauce mixture into the stiffly beaten egg whites.
5. Pour the mixture into a greased 2-quart baking dish. Bake for 30 to 40 minutes or until a knife inserted in the center comes out clean. Serve immediately.

Yield: 8 servings

Oriental Egg Scramble

	Standard	Metric
Fat	2 Tbsp.	30 mL

	Standard	Metric
Chopped green onion	1/4 cup	60 mL
Garlic clove, minced	1/2 clove	1/2 clove
Diced water chestnuts	1/4 cup	60 mL
Shrimp, drained	1 (6-1/2 oz.) can	1 (193 gm)
Fat	2 Tbsp.	30 mL
Eggs, slightly beaten	5	5
Salt	1/2 tsp.	2 mL
White pepper	1/4 tsp.	1 mL

1. Melt fat in a heavy skillet. Sauté onion and garlic until soft. Add chestnuts and shrimp. Cook for 2 minutes.
2. Remove mixture from pan.
3. Melt 2 tablespoons of fat in skillet. Combine the shrimp mixture, salt, pepper, and slightly beaten eggs. Pour the egg mixture into skillet.
4. Cover and cook over low heat until the eggs are set for about 8 minutes. Fold in center, turn out onto a platter, and serve immediately.

Yield: 4 servings

——————— Fruit Meringues ———————

	Standard	Metric
Egg whites	3	3
Sugar	3/4 cup	175 mL
Cream of tartar	1/4 tsp.	1 mL
Peach or pear halves	4	4
Mint jelly	1/4 cup	60 mL

1. Preheat oven to 275° F (135° C).
2. Beat egg whites until frothy. Add cream of tartar and continue beating to the soft peak-foam stage. Gradually add the sugar and beat until stiff peaks are formed and the sugar is dissolved.
3. Fill each of the fruit halves with jelly. Place on a baking sheet and cover the top of the fruit halves with meringue.
4. Bake for 1 hour. Serve hot or chilled.

Yield: 4 servings

LEARNING ACTIVITIES

1. Plan three complete dinner menus applying the knowledge gained from Chapter 1 and the menu-planning points section in this chapter.
   A. Plan a menu with the egg as the entrée.
   B. Plan a menu using the egg as the protein extender in a cereal grain or legume dish.
   C. Plan a menu that incorporates an egg white foam or a custard as part of an entrée or dessert.
2. Survey a local supermarket or food store and write a report on the manner in which eggs are refrigerated, the grades and sizes of eggs available, and the cost per dozen for the sizes and grades available.
3. Prepare two or more of the following egg dishes and compare the finished product for taste, appearance, texture, flavor, and time of preparation.
   A. Eggs baked in tomato juice and in cream.
   B. Eggs scrambled with milk and with water as the liquid ingredient.
   C. Eggs scrambled in a fry pan and scrambled in a double boiler.
   D. One egg cooked to the hard-cooked stage for 15 minutes and another egg cooked for 25 minutes.
   E. One poached egg prepared in continuous boiling water and another poached egg prepared in water that is simmering.
   F. One egg fried in fat and another egg fried in a Teflon-lined or nonstick pan requiring no fat.
4. Beat one egg white that has just been removed from the refrigerator to the

soft peak stage. Beat another egg white that has reached room temperature to the soft peak stage. Analyze the difference in texture and volume between the two.

5. Prepare a stirred custard over low heat in a pan with a heavy bottom. Prepare a stirred custard in a pan with a heavy bottom over high heat. Record the effect of heat on egg cookery.

6. Prepare a hard meringue. Bake one hard meringue according to the recommended procedure for baking hard meringues. Bake the second hard meringue for the same baking time but remove immediately after the oven cooking time has been completed. Examine the difference in texture, taste, and appearance between the two.

7. If a microwave oven is available, prepare an egg by poaching or frying. Prepare another egg on a conventional range. Record the difference in time preparation and cleanup, and note the difference in taste and texture between the two.

8. Prepare a French omelet and choose from a variety of seasonings to alter the flavor slightly.

9. Prepare a fluffy omelet with a sauce accompaniment. Determine the cost per serving.

10. Prepare a green salad and use a form of the hard-cooked egg as the garnish.

11. Investigate the cost of special egg-cooking utensils available on the market and give a report to the class.

12. Investigate the types of convenience egg products that are available on the market. Report to the class on the cost and usability of these products for the home, campers, and hikers.

13. Prepare a dinner with the soufflé as the entrée. Plan to have all components of the meal complete when the soufflé is removed from the oven.

14. Prepare a dish that uses an unsweetened custard as the base, such as a quiche Lorraine. Plan a menu around the entrée and analyze the nutrient content of the meal.

15. Make a list of at least 20 different food dishes that use eggs as a main ingredient. Prepare one of these food dishes as the recipe is stated and prepare it again, omitting the egg. Record the differences between the two dishes in flavor, texture, volume, and appearance.

REVIEW QUESTIONS

1. Why is the egg considered to be a highly nutritious food?
2. Why is the egg considered to be an excellent meat substitute?
3. What is the difference between a brown-shelled and a white-shelled egg?
4. What are the important menu-planning points to remember when planning a menu containing eggs?
5. What basis is used for determining the grade of an egg?
6. What sizes of eggs are available to the consumer?
7. Which size of eggs is recommended for food dishes being prepared from a recipe?
8. Why should eggs with cracks in the shell not be purchased?

9. How long can fresh eggs in the shell be refrigerated?
10. How are egg yolks stored in the refrigerator?
11. What additional ingredients are used when preparing whole eggs or egg yolks for freezer storage?
12. What precautions need to be taken when using frozen eggs?
13. What is the effect of temperature, sugar, salt, and acid on egg coagulation.
14. What happens if a mixture containing egg as a thickening agent is exposed to too high a heat too rapidly?
15. How does an egg serve as a binding and coating agent in food preparation?
16. In what way does the egg serve as an emulsifying agent?
17. What are the characteristics of an overcooked egg?
18. What is the difference in preparation between a French omelet and a fluffy omelet?
19. How hot should the water be to poach an egg?
20. What causes the green discoloration around the yolk of a hard-cooked egg?
21. When are the egg yolks added to the white sauce in preparing a soufflé?
22. What is the best way to tell if a baked custard has completed cooking?
23. How is the best volume achieved in beating egg whites?
24. What are the signs of overbeaten egg whites?
25. What is the reason for not removing a hard meringue from the oven immediately after the cooking time has ended?
26. Why does a soufflé shrink after removal from the oven?
27. How does the presence of fat affect the beating of an egg white foam?
28. Distinguish between the effects of cream of tartar, sugar, and salt in the formation of egg white foams.
29. Name the ingredient proportions for sugar to egg white when making a soft and a hard meringue.
30. What peak of foam development is desirable for a soft meringue and a hard meringue?

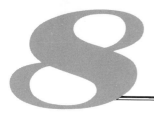

Milk

Milk has been used by people through the centuries both as a beverage and as a basic ingredient in food preparation. Because of its important nutrient composition, milk is the first food of the infant, and it continues to maintain an important role in the growth of children and adolescents. As people mature they continue to require a certain amount of milk in their diet to maintain a state of health and well-being.

Most of the milk consumed in the United States is cow's milk, but in certain geographical areas goat's milk is also available. Many kinds of milk and milk products are available on the market and many food products use milk as a major ingredient, as illustrated in Figure 8–2.

Nutritional Factors to Consider

Carbohydrate

Milk contains a small amount of carbohydrate in the form of lactose, sometimes referred to as "milk sugar." Lactose accounts for the slightly sweet flavor of milk and is important for the body's proper absorption of calcium, phosphorus, and other minerals.

Fat

The milk fat content of milk is dependent upon the form of milk. Fluid whole milk contains a blend of saturated, monosaturated, and

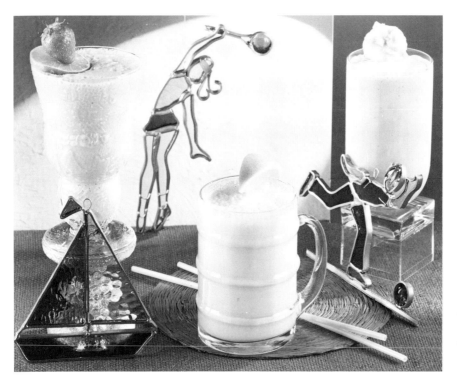

Figure 8-1.
There are many ways to enjoy milk. Try adding various fruits, fruit juices or ingredients such as peanut butter. (United Dairy Industry Association)

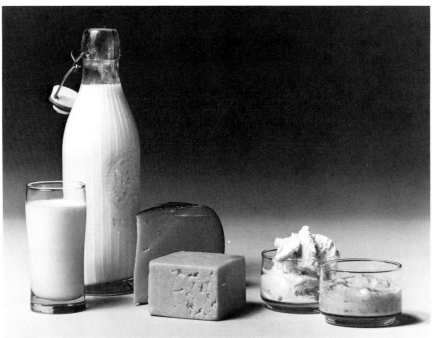

Figure 8-2.
Cheeses, ice cream, and yogurt are examples of the many foods containing milk as a major ingredient.

polyunsaturated fats. Lowfat, nonfat, and nonfat dry milk contain considerably less milk fat. Milk fat is sometimes called "butter fat."

Protein

Milk is a complete protein food because it contains all nine essential amino acids. The principal milk protein is called *casein*. Milk is an economical and highly nutritious food to combine with incomplete protein foods, such as those from the cereal family. Figure 8-3 shows a variety of milk products that can be used as toppings for cereal.

Vitamins and Minerals

Fluid whole milk is a rich source of vitamin A. When the fat is removed from milk in processing, the vitamin A is also removed. However, most nonfat and lowfat milks are fortified with vitamin A. Most forms of milk marketed today are fortified with vitamin D in the amount of 400 U.S.P. units per quart. Vitamin D is added to milk because of its important relationship to the proper absorption of calcium and phosphorus.

Fluid milk forms are excellent sources of riboflavin. Riboflavin is not affected by the removal of milk fat, but it is easily lost when exposed to light.

Milk is the food that provides most of the body's supply of calcium. Phosphorus is also found in milk and, together with vitamin D and calcium, is responsible for the building and maintenance of strong bones and teeth.

Calories

The number of calories in a serving of milk is dependent upon the amount and form of milk being consumed. For example, one 8-ounce serving of fluid whole milk contains 165 calories, whereas, the same-sized serving of fluid nonfat skim milk contains only 85

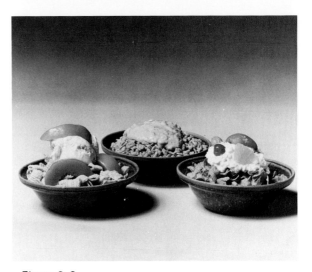

Figure 8-3.
Cereal takes on a special flavor when served with ice cream, ice cream with fruit, yogurt and cottage cheese with fruit.

calories. When a portion of the fat or all the fat is removed from milk, the calorie content of the food is reduced. Table 8-1 shows the nutrient value of milk and some milk products.

Menu-Planning Points

Inherent Factors

Balance. Milk can provide the nutritive balance of any meal because of its high-protein quality and its rich contribution of vitamins and minerals.

Color. The white color of milk and most milk products can be a pleasing contrast to the bright colors of most fruits and vegetables. However, in planning meals care should be taken to see that the milk sauces used with vegetables provide color contrast and not a monotone appearance. For example, creamed potatoes and cauliflower in the same meal would not be aesthetically appealing.

Table 8-1
Nutrient Value of Milk and Some Milk Products

Food	Water Per Cent	Food Energy Calories	Pro-tein gm	Fat gm	Carbo-hydrate gm	Cal-cium mg	Iron mg	Vita-min A I.U.	Thia-mine mg	Ribo-flavin mg	Niacin mg	Ascorbic Acid mg
Milk, whole 3.5% fat, 1 cup	87	159	9	9	12	288	0.1	350	0.07	0.41	0.2	2
Milk, 2% fat 1 cup nonfat milk solids added	87	145	10	5	15	352	0.1	200	0.10	0.52	0.2	2
Milk (nonfat) skim, 1 cup	90	90	9	trace	12	296	0.1	10	0.09	0.44	0.2	2
Chocolate-flavored drink. 2% fat, 1 cup	83	190	8	6	27	270	0.5	210	0.10	0.40	0.3	3
Custard, 1 cup	77	305	14	15	29	297	1.1	930	0.11	0.50	0.3	1
Yogurt, made from whole milk, 1 cup	88	152	7	8	12	272	0.1	340	0.07	0.39	0.2	2

Nutritive Value of American Foods, Agriculture Handbook No. 456, USDA, 1975.

Flavor. Most forms of milk and milk products are rather bland in flavor and they can combine well with more flavorful foods. Certain milk products, such as yogurt and buttermilk, have an acidlike flavor, and sour cream has a tanginess that provides an interesting flavor contrast to a meal. Buttermilk muffins are a tasteful bread to serve with scrambled eggs at breakfast, and sour cream is a flavorful topping for a fruit dessert.

Texture. Both yogurt and sour cream have a custardlike texture, which can be combined with good results with crunchy foods. For example, both yogurt and sour cream may be used as a major ingredient in making salad dressings and dips to be served with crisp, raw vegetables, as illustrated in Figure 8-4.

External Factors

Age and Culture. People of all ages drink milk and enjoy other milk products. Milk is a highly acceptable food in most cultures of the world. Some non-Caucasian peoples are not able to consume milk because their digestive system lacks the enzyme lactase, which is necessary for lactose digestion. However, fermented milk products such as buttermilk, cottage cheese, sour cream and yogurt are tolerated.

Food Availability and Economics. Modern transportation, refrigeration, and milk processing plants make milk readily available. In some remote areas, fresh milk may not be available, but canned and dried forms of milk can be stored for long periods of time.

Owing to the nutritive quality of milk, it is an excellent food buy.

Forms of Milk

Several forms of milk are available to the consumer. With the exception of the raw form,

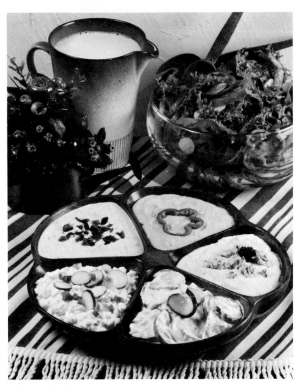

Figure 8-4.
Yogurt, sour cream, and buttermilk help create flavorful and nutritious dips and salad dressings. (United Dairy Industry Association)

all milk, including fresh, canned, dried, and frozen milk, is pasteurized. Pasteurized milk has been heated to just below the boiling point of water, 212° F (100° C), for a certain length of time, depending on the process used, and is then quickly cooled. Milk that is labeled "ultra-pasteurized" has been heated to a temperature of 280° F (138° C) for at least 2 seconds. "Ultra-pasteurization" extends the shelf life of milk under refrigeration. The purpose of pasteurization is to destroy harmful microorganisms that may be present in the milk. Pasteurization also helps to extend the shelf life of milk.

Some forms of milk and milk products have additional milk solids added to improve the product's texture and palatability. Milk solids are the remaining nutrients when the water and milk fat are removed and add to the product's nutrient and calorie content. Milk solids include protein, milk sugar, and minerals.

Fresh Milk

Raw Milk. Milk that has not been pasteurized is called *raw milk.* Some local areas allow the sale of certified raw milk to the public. Even though milk processors who sell certified raw milk are under constant inspection by health departments, milk is highly susceptible to microorganism growth and even certified raw milk can be dangerous.

Homogenized Milk. Most fresh milk and all canned, dried, and frozen milk are homogenized. Homogenization is a process whereby the fat globules are broken into smaller particles that do not rise to the surface and produce a cream layer. This processing is done immediately following the pasteurization of milk. The minimum milk fat content in homogenized milk as set forth by federal law is 3.25 per cent, but individual state laws may require higher minimums.

Lowfat Milk. Lowfat milk must contain not less than 0.5 per cent milk fat nor more than 2 per cent milk fat, and it must contain a minimum of 8.25 per cent milk solids. Lowfat milk must be fortified with 2,000 I.U. of vitamin A but vitamin D fortification is optional. If 10 per cent or more milk solids are added, the product must be labeled "protein-fortified." Nutrition labeling and the percentage of fat contained is mandatory for all lowfat milk.

Nonfat Milk. Nonfat or skim milk has no more than 0.5 per cent milk fat. It must contain a minimum of 8.25 per cent milk solids and it must be fortified with 2,000 I.U. of vitamin A. Nutrition labeling is mandatory.

Chocolate-Flavored Milk. This product is made from pasteurized whole milk to which a sweetener and chocolate or cocoa have been added.

Chocolate-Flavored Milk Drink. This liquid has the same ingredients as chocolate-flavored milk but it is made from pasteurized lowfat milk, which must be fortified with 2,000 I.U. of vitamin A.

Cultured Buttermilk. This product is made by adding a lactic-acid bacterial culture to pasteurized nonfat or lowfat milk. The nutritive value of cultured buttermilk is the same as the kind of milk from which it is made but the flavor is more tart.

Acidophilus Milk. This cultured milk is made by adding the culture *lactobacillus acidophilus* to pasteurized lowfat or nonfat milk. If the milk is unfermented, it has the same flavor as the milk from which it is made.

Yogurt. Yogurt is made from pasteurized nonfat, lowfat, or homogenized milk to which concentrated milk solids and a culture are added. It is available plain or sweetened and fruit-flavored.

Filled Milk. Filled milk is a combination of milk solids, water, and a fat other than milk fat. Filled milk should not be confused with "imitation milk," which contains no dairy products. The use of filled milk is questionable because of the type of fats other than milk fat used in the preparation of the product.

Cream. Cream is the liquid part of milk that is high in fat and is separated from milk. It must contain a minimum of 18 per cent milk fat and come from pasteurized milk. Three kinds of cream are available, based on the milk fat content.

1. Light cream, sometimes referred to as coffee cream or table cream, contains a

minimum of 18 per cent milk fat and a maximum of 30 per cent milk fat.

2. Light whipping cream or whipping cream contains a minimum of 30 per cent milk fat up to a maximum of 36 per cent.

3. Heavy whipping cream or heavy cream contains a minimum of 36 per cent milk fat.

Half-and-Half. Half-and-half is a pasteurized mixture of milk and cream, which must contain a minimum of 10.5 per cent milk fat up to a maximum of 18 per cent milk fat.

Canned Milk

Evaporated. Evaporated milk is milk that has had slightly more than half of the water removed, has been homogenized, and has been sealed in cans and sterilized. It contains not less than 7.5 per cent milk fat and must contain 25.5 per cent total milk solids. It must be fortified with vitamin D. Evaporated milk is available as nonfat evaporated, lowfat evaporated, and evaporated milk.

Sweetened Condensed. This form of evaporated milk is made from pasteurized, homogenized milk with an addition of about 42 per cent sugar.

Canned Whole. This form of canned milk is homogenized milk that has been sterilized and canned. It is available mainly in areas where fresh fluid milk is not available.

Dried Milk

Nonfat Dry. Nonfat dried milk is made from pasteurized skim milk by removing most of the water and the milk fat. Nonfat dried milk, when reconstituted according to the directions, contains the same nutrients as the milk from which it was made. Most nonfat dried milks are fortified with vitamins A and D.

Dry Whole. Dried whole milk is made from pasteurized whole milk and, when reconstituted, has a nutrient content similar to the milk from which it was made. It is available to the consumer only on a limited basis.

Frozen

Frozen milk may be available in certain areas on a very limited basis. The nutritional value of frozen thawed milk is equal to that of fresh milk.

Other Milk Products

Three major milk products, butter, ice cream, and cheese, are discussed in other chapters. Butter is discussed in Chapter 5, ice cream in Chapter 20, and cheese in Chapter 9.

Sour cream is made from pasteurized cream that has been soured by a lactic-acid-producing bacteria.

Acidified sour cream is made by souring pasteurized sour cream with suitable acidifiers. It may or may not contain lactic acid bacteria.

Sour half-and-half is made by souring pasteurized half-and-half with lactic-acid bacteria.

Acidified sour half-and-half is made by souring pasteurized half-and-half with suitable acidifiers.

Grading and Purchasing

Standards for Grade A milk and milk products have been set by the U.S. Public Health Service. Some cities, counties, and states have adopted these standards and others have their own standards. The USDA has established grades for nonfat dry milk and the USDA grade shield on the package signifies that the product was processed under sanitary conditions and meets quality requirements.

The amount and form of milk or a milk product purchased will be influenced by such factors as how it is to be used, the storage facilities available, the time available for food preparation, and the money allotted for food purchasing.

Fresh fluid whole, lowfat, or nonfat milk is most commonly used for drinking. However, to help cut food costs, dry milk which is equally flavorful when reconstituted and chilled thoroughly can be used in place of fresh milk. Another way to cut food costs is to mix equal parts of fresh milk and reconstituted nonfat dry milk.

Both evaporated and nonfat dried milk can be used in place of fresh milk in food preparation and are a more economical purchase. Milk and milk products which are specially flavored, fortified, or cultured are more expensive.

Container Size

Fresh fluid milk is usually a better purchase when it is purchased in half-gallon or gallon containers. If adequate storage facilities are not available, or if the amount purchased cannot be consumed within 3 to 5 days, it is wiser to purchase milk in a smaller size container. Dried milk is usually sold in small and large economy-size packages or in individual packets. The individual packets may be more convenient but will probably be more expensive. Evaporated milk is sold in 5- and 13-fluid-ounce cans. The best size of milk container to buy is determined by the intended use of the milk.

Price

The price of fresh fluid milk will vary as a function of where it is purchased. The price paid for home delivery of milk is usually higher than if it is purchased at a grocery store or at a dairy farm store.

Storage

Fresh milk and milk products need to be refrigerated at a temperature of 40° F (5° C)

immediately after purchase. These foods are not only highly susceptible to microorganism growth but quickly absorb odors and off-flavors. Milk and cream, which have been poured into a separate container for serving, should not be returned to the original container for refrigeration for the same reason.

Canned milk may be stored on the shelf until it is opened. After canned milk is opened, it should be treated as fresh milk, covered and refrigerated in the original container. Dried milk need not be refrigerated unless it has been reconstituted. The dried milk package should be tightly closed after it is opened as dried milk can become lumpy and stale if it is exposed to moisture in the air. However, dried buttermilk will keep better if it is refrigerated after the package is opened.

Fresh milk can be frozen for up to 3 to 4 months but its flavor and appearance may change slightly. Sour cream, yogurt, evaporated milk, and cream should not be frozen.

Some fluid milk and milk products have a date stamped on the container. This date is called the "pull-date" or "sell-by-date" and is the date by which the product should be withdrawn from retail sale.

Milk Cookery

Effect of Heat

When cooking with milk, a low to moderate heat should be used. Milk scorches easily because some of the milk protein settles out and sticks to the bottom and sides of the pan. A heavy pan with a wide bottom surface or a double boiler are the best pans to use for surface cooking. When milk is heated over direct heat, constant stirring will lessen the tendency to scorch.

Other changes that occur when milk is heated include the development of an off-flavor and change in odor. Milk mixtures containing sugar will change to a brownish color, which is desirable in certain desserts.

Milk Curdling

Milk curdles or becomes lumpy when the protein, casein, coagulates. Curdling occurs when a food that has a high acid content such as tomatoes, or lemon is added to milk. The tannins in certain foods, such as potatoes, or foods that have a high salt content, can also cause milk to curdle.

Curdling can be prevented in such mixtures as cream soups by preparing the milk in a white sauce, stirring the milk mixture constantly while adding the vegetable, and heating only briefly before serving.

Milk Scum

A scum or surface skin forms on milk when it is heated. If the scum is not removed, steam builds beneath it and can cause the mixture to boil over. A scum will not form if the mixture is continuously stirred over direct heat or if the mixture is heated in a double boiler.

Recipes often call for scalded milk. To scald means to bring almost to the boiling point. One method to determine if milk is scalded is to check for a slight scum forming on the milk surface, as shown in Figure 8-5.

Functions in Food Preparation

Milk and milk products are used in many types of foods, including baked products, beverages, custards, puddings, and soups, as shown in Figures 8-6, 8-7, and 8-8. The nutritive quality of all foods is increased with the use of milk.

Evaporated milk diluted with an equal amount of water may be used in any recipe calling for fresh milk. Evaporated milk is also used in only partially diluted form or in concentrated form for certain pies, puddings,

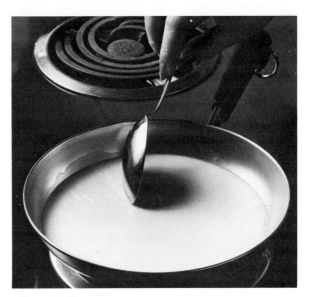

Figure 8-5.

Milk is scalded when a thin film forms on the surface.

candies, icings, and whipping. Recipes using evaporated milk as a major ingredient are shown in Figures 8-9(a) and (b).

Reconstituted dried milk may also be used in place of fresh milk in most recipes calling for fresh milk. For some recipes, dried milk may be mixed in with the dry ingredients and water used as the milk portion of the liquid ingredients. More nutritive quality can be added to baked goods, casseroles, and sauces with an additional portion of dried milk that is not reconstituted.

Sour cream can be used in sauces, salad dressings, casseroles, and some baked dishes. Sour cream will curdle if it is exposed to high temperatures, and should be stirred into hot foods such as beef stroganoff just before serving. Yogurt is used in the preparation of food dishes such as molded salads, salad dressings and desserts. In its ready-to-use form yogurt can serve as a snack or dessert.

Sweetened condensed milk has a high sugar content and is used in the preparation of candies, frosting, and special desserts.

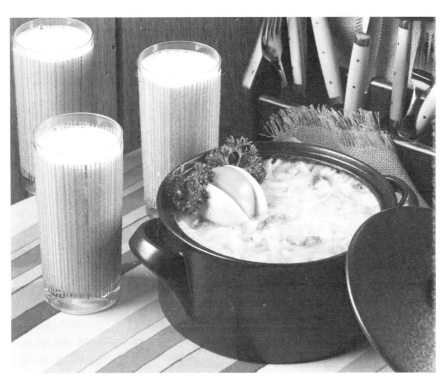

Figure 8-6.
Milk is used in many kinds of casseroles. (United Dairy Industry Association)

Buttermilk cannot be substituted for fresh milk in most recipes. Buttermilk can be used together with milk in the preparation of some baked goods such as cakes and quick breads. The proper proportions are 1/2 cup buttermilk, 1/2 cup regular milk, 1/4 teaspoon baking soda, and no baking powder. If buttermilk is called for in a recipe and none is available, 1 tablespoon of vinegar or lemon juice can be added to the measuring cup and fresh milk, diluted evaporated milk, or reconstituted dried milk added to fill the cup.

Milk Puddings

Milk puddings are a nutritious and flavorful dish that, depending on the ingredient content, can be served as an entrée accompaniment, a flavorful dessert, and sometimes as a snack. The basic ingredients of milk puddings are milk and a starch such as flour, cornstarch, or

Figure 8-7.
Many soups use milk as a main ingredient. (Libby, McNeil, and Libby, Inc.)

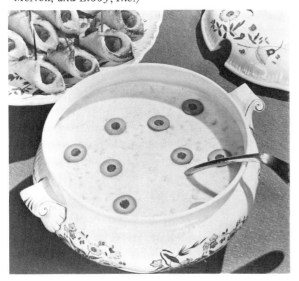

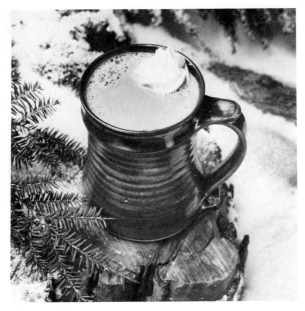

Figure 8-8.
Milk is a part of many beverages. (Sanna Div., Beatrice Foods Co.)

tapioca. Puddings sometime contain egg, a sweetener, and a flavoring. Instant or cooked milk puddings can also be prepared from commercial mixes.

Milk puddings should be refrigerated immediately after being cooked and should be covered with wax paper or plastic wrap to prevent a skin from forming on the surface of the pudding.

Whipping Milk Products

Cream. Either whipping cream or heavy whipping cream must be used for whipping because the fat helps to enclose the air that is beaten into the mixture. Best results are attained when the cream, bowl, and beaters are all chilled. The cream is beaten until it is fairly stiff, and then 1 tablespoon of sugar per 1 cup of unwhipped cream is folded or beaten into the beaten cream. Individual portions of whipped cream can be dropped onto a cookie sheet and

Figure 8-9.
Many foods can use evaporated milk as a main ingredient. (Pet Incorporated)

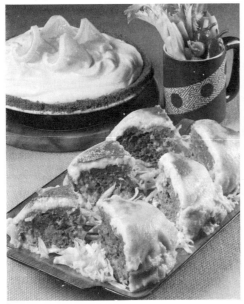

a

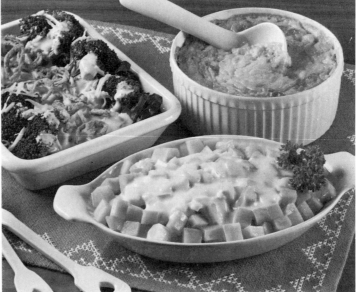

b

frozen for later use. Once the cream has frozen it should be removed from the cookie sheet and wrapped for storing.

Evaporated Milk. Evaporated milk should be whipped in undiluted form. The milk is first poured into an ice-cube tray and frozen until ice crystals form and the mixture is slightly slushy. The mixture is poured into a chilled bowl and whipped with chilled beaters until it is stiff and will hold a peak. The addition of 1 tablespoon of lemon juice to each cup of evaporated milk measured before whipping helps to maintain the whipped product and

improves the flavor. If desired, sugar may be folded into the whipped product. Whipped evaporated milk will hold its form for approximately 1 hour when refrigerated.

Dried Milk. The beaters, bowl, and water must be chilled before dried milk can be whipped. To make 2-1/2 cups of whipped topping, combine in a chilled bowl 1/2 cup cold water with 1 tablespoon of lemon juice and 1/2 cup of nonfat dried milk. The mixture is beaten until stiff and then 2 tablespoons of sugar and 1/4 teaspoon vanilla is beaten in.

RECIPES

Chilled Sour Cream Soup

	Standard	Metric
Cucumber, medium-sized	1	1
Cream of chicken soup	1 (10-3/4 oz.) can	1
Milk	3/4 cup	175 mL
Sour cream	1 cup	250 mL
Garlic salt	1/2 tsp.	2 mL
Cayenne pepper	1/8 tsp.	0.5 mL

1. Peel the cucumber and cut it into chunks and blend in a food blender or finely dice the cucumber and mash with a potato masher.
2. Combine the mashed cucumber with the soup, milk, and sour cream. Add the garlic salt and cayenne pepper.
3. Chill. Serve with a garnish of chopped parsley.

Yield: 4 servings

Clam Chowder

	Standard	Metric
Bacon, chopped	6 slices	6
Onion, small, chopped	1	1
Potato, medium-sized, pared, and chopped	2	2
Carrot, finely minced	1/2 carrot	1/2
Canned clams, drained	1-1/2 cup	375 mL
Liquor from clams		
Worcestershire sauce	1/2 tsp.	2 mL
Milk	1 qt.	1000 mL
Salt	1 tsp.	5 mL

1. Fry bacon until crisp. Remove from pan and drain.
2. Add the onion to the bacon fat and sauté in the fry pan.
3. Add the potato, carrot, and clam liquor. Bring the mixture to a boil; turn heat to simmer and cook until the vegetables are just tender. If desired, mixture may be lightly mashed.
4. Add the clams, milk, seasonings and bacon. Heat over a low heat until thoroughly heated.

Yield: 4 servings

Cream of Tomato Soup

	Standard	Metric
Canned tomatoes	2 cups	500 mL

	Standard	Metric
Minced onion	2 tsp.	10 mL
Salt	1 tsp.	5 mL
White pepper	1/4 tsp.	1 mL
Sugar	2 tsp.	10 mL
Butter or margarine	2 Tbsp.	30 mL
Flour	2 Tbsp.	30 mL
Milk, scalded	1 qt.	1000 mL

1. Cook the tomatoes, onion, salt, pepper, and sugar in a saucepan for 15 minutes over low heat.
2. Strain the tomato mixture.
3. In another saucepan melt the butter or margarine; stir in flour, and gradually add milk, stirring constantly.
4. Add the tomato mixture gradually to the milk mixture, stirring constantly.
5. Serve immediately. Garnish with croutons or chopped chives.

Yield: 4 to 6 servings

───────── Corn Pudding ─────────

	Standard	Metric
Butter or margarine	2 Tbsp.	30 mL
Flour	2 Tbsp.	30 mL
Evaporated milk	1/2 cup	125 mL
Water	1/2 cup	125 mL
Salt	1 tsp.	5 mL
Whole kernel corn, drained	2 cups	500 mL
Sugar	2 tsp.	10 mL
Eggs, well-beaten	2	2
Dry bread crumbs	1/2 cup	125 mL

1. Preheat oven to 350° F (175° C).
2. Melt the butter or margarine in a heavy saucepan; blend in the flour. Mix the milk and water together.
3. Gradually add the milk, stirring constantly. Cook until the mixture thickens.
4. Stir in the salt, corn, and sugar, and cook the mixture to heat the ingredients thoroughly.
5. Remove from heat and add the eggs.

6. Pour into greased baking dish and top with crumbs.
7. Bake for 25 minutes.

Yield: 6 servings

───────── Scalloped Potatoes ─────────

	Standard	Metric
Potatoes, medium-sized	4	4
Butter or margarine	3 Tbsp.	45 mL
Flour	3 Tbsp.	45 mL
Milk	2 cups	500 mL
Salt	1-1/2 tsp.	7 mL
Dehydrated onion flakes	1 tsp.	5 mL

1. Preheat oven to 350° F (175° C).
2. Peel the potatoes. Slice crosswise into 1/8-inch thick slices.
3. Melt the butter or margarine in a heavy saucepan. Blend in the flour. Add the milk gradually, stirring constantly and cook until thickened. Stir in the salt and onion flakes.
4. Place the sliced potatoes in a lightly greased casserole and pour over the white sauce. Bake for approximately 1 hour or until tender.

Yield: 4 servings

Variations
1. Add 1 cup of grated cheese to the white sauce.
2. Use 1 can cream of mushroom soup diluted with 1/2 cup milk in place of the white sauce.

───────── Orange Cream Dessert ─────────

	Standard	Metric
Cold water	1 cup	250 mL
Nonfat dry milk	1 cup	250 mL
Sugar	1/3 cup	75 mL
Frozen orange juice	1 (6 oz.) can	1 (177 mL)

1. Chill the water, mixing bowl, and beaters.
2. Put the cold water in the mixing bowl and sprinkle the dry milk over it. Beat until stiff.

3. Beat in the sugar and orange juice; turn into refrigerator trays or sherbet glasses and freeze.

Yield: 6 servings

—————————— Fruity Milk Shakes ——————————

	Standard	Metric
Milk	1 cup	250 mL
Crushed pineapple, undrained, or 1/2 cup fresh or frozen strawberries or 1 banana, mashed	1/2 cup	125 mL

1. Blend milk and fruit in a blender, electric mixer, or a jar with a lid.
2. If desired, 1/4 cup of ice cream may be added.

Yield: 1 serving

—————————— Peach Yogurt ——————————

	Standard	Metric
Canned peach halves or 1 cup peach sections, drained	6	6 or 250 mL
Peach liquid	1/4 cup	60 mL
Plain yogurt	1 cup	250 mL
Cinnamon	1 tsp.	5 mL

1. Blend the peaches and liquid in a food blender or mash completely.
2. Stir in the yogurt and cinnamon. Chill.

Yield: 4 servings

—————————— Basic Dessert Milk Pudding ——————————

	Standard	Metric
Cornstarch	3 Tbsp.	45 mL
Sugar	5 Tbsp.	75 mL
Salt	1/4 tsp.	1 mL
Cold milk	1/4 cup	60 mL
Scalded milk	1-3/4 cups	425 mL
Vanilla extract	1 tsp.	5 mL
Egg whites, beaten stiff	2	2

1. Mix the cornstarch, sugar, and salt with the cold milk.
2. Add to the scalded milk and cook over medium heat, stirring frequently, until thickened. Cook an additional 3 minutes.
3. Cool the mixture slightly; add the vanilla extract.
4. Fold in the egg whites until thoroughly mixed.
5. Pour into individual molds and chill.

Yield: 4 servings

Variations

1. For a creamier pudding use only 2 Tbsp. of cornstarch and eliminate the egg whites.
2. For butterscotch pudding use 5 Tbsp. of brown sugar, firmly packed, in place of the white sugar.
3. For chocolate pudding, melt 1-1/2 squares of chocolate in the scalded milk, and increase the sugar to 1/2 cup.
4. For coconut pudding, fold in 1/2 cup of shredded coconut.
5. For fruit pudding, add 3/4 to 1 cup of minced fruit such as bananas, raisins, or dates to the cooked pudding.

—————————— Chocolate Pudding Mix ——————————

	Standard	Metric
Flour, sifted	1-1/3 cups	325 mL
Dry nonfat dry milk	2 cups	500 mL
Salt	2 tsp.	10 mL
Sugar	2 cups	500 mL
Cocoa	2 cups	500 mL

1. Mix all ingredients thoroughly and sift three times.
2. Store in a covered glass or metal container at room temperature.

Chocolate Pudding

1. Add 1-1/2 cups of water to 1 cup of mix and cook over boiling water or in a saucepan over moderate

heat, stirring constantly. Stir in 1 tsp. fat and 1/2 tsp. vanilla.

Yield: 3 servings

Chocolate Sauce

1. Add 2 cups of water and 1/4 cup sugar to 1 cup of mix. Cook over boiling water or in a saucepan over moderate heat, stirring constantly. Add 2 Tbsp. of fat and 1/2 tsp. vanilla to the cooked sauce.

Yield: 2 cups

─────────── Bread Pudding ───────────

	Standard	Metric
Dry bread cubes	1 cup	250 mL
Milk, scalded	2 cups	500 mL
Sugar	1/4 cup	60 mL
Butter	1 tsp.	5 mL
Salt	1/8 tsp.	0.5 mL
Eggs, slightly beaten	2	2
Vanilla extract	1 tsp.	5 mL
Sugar	2 Tbsp.	30 mL
Cinnamon	1 tsp.	5 mL

1. Preheat oven to 350° F (175° C).
2. Place the bread cubes in a large mixing bowl and pour the scalded milk over them. Let stand for 3 minutes.

3. Add sugar, butter, and salt, and lightly mix.
4. Add the eggs and vanilla and mix thoroughly.
5. Pour into a greased baking dish. Sprinkle with the sugar and cinnamon.
6. Bake in a pan of hot water for 1 hour or until firm.

Yield: 4 servings

─────────── Fruit Confections ───────────

	Standard	Metric
Chopped dried apricots	1/2 cup	125 mL
Chopped dried prunes	1/2 cup	125 mL
Chopped dried dates	1/2 cup	125 mL
Raisins	1/2 cup	125 mL
Sweetened condensed milk	1-1/3 cups	325 mL

1. Preheat oven to 375° F (190° C).
2. In a bowl combine the apricots, prunes, dates, and raisins.
3. Add the milk and mix thoroughly.
4. Drop by teaspoonful onto a greased cookie sheet and bake for 15 minutes. Remove from the pan while still hot.

Yield: 30 cookies

LEARNING ACTIVITIES

1. Compare the price of fresh homogenized milk in a quart, half-gallon, and gallon container to determine which size would be the best buy for a family and for an individual living alone.
2. Calculate the difference in cost between a quart of fresh milk and a quart of reconstituted dried milk.
3. Serve a glass of chilled reconstituted dried milk, a glass of milk that is one-half fresh homogenized and one-half reconstituted dried milk, and a glass of fresh homogenized milk to four class members. Have them write their taste preferences. Evaluate the results.
4. Make a list of food products in which dried milk could be stirred into the other dry ingredients and in which water could be used as the liquid.
5. Read the label of as many milks and milk products as you can find at the grocery store and prepare a report on

how the information would help you in making a purchasing decision.

6. Prepare milk puddings from an instant and a cooked commercial mix. Prepare a milk pudding from the basic recipe in this chapter. Keep track of the time involved for each of the three preparations and compare the flavor of each of the three products. Based on the time and flavor study, report on which would be the wisest choice to serve to guests, on the basis of time, cost, and flavor.

7. Prepare three whipped foams from fresh whipping cream, evaporated milk, and dried milk. Chill in the refrigerator for 1 hour. Compare the difference in holding ability between each of the three foams.

8. Make a cost and calorie chart for the three whipped products and indicate when each whipped product would be the best to use.

9. Plan a day's menu for an adult who does not drink milk so that the adult would get the needed daily food requirement of two glasses of milk.

10. Develop a recipe for a milk punch that would be suitable for a children's party.

11. Prepare three medium white sauces for a vegetable using fresh homogenized milk, reconstituted dried milk, and diluted evaporated milk as the liquid. Compare the difference in flavor and cost between the three sauces.

12. Make a list of snacks containing milk that would be used for children.

REVIEW QUESTIONS

1. Why is lactose important in the human diet?
2. Why is milk considered a complete protein food?
3. What is the principal protein in milk called?
4. Of which B vitamin is milk an excellent source?
5. Which three nutrients are responsible for building strong bones and strong teeth?
6. How can the number of calories in a serving of milk be controlled?
7. What should be remembered about the color of milk in relation to menu planning?
8. What is the purpose of "ultrapasteurization?"
9. Why is it not advisable to drink raw milk?
10. What does homogenization mean?
11. What is the minimum milk fat content of fluid whole milk?
12. Which forms of fresh milk must be fortified with vitamin A?
13. What is the difference between lowfat and nonfat milk in relation to milk fat content?
14. What is the difference between filled milk and other milk?
15. How is evaporated milk processed?
16. Which two federal agencies are responsible for the grading standards for milk?
17. What are two ways by which the cost of milk can be reduced?
18. When might an individual choose to have milk delivered to the home?
19. Why should milk be refrigerated?
20. What should be remembered about the storage of dried milk?
21. How can the "pull date" on the milk container be used by the consumer?

22. Why does milk scorch?
23. What causes milk to curdle?
24. Which three groups of foods are likely to cause milk to curdle?
25. How can curdling of milk be prevented?
26. How can one tell if milk is scalded?
27. How is evaporated milk substituted for fresh milk in a recipe?
28. What prepreparation is necessary to make cream whip properly?

Cheese

Cheese is made from the curd of milk and is chiefly composed of the milk protein, casein. The curd is separated from the liquid portion of milk by adding rennet or acidifying the milk after which the milk is heated. Rennet is an enzyme that comes from the stomach of young calves and the acid is made from lactose, milk sugar. Most cheeses are made from one or a combination of the several forms of cow's milk although some kinds of cheese are made from sheep or goat's milk. Whey, the liquid portion of the milk that is drained off to attain the curd, is composed of lactose and water-soluble vitamins and minerals. It is used as an ingredient in many food products.

Cheese is a healthy and nutritious snack food and serves equally well as an accompaniment or entrée dish. Many recipes use cheese as an additional ingredient to enhance the flavor, texture, color, and nutrition of a product.

In the past cheese-making was a method of preserving milk. Today over 400 varieties of cheese are made all over the world.

Nutritional Factors to Consider

Carbohydrate

Cheese is not a supplier of carbohydrate because the lactose remains in the whey when the curd is separated out. Cheese is thus permitted as a food for those who cannot digest milk because they lack the necessary lactose enzyme. However, processed cheese foods may contain carbohydrate if whey solids are added when the product is made.

Protein and Fat

Cheese is a concentrated source of complete protein. A 1-ounce slice of cheddar cheese supplies approximately 12 per cent of the RDA for protein or an amount approximately equivalent to one 8-ounce glass of milk.

The fat content of cheese will vary with the form of milk used in making the cheese. For example, cheese made from lowfat milk contains less fat than cheese made from whole milk. Many lowfat cheeses are available, and some cheese manufacturers show the amount and type of fat present in the product in the nutritional labeling.

Vitamins and Minerals

Most of the water-soluble vitamins are lost with the whey but vitamin A remains in the curd of cheese that is made from whole milk. Whole-milk cheeses, which are made from rennet-started curd, have a high proportion of calcium and phosphorus, whereas cottage cheese, which is made from a lactic acid starter, is not as high in calcium and phosphorus.

Calories

The calorie content of cheese will vary slightly with the kind of milk from which it is made. For example, 1/2 cup of creamed cottage cheese with a 4 per cent milkfat content equals approximately 112 calories, and 1/2 cup of uncreamed cottage cheese equals approximately 63 calories.

Menu-Planning Points

Inherent Factors

Balance. Because of its many flavors and textures along with its high nutritional value, cheese can serve to balance any meal. For example, the mild flavor, soft texture, and high protein quality of cottage cheese can balance a meal that features a less complete protein food such as baked beans. The dinner can be more balanced by combining the cottage cheese with fruit for a salad accompaniment.

Color. The addition of a yellow cheese to a white sauce served with a vegetable such as broccoli adds both color and nutrients. Cream cheese, which is white in color, is a good contrast to serve with a brightly colored molded salad such as cherries in a cherry-flavored gelatin base.

Shape. Most hard and semihard cheeses can be cut into various geometric shapes for serving, and the softer cheeses can be shaped into balls to give added dimension to a meal. Figure 9–1 illustrates cheeses of varying shapes.

Flavor. Cheeses can be classified as mild, medium, and strong flavored. The more strongly flavored cheeses add a pleasing contrast to bland foods. For example, strong flavored cheeses such as Roquefort and Gruyère are pleasing complements to fruits, and sharp cheddar adds a tangy contrast to vegetables such as broccoli or asparagus. Other cheeses such as the sharp flavored Parmesan and Romano are good seasonings to use with mild flavored pasta dishes such as noodles served with a white sauce or butter-coated spaghetti.

Texture. The texture of cheese varies with the extent to which a cheese is ripened and aged. Soft textured cheeses that have a short ripening and aging process include Brie, Camembert, cottage cheese, cream cheese, Limburger, Neufchatel, and Ricotta. Semisoft cheeses include Muenster, Mozzarella, and Port du Salut. Hard textured cheeses include Parmesan and Romano. The textural firmness of a cheese as well as its perishability will affect the way the cheese is used in food preparation. For example, hard cheeses are grated and used as food toppings, whereas softer cheeses are eaten plain or melted in certain types of food preparation.

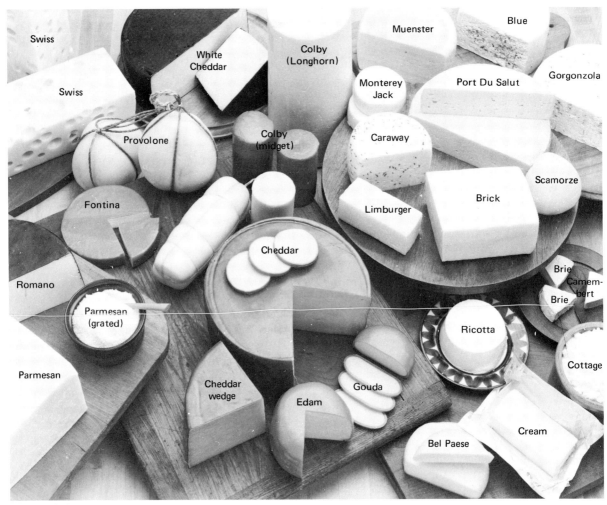

Figure 9-1.

Cheeses are arranged from very hard (left) to hard, to semi-soft to soft (right). (United Dairy Industry Association)

External Factors

Age. Cheese is accepted by various age groups according to the kinds of cheese to which they were introduced at an early age and according to their personal flavor preferences. For example, most children like the bland flavor and soft texture of cottage cheese, but do not accept more strongly flavored cheeses such as Roquefort or blue cheese until they are adults.

Culture. Culture too plays a large part in cheese acceptance. Most cheeses originated in distant parts of the world, and cheese, probably more than any other food, is passed down by succeeding generations of a culture. Cheese is an excellent source of calcium for all peoples of certain cultures who have a lactose intolerance.

Economics. Compared to the high cost of other complete protein foods, cheese is an excellent buy and combines readily with other foods that are of poorer quality protein.

Cheese is readily available in food markets and is seldom affected by crop failures and adverse climatic conditions. It takes up little storage space, and with the exception of the soft, unripened cheeses such as cottage or cream cheese, cheese can be stored for periods of 2 weeks to several months. Cheese is often served without any preliminary preparation, which makes it an excellent food to serve for snacks and as an additional ingredient in many food dishes.

Types of Cheese

Cheese is most often classified on its moisture content and the length of time it is ripened. The less moisture present, the firmer is the cheese; the longer a cheese ripens, the stronger is its flavor. Characteristics of low-moisture cheeses include a firm texture, a slow ripening stage, and a longer storage ability.

Cottage cheese, cream cheese, and Ricotta cheese are unripened cheeses that are acid-cured, meaning that an acid is used to curdle the milk. Cottage cheese is further classified according to its curd size and is sold as small or large curd cottage cheese.

Other cheeses are ripened by the addition of bacteria, molds, or a combination of both. Unripened and ripened cheeses are called natural cheeses and are classified as very hard, hard, semisoft, and soft according to texture. Processed cheeses are natural cheeses that have undergone further production steps. The following discussion explains some of the cheeses found in each classification.

Very Hard

Very hard cheeses must have a moisture content of less than 32 per cent. Parmesan and Romano cheeses are examples of very hard cheese that have a brittle, granular texture with a sharp, tangy flavor. They are grated and used as an additional seasoning and topping for casseroles or salads.

Hard

Hard cheeses have a moisture content of up to 41 per cent. Their flavor is dependent upon the length of ripening. One of the most popular cheeses in the United States is cheddar, which is available in a mild, medium, or sharp flavor. Cheddar cheese is sometimes called American cheese. Other examples of hard cheese include Colby, Edam, Gouda, provolone, and Swiss. Cheddar and Colby are the kinds of hard cheeses that are most often used in prepared dishes and all kinds are good when they are eaten plain.

Semisoft

Semisoft cheeses contain no more than 50 per cent moisture and have a variety of flavors. Blue and Roquefort cheeses are ripened with a mold culture and have a pungent flavor and a low-moisture content. Roquefort cheese is made only in southern France but blue cheese is made in several parts of the world, including the United States. Mild flavored semisoft cheeses used in cooking and eaten plain include Monterey Jack, mozzarella, and Muenster. Semisoft cheeses that are often served with fruit for a dessert include Bel Paese and Port du Salut.

Soft

Soft ripened cheeses, which include Brie, Camembert, Limburger, and Neufchatel, contain 50 to 55 per cent moisture. These are excellent dessert cheeses. Unripened cheeses that are soft include cottage, cream, and Ricotta cheeses. Cottage cheese has a moisture content of 80 per cent.

Processed Cheese

Processed cheeses are natural cheeses that have been grated or ground. They are sometimes mixed with other natural cheeses or with additional ingredients and are heated to produce a softer textured cheese. Processed cheeses usually have a slightly modified flavor and have a smooth consistency when melted, because of the addition of an emulsifier that helps to prevent the fat from separating from the protein.

Pasteurized Processed Cheese. The fat and moisture content of pasteurized processed cheese must be equal to the cheeses from which it is made. This cheese may be a combination of several different cheeses such as cheddar and Swiss, or it may be a combination of the same cheese selected at different stages of ripening.

Pasteurized Processed Cheese Food. Cheese food can contain as much as 44 per cent moisture, but must contain not less than 23 per cent milkfat. Cheese foods contain less cheese and more milk solids, whey solids, or water. The higher moisture content of cheese foods accounts for their softer texture and a product that melts more rapidly than process cheese. Cheese food has a mild flavor.

Pasteurized Processed Cheese Spread. These cheese products cannot contain more than 60 per cent moisture nor less than 20 per cent milkfat. Many flavor combinations are achieved by the addition of other ingredients.

Cold Pack or Club Cheese. These cheeses are similar to the pasteurized cheese products except that they are blended without heating. These cheeses may have additional ingredients added for flavoring and textural quality, and they have a soft, easy spreading consistency.

Grading

Only a few cheeses have grade standards as established by the USDA. If standards for cheese do exist, the grading is based on such factors as flavor, texture, and color of the cheese. The grade marks used are US Grade AA and US Grade A, but these grade marks do not usually appear on the retail package in which the cheese is sold. Cottage cheese and pasteurized process cheese may bear the label "Quality Approved" by the USDA, which means that the plant was inspected and the cheese was processed under sanitary conditions.

Purchasing

When purchasing cheese and cheese products, the label must be read to find out the kind of cheese being purchased. Labels of natural cheeses will give the variety of the cheese, such as Brie or Swiss, and, in the case of cheddar cheese, will also tell the age and ripening stage of the cheese that provides some information as to its flavor. For example, sharp cheddar cheese has been aged for 8 to 12 months; medium cheddar, for 4 to 7 months; and mild cheddar, for 2 to 3 months.

The labels on pasteurized cheese products include the kind of cheeses used in the processing and usually give some indication as to the flavor of the product. The labels also include a list of the additional ingredients.

Cheese is sold on a basic price per pound or, in the case of various cheese products, may be sold at a container price. Pasteurized cheese products are usually less expensive than natural cheeses, but some that are packaged in decorative containers are more expensive because the consumer pays for the container. Processed cheese spread is less expensive than other processed cheeses because the spread has a higher moisture content, but it does not have as high a nutritional value.

The harder cheeses, which are aged for long periods, are more costly than the mild and unripened varieties, which have no aging or else age in a shorter period of time. Imported cheeses are more costly than domestic cheeses. Whenever cheeses are specially cut, such as in cubes or slices, or when they are specially wrapped or have additional ingredients added, such as fruit to cottage cheese, they will be more expensive than the unseasoned and uncut varieties.

Large supermarkets frequently purchase bulk cheese and cut and package it into smaller portions. This form of cheese is less expensive than the precut cheeses that are packaged under national brand labels.

Storage

All cheeses need to be refrigerated. Processed cheese food and cheese spread may be stored at room temperature until they are opened, but after opening, the cheese must be refrigerated.

Soft, unripened cheeses such as cottage cheese and Ricotta are stored in the refrigerator and should be used within 2 to 3 days. Many of these cheeses are "use-dated," which helps to determine the length of storage times. Soft cheeses, like cream cheese and Brie, will keep for about a 2-week period.

Harder varieties of cheese can be stored for several months if they are properly wrapped. Cheese that is not properly covered will dry out and can become infected with mold growth.

Most cheese is sold in a plastic or foil wrap. Some cheese specialty stores cut the cheese in bulk at purchase and wrap it only in paper for the sale. These cheeses and those that have been opened should be completely wrapped in foil, plastic wrap, or waxed paper. Cheese may

also be stored in a covered container, which is particularly advisable for strong-smelling cheeses like blue or Roquefort.

Cheeses do not freeze well because of the change in texture, but for some types of food preparation this factor is not objectionable. Hard cheeses will become more crumbly and soft cheeses will become more watery when frozen. The most acceptable cheeses for freezing are cheddar, Edam, Swiss, mozzarella, and Parmesan. If cheese is to be frozen, it should be frozen in amounts less than 1 pound and not be more than 1 inch thick. The cheese should be chilled before it is frozen.

Cheese Preparation

All kinds of cheese can be eaten and enjoyed without further cooking. Cheese, that is to be served in uncooked form will have its best flavor and texture when it is brought to room temperature before it is served. This usually takes about 1 hour after the cheese is removed from the refrigerator. Exceptions are the soft, unripened cheeses, such as cream cheese and cottage cheese, that are kept chilled until it is time for them to be served. Cheeses are easier to grate if they are chilled. Some cheeses are easier to slice if chilled, and this depends on the texture of the cheese.

Plain cheeses are best when they are served with crisp crackers, hard rolls, various breads, or fresh fruits. Cheese can be sliced, cubed, cut in wedges, or made into balls as with soft cream cheese. A cheese tray is best when it contains a variety of cheeses with different flavors and textures.

Cheeses are often softened or grated and combined with other ingredients to make flavorful dips and spreads. Using a combination of cheeses in food preparation makes many interesting textures and flavors.

Cheese is sometimes heated or cooked with other ingredients. When cheese is heated, it melts. If it is overheated, it will become tough, stringy, and rubbery, because cheese is a protein food and overcooking causes the fat to separate out and a tough curd to develop. Best results are attained when cheese that is to be cooked is cubed or grated before it is mixed with other ingredients. If a mixture that includes a cheese is cooked on top of the stove, a low heat is used and the mixture is stirred constantly during the melting process, as when cheese is added to a white sauce.

Processed cheeses will produce a creamy, satiny texture when they are cooked, and because of the added emulsifier, they will not tend to separate. However, natural aged cheeses are sometimes preferred because of their more pungent flavor. Mild-flavored cheeses tend to become stringy more rapidly than the stronger-flavored varieties do.

A microwave oven quickly melts cheese. Many cooked food dishes can be quickly garnished with a slice of cheese or a sprinkling of grated cheese and placed in a microwave oven for a few seconds to melt the cheese.

Convenience Cheese Food Products

Several kinds of cheese are available in a convenience form but these kinds are more expensive. Grated cheese and many presliced cheeses can save steps in food preparation. Some cheeses are packaged in chunks with crackers for quick snacking. Processed cheeses come in tubes or cans for easy spreading on crackers. The best purchase in cheese convenience foods is probably the pregrated Parmesan or Romano because it is expensive in bulk form and sometimes is not available. It can also be used as a quick topping for many food dishes.

RECIPES

Nachos

	Standard	Metric
Corn chips	3 cups (12 oz.)	750 mL
Taco sauce	1 cup	250 mL
Grated sharp cheddar cheese	1 cup	250 mL

1. Preheat oven to broil.
2. Place the corn chips in a shallow baking pan; pour taco sauce over the corn chips; sprinkle with the grated cheese.
3. Place 3 inches from the broiler unit and heat until the cheese melts.
4. Microwave Oven: Place ingredients on paper plate, following procedure in step number 2. Heat 2-1/2 minutes, rotating dish 1/4 turn at 1-1/4 minutes.

Yield: Snack for 6 to 10 people

Cheese Wafers

	Standard	Metric
Flour, sifted	1-1/2 cup	375 mL
Salt	3/4 tsp.	4 mL
Cayenne pepper	1/8 tsp.	0.5 mL
Grated sharp cheddar cheese	1 cup (4 oz.)	250 mL
Butter or margarine	1/2 cup	125 mL

1. Sift the flour with the salt and cayenne pepper.
2. Combine the flour mixture with the grated cheese.
3. Cream the butter until it is fluffy; add the flour-cheese mixture; blend thoroughly. Mold the mixture with a spoon until the mixture is smooth and creamy.
4. Shape the mixture into a roll 2 inches in diameter and chill in the refrigerator for 1 to 2 hours.
5. Preheat the oven to 400° F (205° C).

6. Slice the cheese roll into 1/4-inch thick slices and bake on an ungreased baking sheet for 10 minutes.

Yield: 6 dozen

1. Soften the cream cheese to room temperature.
2. Thoroughly blend the cottage and cream cheeses with a spoon or with an electric mixer or blender until smooth.
3. Add the Worcestershire sauce, garlic and celery salts, and dill weed. Mix to blend thoroughly.
4. Chill for 2 hours or longer in refrigerator before serving with crackers.

Yield: 1-1/2 cups

——————— Cheese Soup ———————

	Standard	Metric
Butter or margarine	2 Tbsp.	30 mL
Flour	2 Tbsp.	30 mL
Milk	3 cups	750 mL
Chicken stock or bouillon	1 cup	250 mL
Dehydrated minced garlic	1 tsp.	5 mL
Dehydrated minced onion	1 tsp.	5 mL
Pepper	1/4 tsp.	1 mL
Grated sharp cheddar cheese	2 cups	500 mL
Egg yolks, slightly beaten	2	2

1. Melt the butter in a large heavy saucepan; blend in the flour.
2. Add the milk, chicken stock, dehydrated garlic, and onion and pepper; bring to a boil, stirring constantly.
3. Add the cheese and stir until melted.
4. Remove from the heat. Add a small amount to the egg yolks and blend together. Return the egg yolk mixture to the soup and cook an additional 2 minutes.

Yield: 6 servings

——————— Welsh Rarebit ———————

	Standard	Metric
Butter or margarine	1 Tbsp.	15 mL
Flour	1 Tbsp.	15 mL
Milk	1 cup	250 mL
Processed American cheese, diced	1/2 pound	227 mL
Dry mustard	1/2 tsp.	2 mL
Cayenne	1/4 tsp.	1 mL

1. Melt the butter or margarine; add the flour and stir to blend. Add the milk and cook over low heat, stirring constantly, until thick.
2. Stir in seasonings and add cheese; stir until just melted.
3. Serve over toast.

Yield: 4 to 6 servings

——————— Creamy Dip ———————

	Standard	Metric
Cream cheese	1 (3 oz.) pkg.	1 (85 gm)
Cottage cheese	1 cup	250 mL
Worcestershire sauce	1 tsp.	5 mL
Garlic salt	1/2 tsp.	2 mL
Celery salt	1/2 tsp.	2 mL
Dill weed	1 tsp.	5 mL

——————— Baked Cheese Fondue ———————

	Standard	Metric
Butter or margarine	1/3 cup	75 mL
White bread	8 slices	8
Gruyère cheese	6 oz.	170 gm
Eggs	2	2
Salt	1 tsp.	5 mL
Pepper	1/4 tsp.	1 mL
Milk	1-1/2 cup	375 mL

1. Preheat oven to 375° F (190° C).

2. Spread one side of the bread with butter or margarine and cut into 1-inch strips.

3. Cut the cheese into 1-inch strips.

4. Place a layer of bread in a greased 9-inch square baking pan; add a layer of cheese; add another layer of bread and another layer of cheese.

5. Put the eggs, salt, pepper, and milk into a bowl and beat slightly to mix.

6. Pour the mixture over the bread and cheese.

7. Bake for 35 minutes or until the fondue is golden brown.

8. Cut into squares and serve immediately.

Yield: 4 servings

——————————— Cheddar Fondue ———————————

	Standard	Metric
Butter or margarine	2 Tbsp.	30 mL
Flour	2 Tbsp.	30 mL
Garlic salt	1/2 tsp.	2 mL
Onion salt	1/2 tsp.	2 mL
Milk	1/2 cup	125 mL
Grated sharp cheddar cheese	1/2 pound	227 gm
Cubed French bread	3 cups	750 mL

1. Melt the butter or margarine in a heavy saucepan, an electric fry pan, or a chafing dish. Stir in the flour and garlic and onion salt.

2. Stir until smooth.

3. Add the milk and stir to blend. Add the cheese and stir until it is melted over low heat.

4. Serve warm with bread cubes and wooden sticks or forks for dipping.

Yield: 2 cups

——————————— Baked Cheese Sandwiches ———————————

	Standard	Metric
Bread	8 slices	8
Butter or margarine	2 Tbsp.	30 mL

Tuna fish	1 (7 oz.) can	1 (198 gm)
Mayonnaise	1/4 cup	60 mL
Roquefort or blue cheese, optional	2 Tbsp.	30 mL
Finely chopped celery	1/4 cup	60 mL
American cheese	4 slices	4
Tomato	4 slices	4
Cream of mushroom soup	1 can	1
Milk	1/2 cup	125 mL

1. Preheat the oven to 350° F (175° C).

2. Butter one side of each slice of bread.

3. Combine the tuna fish, mayonnaise, Roquefort or blue cheese, and celery. Divide equally among four slices of bread; spread evenly. Top each with a cheese and tomato slice; add the other piece of bread.

4. Place the sandwiches in a buttered 9 × 12 × 2-inch baking dish.

5. Combine the mushroom soup and the milk and pour over the top.

6. Bake for 25 minutes.

Yield: 4 servings

——————————— Swiss Cheese Loaf ———————————

	Standard	Metric
Butter or margarine, softened	1/2 cup	125 mL
Minced onion	1/3 cup	75 mL
Prepared mustard	3 Tbsp.	45 mL
Poppy seeds	1 Tbsp.	15 mL
Lemon juice	2 tsp.	10 mL
Loaf bread, unsliced	1	1
Processed Swiss cheese, sliced	1/2 pound (8 slices)	227 gm
Bacon, halved	3 slices	3

1. Preheat the oven to 350° F (175° C).

2. Mix together in a bowl the butter, onion, mustard, poppy seeds, and lemon juice.

3. Make eight diagonal cuts, evenly spaced, from the

top to the bottom of the bread, cutting only to the bottom crust.

4. Reserve 3 tablespoons of the butter mixture and spread the rest on the cut surfaces of the bread.

5. Place one slice of cheese between each cut and set the filled loaf in a loaf baking pan.

6. Spread the reserved butter mixture on top of the loaf and add the bacon slices.

7. Bake for 20 minutes or when the bacon is cooked and the loaf is slightly browned.

Yield: 6 to 8 servings

Miniature Pizza

	Standard	Metric
English muffins, split	4	4
Sieved canned tomatoes	1/2 cup	125 mL
Oregano	1/4 tsp.	1 mL
Garlic salt	1/2 tsp.	2 mL
Mozzarella cheese	8 slices	8
Olive oil or other cooking oil	4 tsp.	20 mL
Grated Parmesan cheese	4 tsp.	20 mL

1. Preheat the oven to 400° F (205° C).

2. Mix the tomatoes with oregano and garlic salt.

3. Spread each muffin half with 2 Tbsp. of the tomato mixture.

4. Top each half with a slice of mozzarella cheese and sprinkle each half with 1/2 tsp. Parmesan cheese and 1/2 tsp. olive oil.

5. Bake in the oven for 5 to 8 minutes or until bubbly.

Yield: 8 miniature pizzas

Cheese Spoon Bread

	Standard	Metric
Milk, scalded	2 cups	500 mL
Yellow cornmeal	1 cup	250 mL
Eggs, separated	4	4
Cheddar cheese, grated	1-1/2 cups (6 oz.)	375 mL
Butter	1/4 cup	60 mL
Sugar	1 tsp.	5 mL
Salt	1/2 tsp.	2 mL

1. Preheat the oven to 375° F (190° C).

2. To the hot scalded milk add the cornmeal gradually, stirring constantly over low heat until the mixture thickens and is smooth.

3. Beat the egg yolks slightly. Stir 2 Tbsp. of the cornmeal mixture into the egg yolks and then add the egg yolks to the cornmeal mixture.

4. Add the grated cheese, butter, sugar, and salt. Mix until well blended.

5. Beat the egg whites until stiff and fold into the cornmeal mixture until blended.

6. Turn the mixture into a 1-1/2 quart, greased casserole and bake for 35 to 40 minutes or until a knife inserted near the center comes out clean.

7. Serve with butter.

Yield: 6 servings

Cheesecake

	Standard	Metric
Graham cracker crumbs	1-1/2 cups	375 mL
Sugar	1/4 cup	60 mL
Butter or margarine	1/2 cup	125 mL
Cottage cheese	1 cup	250 mL
Cream cheese	2 (3 oz.) pkgs.	170 gm
Eggs	2	2
Sugar	1/2 cup	125 mL
Vanilla extract	1 tsp.	5 mL
Salt	1/4 tsp.	1 mL
Sour cream	1/2 cup	125 mL
Sugar	2 Tbsp.	30 mL
Vanilla extract	1/2 tsp.	2 mL

1. Preheat the oven to 350° F (175° C).

2. Melt the butter or margarine and combine the crumbs and 1/4 cup sugar. Press the mixture into

a greased 9-inch round springform pan with 3-inch sides.

3. Bake for 8 minutes. Let cool.
4. Press the cottage cheese through a sieve and mix with the cream cheese, eggs, 1/2 cup sugar, 1 tsp. vanilla extract, and salt. Blend until smooth.
5. Pour the mixture into the crust and bake at 350° F (175° C) for 20 minutes or until set.
6. Blend together the sour cream, 2 Tbsp. sugar, and 1/2 tsp. vanilla.
7. Spread over the cheesecake and chill thoroughly.

Yield: 8 servings

——————— Cream Cheese Topping ———————

	Standard	Metric
Cream cheese	6 oz.	170 gm
Confectioners' sugar, sifted	1 cup	250 mL
Milk	5 Tbsp.	75 mL
Vanilla extract	1/2 tsp.	2 mL

1. Beat the cream cheese until it is fluffy.
2. Add the confectioners' sugar to the cream cheese gradually, beating after each addition.
3. Add the milk and vanilla and beat until smooth.
4. Chill. Serve as a dessert topping or a frosting.

Yield: 1–1/3 cups

LEARNING ACTIVITIES

1. Investigate the local grocery store to determine the kinds of natural cheeses that are available and the forms in which they are sold. Do a price comparison between convenience and bulk forms of the same type of cheese and determine which form would be the best buy for a family and a single person.
2. Investigate a local grocery store to find the kinds of processed cheeses that are available there. Read the labels to see what additional ingredients have been used, if any. Compare the price of processed cheese, cheese food, and cheese spread and decide which would be the best buy for making a cheese sauce and for snacking.
3. Plan a menu for breakfast that includes cheese. Calculate the amount of protein the menu contains.
4. Plan a luncheon menu with an entrée of cheese salad.
5. Plan a dinner menu that uses cheese in some cooked form.
6. Plan a dessert cheese and fruit tray using four different kinds of cheese that range in flavor from mild to strong.
7. Prepare two medium white sauces using sharp cheddar cheese and a processed cheese. Compare the cost, flavor, and texture of the two sauces.
8. Prepare a medium white sauce that uses a cheese other than cheddar or a processed cheese for flavoring. Note the difference between the results obtained in number 7 and this sauce. Determine when this sauce would be a suitable substitute for the other sauces.
9. Plan and present a cheese-sampling demonstration to the class. Discuss the various kinds of cheese that you are using relative to the use of the cheeses in cooking and eating.
10. Develop a baked cheese sandwich of your own liking and prepare it.
11. Plan a menu with a meat alternate that uses cheese as the complete protein food.
12. Make a list of the various ways that

cottage cheese can be used in food preparation.

13. Develop a dip or spread recipe that uses cheese as the main ingredient.

14. Freeze 1/2 cup of cottage cheese; thaw in the refrigerator and note the textural changes.

REVIEW QUESTIONS

1. How is the curd of milk attained?
2. Of what is the whey of milk composed?
3. Why does cheese not contain carbohydrate when milk does?
4. What determines the mineral content of cheese?
5. Why is cottage cheese a good source of protein and a poor substitute for the calcium that is present in milk?
6. What kinds of cheese would be good flavorings for milk-flavored food dishes?
7. What are the characteristics of low-moisture cheeses?
8. What are the four general classifications of cheeses?
9. What is another name for cheddar cheese?
10. What is the main difference between Roquefort cheese and blue cheese?
11. What are processed cheeses?
12. What is the difference between a process cheese food and cheese spread?
13. How does a club cheese differ from a process cheese?
14. What does a label on cheese bearing "Quality Approved" by the USDA signify?
15. What is the most expensive form of natural cheese?
16. What is the most costly of processed cheeses?
17. How long can cottage cheese be stored in the refrigerator?
18. How should cheese be wrapped for storage?
19. What happens when cheese is frozen?
20. At what temperature should cheese be served when it is eaten plain?
21. What happens when cheese is overheated?
22. How should cheese be prepared when it is to be added to a white sauce.
23. What is the difference between using a processed cheese and a natural cheese in a white sauce?
24. Why does natural cheese become tough and stringy when it is overcooked?
25. When would it be desirable to purchase a convenience cheese food?

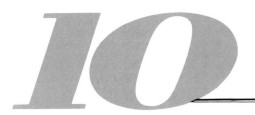

Meat Alternates

Meat alternates are foods that can be served in place of meat or other complete protein foods in a meal. They also can be used as meat extenders so that a lesser amount of a complete protein food is needed in a food product. Legumes, pastas, rice, and nuts are foods that make suitable meat alternates. Although they are not satisfactory substitutes for complete protein foods because they lack some of the nine essential amino acids, meat alternates become of higher protein value when they are combined with a small amount of a complete protein food. As food technology increases, many more nontraditional meat alternates will probably be available from such food sources as plants, algae, and fish concentrates.

There are several reasons for incorporating meat alternates into an eating plan. First, as the population in many areas of the world continues to increase, the once abundant food supply is beginning to lessen. We need to balance the world's protein intake from many sources and not depend on meat alone. Further, the cost of meat has risen rapidly over the past few years and the use of meat alternates can help reduce the food budget.

Nutritional Factors to Consider

Carbohydrate and Fat

Legumes, pastas, rice, and nuts are all moderately high in carbohydrate, which makes them a good source of energy. Starch is the form of carbohydrate found in these foods.

Pasta, rice, and legumes, with the exception of soybeans, contain only a trace of fat. Nuts and soybeans are high in fat as shown in Table 10-1.

130

Protein

All meat alternates discussed in this chapter are incomplete protein foods because they either lack one or more of the nine essential amino acids or do not contain enough of one essential amino acid to classify them as complete protein foods. The soybean is the most complete of the plant proteins, only lacking an adequate amount of the amino acid, methionine. Rice is the best source of protein from the cereal grains, and peanuts have the highest value of protein from the nut group. Two tablespoons of peanut butter contain as much protein as a medium-sized egg, 1 ounce of cooked hamburger, or 6 ounces of milk. Figure 10-1 illustrates the portions of meat alternates that must be consumed to meet approximately one third of the daily protein requirement. Meat alternates need only a small amount of a complete protein food to raise the protein value. For example, a serving of macaroni and cheese or rice pudding made with milk provides ample protein in a meal.

Vitamins and Minerals

Legumes, rice, and nuts are fair sources of the B vitamins, and enriched pasta and rice products are excellent sources of thiamine, riboflavin, and niacin. Legumes, rice, nuts, and enriched pasta products are excellent sources of iron.

Calories

Meat alternates are not high in calories. One-half cup servings of legumes average 120 calories; rice has 82 calories per 1/2 cup serving; macaroni has 105 calories per 1/2 cup serving; and peanut butter averages 180 calories for 2 tablespoons. Nuts, because of their fat content, are higher in calories than other meat alternates. Table 10-1 gives the content of some meat alternates.

Menu-Planning Points

Inherent Factors

Balance. Meat alternates are all rather bland in taste, making them a good combination to serve with more flavorful and spicy foods. They provide a good nutritional balance for meals that may be short of complete protein foods.

Color. The color of meat alternates often depends upon the variety of the food used. Most pasta products are a creamy-white with the exception of spinach egg noodles. Legumes,

Table 10-1

Fat, Protein, and Calorie Content of Some Meat Alternates

Food	Fat gm	Protein gm	Food Energy Calories
Almonds, shelled, 1/2 cup	39	13	425
Beans, cooked, Great Northern, 1/2 cup	.6	7	106
Macaroni, cooked, 1 cup	.7	6.5	192
Peanut butter, 2-1/2 Tbsp.	20.2	10	235
Rice, cooked, 1 cup	Trace	4	180
Soybeans, cooked, 1/2 cup	5	10	117
Split peas, cooked, 2/3 cup	Trace	11	153

Nutritive Value of American Foods, Agriculture Handbook No. 456, USDA, 1975.

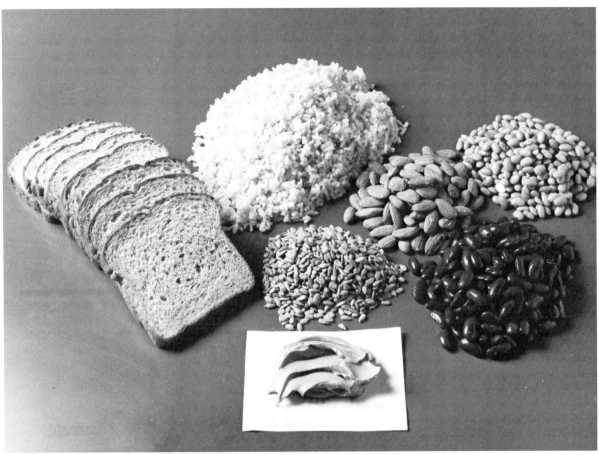

Figure 10-1.
Eight slices of whole wheat bread, 4 cups of brown rice, 1 cup of almonds, 1 cup of soybeans, 1-1/3 cup kidney beans, 1 cup sunflower seeds, or 5 tablespoons of peanut butter can each meet approximately 1/3 of the day's protein requirement.

such as lima beans and split green peas, are of a green color. Rice is either a creamy white or a light brown. Nuts vary according to whether they are blanched or used in the skin.

Shape. The small delicate shape of legumes and rice is a pleasant contrast to larger chunks of food. Pastas come in a wide variety of shapes including flat noodles, tubular and seashell macaroni, and rod-shaped spaghetti.

Figure 10-2 shows a variety of pasta shapes. Nuts can be left whole, ground, or chopped to add more shape variety to a food dish.

Flavor. The flavor of meat alternates is enhanced with additional spices, herbs, or liquid flavoring used in cooking them. Rice has an enriched flavor when it is cooked in a chicken broth or beef bouillon, and brown rice has a nutty flavor that is a good complement to many meat dishes. Roasted nuts are a flavorful addition to a dish such as creamed noodles and tuna fish.

Texture. Legumes, pastas, and rice when they are properly cooked have a soft texture. Nuts are crunchy and crisp and add not only nutrients but additional texture when they are used in baked goods, such as the bread shown in Figure 10-3.

External Factors

Age. Some legumes cause a flatulent condition in some individuals. This problem can be partially eliminated by discarding the water used for soaking legumes and using fresh water for cooking. It also is advisable to drain off the liquid from cooking. Caution should be used in serving nuts to young children because of the danger of their choking on the nuts.

Figure 10-2.
Pastas come in a variety of shapes. (National Macaroni Institute)

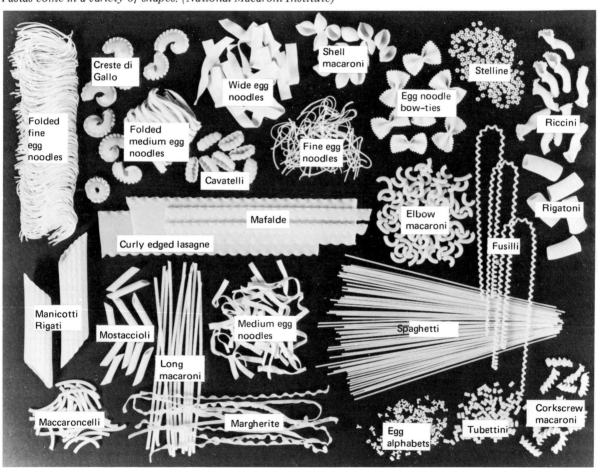

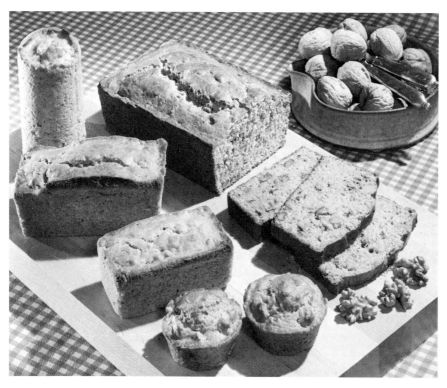

Culture and Economics. Meat alternates are the main food source available for many cultures. One of the advantages of using meat alternates in food preparation is the comparatively low cost of meat alternates in relation to other high-protein foods.

Space and Equipment. All uncooked meat alternates can be stored at room temperature and thus do not take up storage space needed for perishable foods. The main equipment needed for cooking legumes and pastas is a large saucepan with a lid. Smaller saucepans are used for cooking rice.

Time Scheduling. The main disadvantage of using legumes in food preparation is the long time required to cook them. For example, beans need to be boiled and soaked for 1 hour or soaked overnight before the additional

cooking with other ingredients of approximately 2 hours. However, quantities of legumes can be cooked ahead of time and stored in the refrigerator for up to 1 week, or up to 1 year in the freezer. In the future, more quick-cooking legumes will probably become available. Regular rice requires an average of only 15 minutes cooking time and the precooked varieties of rice cook in less time. Legumes, pastas, and rice can be held for short periods of time before serving, which is an advantage in meal scheduling.

Types of Legumes, Pastas, Rice, and Nuts

Many types and varieties of these foods are available today, and food technology continues to discover new methods of processing and converting these foods into even more "convenient-to-use" forms. Many of the food products purchased contain some form of plant protein.

Legumes

Legumes are the dried seeds of pod vegetables. They include beans, peas, and lentils.

Dried Beans. Common varieties of dried beans include garbanzo, kidney, lima, pinto, navy, soybeans, and white beans. The soybean is the most widely developed and used dried bean in the world. In addition to being cooked, the soybean is found in food products in three forms.

1. Soy flour is made by grinding the bean solid after the seed covering and oil are removed. The protein content of the flour is 50 to 52 per cent.
2. Soy concentrate is made by removing the oil and most of the soluble carbohydrate from the bean. It is approximately 70 per cent protein.
3. Soy isolate is obtained by removing the fat and carbohydrate from soy flour. It contains 90 per cent or more protein.

Dried Peas and Lentils. Marketed forms include the yellow or split green pea. Lentils are similar to a pea in appearance but are thinner and smaller.

Pasta

Pasta is an Italian generic term now commonly used in the United States to encompass all macaroni products including macaroni, spaghetti, and egg noodles. Pasta products are made from semolina, the heart of durum wheat, which is the hardest wheat grown. Pasta products are made in varying lengths, sizes, and shapes.

Macaroni is a hollow pasta form made in varying widths, lengths, and shapes. In addition to the popular elbow macaroni, rigatoni, mostacolli, and manicotti are frequently used in food preparation.

Noodles contain a minimum of 5.5 per cent egg solids, along with the semolina and water used in making pastas. Noodles are flat and are made in varying widths and lengths. Commonly used noodles include the egg noodle and fettuccine.

Spaghetti is a solid rod pasta made into varying degrees of thickness and length. In addition to the popular pasta termed "spaghetti" other commonly used forms include spaghettini and vermicelli.

Rice

Rice is a grain just as wheat or oats are classified. Three different types of rice are available as shown in Figure 10-4.

1. Long-grain rice has a long, narrow kernel. When it is cooked, the long-grain rice is fluffy and dry with kernels that do not cling together.
2. Short- and medium-grain rice when cooked are more tender and moist with kernels that tend to cling together.

Available forms of rice for purchase include brown, parboiled, converted, regular-milled, and precooked. Brown rice has had only the outer hull and a small portion of the bran removed. Regular-milled rice has had the bran completely removed and is a white rice. Parboiled rice is the rice kernel that has been subjected to steam and pressure prior to hulling. The processing of converted rice is similar to that of parboiled rice. Precooked rice is rice that has been cooked and then dehydrated.

Wild rice is not a rice but the seed of a wild grass. It is expensive.

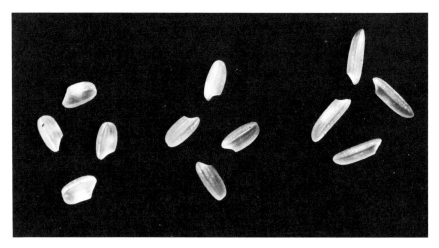

Figure 10-4.
From left to right, short, medium, and long grain rice kernels are shown. (Rice Council)

Nuts

A nut is the fruit of a tree. It grows in a hard or semihard shell. Peanuts are actually legumes but are most commonly associated with nuts. Many types of nuts are available in the shell and as raw nut meats.

Nuts sold in the shell include almonds, brazils, coconuts, peanuts, pecans, pines, and pistachios. These nuts are often available in a mixed variety. Almonds, pecans, and walnuts are the most common nutmeats available shelled and in raw form. Almonds, brazils, cashews, filberts, and peanuts are available roasted and in a salted, mixed nut-meat combination. Dry roasted nut meats are also sold. The term *dry roasted* means that no fat was added to the nuts in the roasting process.

Peanut butter is a popular spread made from roasted and ground peanuts. Some types of peanut butter, which contain small pieces of peanuts, are labeled "chunky."

Textured Vegetable Protein

Textured vegetable protein (TVP) refers to foods and ingredients made from soy, wheat, oats, and cottonseed. The principal vegetable protein source used is the soybean. TVP has been available to the consumer for several years. Modern food processing has developed a variety of shapes, sizes, flakes, and fibrous characteristics of TVP as shown in Figure 10-5. The most acceptable products have been in bits and chunks and in granular form.

TVP is principally available in two forms. As a meat extender, it is used in combination with various meat products to extend the number of servings. A meat analog is a textured vegetable protein that has been processed to have the same taste, color, and fiber characteristics as the meat product for which it is a substitute. Meat analogs currently on the market include ham and chicken chunks, granular form ground beef, and sausage patties.

Purchasing

Legumes should be selected that are even in size, have good color for the variety chosen, and do not have broken seeds. Legumes are usually sold in see-through packages or in bulk so that it is easy to check their appearance. Broken packages of legumes may be contaminated and should not be purchased.

Various legumes are also available in canned cooked form. Although they are more expensive than the dried legumes, the cost of cooked legumes may be justified by the time saved in their preparation. Some quick-cooking beans are available as a refrigerated product.

Different varieties of pasta vary in cost, which is also determined by the size of package purchased. Comparing the cost per quantity in the package can help to determine the best buy.

Precooked and specially flavored rices are more costly than brown and regular rice. However, if time is a valuable commodity, the more convenient form of rice may be a better buy.

Unshelled nuts cost less than shelled nuts. The shell of the nut should not be broken and should have a good color for the variety. Specially processed and mixed nuts are more expensive than the plain, unshelled nuts. An oily, yellowish-colored nut may be stale or rancid.

The cost of mixed nuts is often determined by the percentage of peanuts the mixture contains. Because peanuts are less costly than other nuts, the more peanuts in the mixture the less expensive is the product. Broken nut meats are less expensive than whole or halves of nuts.

Storage

Legumes, pastas, and rice can all be stored at room temperature. They should either be properly sealed in the package in which they are purchased or stored in another container with a tight cover to prevent insects from entering. These foods if properly covered do not deteriorate and can be stored for long periods of time. Brown rice, because of the fat content in the germ layer, and rice mixes with special flavorings that deteriorate over a period of time should be stored for a maximum of 4 to 6 months.

Nuts will keep for long periods of time if they are properly stored. Because nuts have a high fat content they may become rancid when

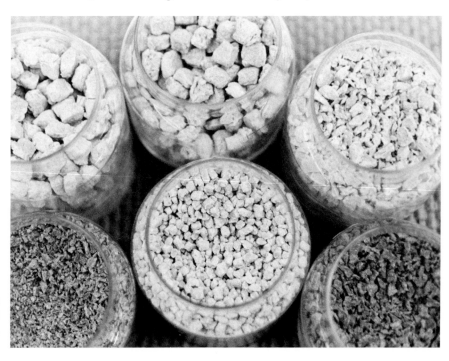

Figure 10-5.
Textured vegetable protein can be made into a variety of shapes. (Archer Daniels, Midland Company)

they are exposed to air. It is thus important to keep shelled nuts in a tightly closed container and store them in the refrigerator or freezer. Nuts, which are vacuum-packed or packaged with a preservative, will keep longer than shelled nuts kept in a cellophane bag.

Unshelled nuts can be stored in a cool, dry area for several months.

Basic Methods of Legume Cookery

Since legumes develop a tough fibrous structure during the drying process, legumes should be soaked in water prior to cooking to help soften the structure. Exceptions to this are split peas and lentils that are not soaked. The first step in preparing legumes for soaking is to sort through them to remove any broken seeds or foreign material. The legumes are then washed thoroughly in water, preferably in a sieve or colander for washing. The two basic methods for soaking legumes are as follows:

1. Three cups of water are added to 1 cup of legumes in a large saucepan, and the mixture is brought to a boil and boiled uncovered for 2 minutes. The pan is removed from the heat and covered and the beans are then soaked for 1 hour.

2. Three cups of water are added to 1 cup of legumes; they are covered and soaked overnight.

The first method of soaking is preferred because beans rehydrate faster in hot water. If hard water is used for soaking, 1/8 teaspoon baking soda per pint of water may be used to hasten the softening process. The minerals in hard water prevent the proper softening and even cooking of legumes, and the alkalinity of baking soda helps to counteract this.

Soaked dried legumes are best cooked in the same liquid in which they are soaked. To eliminate the flatulence factor, they may be drained and fresh water used for cooking.

There is some reduction in nutrients, however, when the soaking liquid is discarded. The beans are cooked with 1 teaspoon salt per cup of beans in a covered saucepan at a slow boil for 1 to 2 hours or until the beans are tender. Additional water may have to be added during the cooking. Because legumes have a tendency to foam while cooking, the lid of the saucepan should be left slightly ajar. A small amount of cooking oil also helps to reduce foaming.

Dried beans may also be cooked in a pressure cooker. It is not recommended that dried peas be cooked by this method because they foam readily when they are boiled and may clog the vent pipe. At the start of cooking, the dried beans and water should not fill the cooker by more than 1/3 of the total capacity, because the beans will expand while cooking.

The cooking procedure for lentils and split peas is the same as for other legumes except that lentils will cook to the tender stage in about 30 minutes and split peas in 45 minutes.

One cup of uncooked legumes will yield approximately 2-1/2 cups when cooked, as shown in Figure 10-6.

Figure 10-6.
One cup of uncooked legumes will yield 2-1/2 cups when cooked.

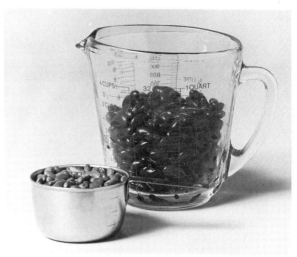

Legumes are used in soups, chowders, stews, and casseroles, and they can be baked. The bland flavor of legumes adapts well to being cooked with meats such as bacon and ham hocks. Additional flavor can be attained by cooking legumes with onion, garlic, carrot, and celery, and herbs such as thyme, basil, and oregano.

Acidic foods such as tomatoes should be added after the legumes are tender as the acid prohibits the softening of the legumes' fibrous structure.

Basic Method of Pasta Cookery

Pasta products should not be washed or soaked before they are cooked. The basic method is to drop the pasta product into boiling salted water and to boil uncovered for approximately 15 minutes or until the pasta is tender. The usual proportion is 1 cup of pasta to 2 quarts of boiling water to which 1 tablespoon of salt has been added. Pasta products have a tendency to stick to the bottom of the pan when they are being cooked. To eliminate this, 1 tablespoon of fat may be added at the start of cooking and the pasta can be lightly stirred once or twice during the cooking time.

After the pasta is cooked the water is drained off. The pasta should not be rinsed after it is cooked because there is a considerable loss of nutrients with this procedure.

One cup or 4 ounces of uncooked macaroni or spaghetti will yield approximately 2 cups of cooked pasta, and 1 cup or 2 ounces of noodles yields 1 cup of cooked noodles.

Pastas are served in many ways to provide wholesome main dish entrées. The way in which pastas are served depends on the variety of pasta used. Spaghetti and noodle forms are served with sauces or baked with various ingredients in casseroles as illustrated in Figure 10-7. They can also be a nutritious addition to soups and can be used as the main ingredient

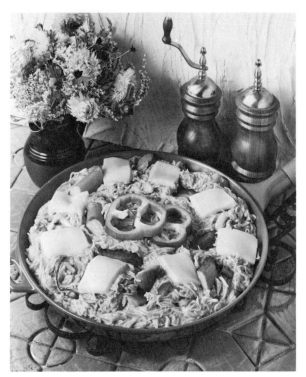

Figure 10-7.
Spaghetti, frankfurters, and cheese combine to make a hearty casserole. (National Macaroni Institute)

in salads. Tubular macaroni can be stuffed with a small portion of a complete protein and baked with a sauce. Figure 10-8 shows the filling of manicotti shells with a meat stuffing. Other macaroni products are used in salads, soups, and casseroles.

Basic Methods of Rice Cookery

As with pastas, rice is not washed or soaked prior to cooking. Although rice may be started to cook in cold water, most people prefer to start the rice cooking in boiling water. Cold water makes rice very gummy. Adding a small amount of fat helps to keep the rice granules separated. Rice can be cooked by several methods.

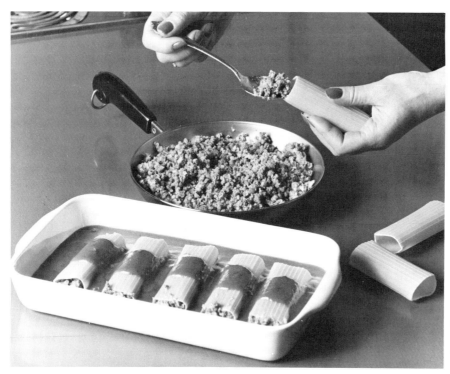

Figure 10-8.
Manicotti shells may be uncooked or partially cooked and then filled with a meat or cheese filling.

Saucepan Method

The package directions should be followed for the amounts of liquid and rice to use for the desired number of servings. The length of cooking time will vary with the type of rice used and this will be noted in the directions. The rice is added to boiling salted water, and the mixture is brought back to a boil and stirred once or twice. The rice is cooked covered over a low heat until all the liquid is absorbed into the rice. Figure 10-9 shows the proper equipment to use for the saucepan method.

Baking Method

The rice is added to boiling, salted water in a baking dish and is then stirred, covered, and baked at 350° F (175° C). Regular rice takes approximately 25 minutes; parboiled rice bakes in 35-40 minutes; and brown rice cooks in 1 hour.

Figure 10-9.
The correct equipment is necessary for the proper cooking of rice. (Rice Council)

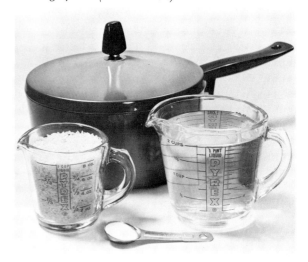

Double-Boiler Method

This method is used most often when cooking rice in milk. The milk and rice are brought to boiling in the top of the double boiler and are then placed over boiling water and cooked for approximately 40 minutes or until the milk is absorbed by the rice.

Fried Method

There are two ways to fry rice. The first is to use cooked rice, which is heated in a small amount of fat in a heavy fry pan. Slightly beaten eggs are stirred into the cooked rice, and the mixture is cooked until the eggs are done. Small pieces of meat and vegetables may also be added to the mixture. For 2 cups of cooked rice, three eggs are used.

The second method is to fry the kernels of rice in fat in a fry pan until the rice turns light brown in color. The liquid is then added and the rice is cooked in a covered saucepan by the saucepan or baking method.

Special rice cookers are available on the market that allow rice to cook by the steam which comes in contact with the pan holding the rice, or the steam may come in direct contact with the rice.

One cup of uncooked regular milled rice will yield 3 cups when cooked; brown and parboiled rice will yield 3 to 4 cups; and precooked rice yields 1 to 2 cups.

Rice should not be stirred while it is cooking nor should it be left in the pan in which it was cooked as it will become gummy. The rice is removed from the pan and fluffed with a fork to separate the rice kernels. Rice may be refrigerated and reheated by adding 2 tablespoons of liquid per cup of rice and heating in a covered saucepan.

The flavor of rice may be varied by the addition of ingredients to the cooking liquid such as chopped onion, parsley, mushrooms, crushed garlic, or green pepper. Other ingredients that may be added include raisins or the grated rind

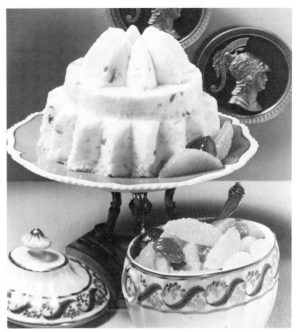

Figure 10-10.
Rice can be cooked and molded for an elegant dessert. (Florida Citrus Commission)

of a lemon or orange. The liquid may be varied by cooking the rice in a chicken broth or beef bouillon, or in a mixture of part tomato juice and part water. Figure 10-10 shows rice as part of a molded dessert.

Rice is prepared in many ways to serve as a meat alternate or as a separate accompaniment to a meal. It can be cooked and served with milk, sugar, and cinnamon for the main protein food at breakfast; combined with a small portion of meat for a hearty and complete luncheon salad; or combined with a small amount of cheese, eggs, meat, or fish for a dinner casserole. Rice is used in soups, stews, and desserts and as a meat extender in such food dishes as meat loaf. Rice can also be molded into an attractive ring shape to serve as the container for another food dish such as lamb curry. As the main ingredient of many parfaits, puddings, and pies, rice is a nutritious dessert.

Basic Methods of Nut Cookery

Many nuts are ready to eat or use in other cookery when they are purchased. Time is saved by using preshelled nuts, but they are more expensive than those in the shell.

A recipe often calls for a blanched nut—one that has had the outer skin removed. The easiest way to remove the outer skin of raw nuts, such as almonds and peanuts, is to let them stand in boiling water for 2 to 3 minutes. The skin should then easily slide off.

Nuts may also be roasted for a richer flavor and color. They are spread in a shallow baking pan and baked at 350° F (175° C) for 5 to 15 minutes or until they are lightly browned. They should be stirred frequently. One teaspoon of fat per one cup of nut meats may be added for additional flavor. The nuts may be salted at the end of the cooking time.

When nuts are added to other foods for additional flavor and texture, they should always be added near the end of the cooking time so that they maintain their crispness.

Microwave Cookery

Legumes are not satisfactory when cooked in a microwave. Pastas and rice can be cooked in the microwave, but the cooking time is approximately the same as for conventional cooking. A sauce can often be quickly prepared in the microwave oven while the pasta or rice is being cooked in the regular manner. Most casserole dishes containing pastas, rice, and cooked legumes are excellent when cooked in a microwave oven.

Nuts can very easily and very quickly be blanched, toasted, or roasted by microwave cooking.

Convenience Meat Alternate Food Products

Many forms of legumes, pastas, and rice are available in convenience forms. Several varieties of cooked and canned beans can be purchased. Ravioli and various kinds of spaghetti come prepared in a sauce and ready to heat and eat, and various other noodle and bean dishes are also canned. Macaroni and cheese are sold in packaged or canned form, and many flavorful precooked rice and noodle products are available that just need water for cooking. Other convenience rice products include ready-to-eat cereal, instant cooked cereal, and rice pudding. Several different types of dried soup mixes containing meat alternates may be purchased. Some are quick-cooking and some are cooked in the way legumes are cooked.

RECIPES

Bean Sandwiches

	Standard	Metric
Cooked navy beans	1/2 cup	125 mL
Catsup	2 Tbsp.	30 mL
Mayonnaise	1 Tbsp.	15 mL
Bread, buttered	8 slices	8

1. Mash the beans or press through a sieve.
2. Combine beans with catsup and mayonnaise.
3. Put the bean spread on four slices of buttered bread and top with remaining slices.

Yield: 4 servings

Baked Beans

	Standard	Metric
Navy beans	1 cup	250 mL
Salt	1 tsp.	5 mL
Molasses	2 Tbsp.	30 mL
Brown sugar	2 Tbsp.	30 mL
Dry mustard	1/4 tsp.	1 mL
Salt pork or 1 small ham hock	1/4 pound	113 gm

1. Wash, cover with water, and soak the beans overnight or bring to a boil; boil 2 minutes and let stand for 1 hour. Do not drain.
2. Combine the soaked beans with the salt, molasses, brown sugar, dry mustard, and salt pork and pour into a casserole dish; cover and bake at 325° F (165° C) for 2 hours or until tender. If beans become dry, add water to keep them moist.

Yield: 4 servings

Hearty Bean Casserole

	Standard	Metric
Beans, any variety	1 cup	250 mL
Dry onion, peeled	1	1
White sauce	1-1/2 cup	375 mL
Cooked meat or seafood	1 cup	250 mL
Shredded cheddar cheese	1/2 cup	125 mL
Thyme	1/2 tsp.	2 mL

1. Wash, cover with water, soak the beans overnight or bring to a boil, boil 2 minutes, and let stand covered for 1 hour. Do not drain.
2. Simmer the beans in soaking liquid with onion for 2 hours or until tender.
3. Drain the beans and combine with 1 cup of cooked meat or seafood. Mix in the white sauce, shredded cheese, and thyme.
4. Pour the mixture into a buttered casserole and bake at 350° F (175° C) for 30 minutes, or in the microwave oven for approximately 12 minutes, rotating 1/2 turn after 6 minutes cooking time. Let stand 5 minutes before serving.

Yield: 4 servings

Variations

1. Two cups of canned, drained beans may be used in place of the dried beans and the recipe is followed beginning with step 3.
2. Add 1/2 cup dehydrated onion when combining the ingredients in place of the raw onion listed in the dry ingredients.
3. One-third cup chopped green pepper sautéed in butter may be added to the ingredients.

Lentil Casserole

	Standard	Metric
Lentils	2 cups	500 mL
Salt	1 tsp.	5 mL
Onion, stuck with two cloves	1	1
Carrot, medium-sized, chopped	1	1
Frankfurters, sliced, or one Polish sausage, sliced	4	4

1. Sort and wash the lentils; drain.
2. Place in a saucepan with salt, onion, and carrot; add water to cover. Bring to a boil; cover and simmer for 30 minutes. Remove the onion.
3. Drain the lentils, saving the liquid.
4. Combine the lentils with the frankfurters or sausage in a casserole dish. Pour the lentil liquid over the mixture in the casserole dish.
5. Bake at 350° F (175° C) for 35 minutes, or in the microwave oven for 18 minutes. Stir and rotate 1/2 turn after 9 minutes cooking time. Let stand 5 minutes before serving.

Yield: 4 servings

Split Pea Soup

	Standard	Metric
Green or yellow split peas	1 cup	250 mL
Water	5 cups	1250 mL
Consommé	1/2 cup	125 mL
Smoked ham hock	1	1
Onion, chopped	1	1
Parsley	1 tsp.	5 mL

	Standard	Metric
Thyme	1/4 tsp.	1 mL
Diced carrot	1/4 cup	60 mL

1. Combine the peas, water, consommé, ham hock, onion, parsley, thyme, and carrot in a large saucepan. Bring to a boil; cover and simmer for 2 hours.
2. Remove the ham hock from the mixture; skin; dice the meat and return to the mixture.

Yield: 4 servings

---------- Macaroni Loaf ----------

	Standard	Metric
Butter or margarine	1/4 cup	60 mL
Flour	1/4 cup	60 mL
Milk	1-1/2 cups	375 mL
Seasoning salt	1 tsp.	5 mL
Pepper	1/4 tsp.	1 mL
Elbow macaroni	2 cups (8 oz.)	500 mL (227 gm)
Grated sharp cheddar cheese	2 cups	500 mL
Cracker crumbs	1/2 cup	125 mL
Chopped parsley	1 Tbsp.	15 mL

1. Preheat the oven to 350° F (175° C).
2. Cook the macaroni in boiling salted water according to the package directions. Drain.
3. Melt the butter or margarine in a heavy saucepan. Stir in the flour, seasoning salt, and pepper. Cook 1 minute. Gradually add the milk, stirring constantly, and cook over low heat until thickened. Add the grated cheese and allow to melt.
4. Combine the cheese sauce, macaroni, cracker crumbs, and parsley. Pour into a buttered 8 × 5-inch loaf pan and bake for 30 minutes. Allow to stand for 10 minutes and turn out onto a serving platter.

Yield: 4 to 6 servings

---------- Stuffed Manicotti ----------

	Standard	Metric
Ricotta or cottage cheese	1 cup	250 mL
Chopped cooked spinach, drained	1 cup	250 mL
Ground beef	1/2 pound	227 mL
Garlic salt	1/2 tsp.	2 mL
Oregano	1/2 tsp.	2 mL
Manicotti shells	8	8
Canned Italian-style spaghetti sauce	4 cups	1000 mL

1. Preheat the oven to 375° F (190° C).
2. Brown the ground beef in a heavy fry pan until the pink is gone.
3. Cook the manicotti shells in boiling salted water for 6 minutes or until just barely tender. Drain.
4. Combine ricotta, spinach, ground beef, garlic salt, and oregano in a dish.
5. Gently stuff the meat-cheese mixture into the shells.
6. Pour 3 cups of the sauce into the bottom of a 12 × 9 × 2-inch oblong baking dish. Place the manicotti shells on top of the sauce. Cover with the remaining sauce.
7. Bake for 30 minutes or in the microwave oven for 14 minutes, rotating dish 1/2 turn after 7 minutes cooking time. Let stand 5 minutes before serving.
8. Manicotti shells may be stuffed uncooked. Cover the baking dish with foil and bake 40 minutes at 400° F (205° C). Bake 10 minutes longer uncovered.

Yield: 4 to 6 servings

---------- Baked Noodles ----------

	Standard	Metric
Egg noodles	4 cups (8 oz.)	1000 mL (227 gm)
Cottage cheese, large curd	1-1/2 cup	375 mL
Dehydrated onion	1 Tbsp.	15 mL
Sour cream	1 cup	250 mL
Green onions, chopped	3	3
Chopped green pepper	1/2 cup	125 mL
Frankfurters, chopped	2	2

Grated Parmesan cheese	1/2 cup	125 mL

1. Preheat the oven to 350° F (175° C).
2. Cook the noodles in boiling salted water according to the package directions. Drain.
3. Combine the noodles, cottage cheese, onion, sour cream, green onions, green pepper, and frankfurters.
4. Turn into a buttered 12 × 9 × 2-inch casserole dish. Sprinkle with the Parmesan cheese.
5. Bake for 25 minutes, or bake in microwave oven for 12 minutes, rotating 1/2 turn after 6 minutes cooking time. Let stand 5 minutes before serving.

Yield: 6 to 8 servings

Spaghetti with Clam Sauce

	Standard	Metric
Chopped onion	1/4 cup	60 mL
Garlic cloves, minced	2	2
Olive oil	1/3 cup	75 mL
Minced clams, drained, saving liquor	2 cans (7 oz.)	2 (198 gm)
Chopped parsley	3 Tbsp.	45 mL
Spaghetti	2 cups (8 oz.)	2 (227 gm)
Grated Parmesan cheese	1/2 cup	125 mL

1. Sauté the onion and garlic in the olive oil over low heat in a fry pan just until tender; do not let brown.
2. Cook the spaghetti according to the package directions. Drain.
3. Add the liquor from the clams and the parsley to the onion mixture and heat to the boiling point. Cook over low heat while the spaghetti is cooking. Add the clams and cook just until heated through.
4. Serve the clam sauce over the spaghetti and sprinkle with Parmesan cheese.

Yield: 4 servings

Quick Spanish Rice

	Standard	Metric
Fat	2 Tbsp.	30 mL
Chopped onion	1/4 cup	60 mL
Chopped celery	1/4 cup	60 mL
Chopped green pepper	1/4 cup	60 mL
Cooked tomatoes	1 cup	250 mL
Water	1 cup	250 mL
Salt	1 tsp.	5 mL
Worcestershire sauce	1/2 tsp.	2 mL
Paprika	1/4 tsp.	1 mL
Precooked rice, uncooked	1 cup	250 mL

1. Melt the fat in a heavy skillet and cook the onion, celery, and green pepper in fat over low heat until transparent.
2. Add the tomatoes, water, salt, Worcestershire sauce, and paprika to the vegetables in a skillet and heat to the boiling point. Stir in rice; cover; reduce heat to low and cook for 15 minutes.

Yield: 4 servings

Variations
1. Consommé may be used in place of one half the water.
2. One cup of chopped cooked meat or seafood may be added to the mixture.

Brown Rice Supper

	Standard	Metric
Eggs, separated	3	3
Salt	1/2 tsp.	2 mL
Milk	1/2 cup	125 mL
Cooked brown rice	1 cup	250 mL
Cooked meat or seafood	1 cup	250 mL
Grated cheddar cheese	1 cup	250 mL
Butter, melted	2 Tbsp.	30 mL

1. Preheat the oven to 300° F (150° C).
2. Beat the egg whites with salt until stiff.
3. Beat the egg yolks slightly.
4. Combine the egg yolks, milk, rice, meat, cheese, and butter. Fold in the egg whites.

5. Pour into a 1-quart baking dish. Bake for 40 minutes or until the mixture is a light brown on top.

Yield: 4 servings

—————————— Rice Pancakes ——————————

	Standard	Metric
Egg, slightly beaten	1	1
Milk	1-1/2 cup	375 mL
Pancake mix	1 cup	250 mL
Cooked rice	1 cup	250 mL

1. Combine the egg, milk, and pancake mix, stirring to thoroughly mix the ingredients. Stir in the rice.
2. Fry on a hot well-greased griddle until brown on both sides.

Yield: 12 average sized pancakes

—————————— Rice Pudding ——————————

	Standard	Metric
Regular milled rice	1 cup	250 mL
Salt	1/4 tsp.	1 mL
Sugar	1 cup	250 mL
Milk	3 cups	750 mL
Chopped nuts	2 Tbsp.	30 mL
Grated orange rind	1 Tbsp.	15 mL
Raisins	1/4 cup	60 mL
Cinnamon		

1. Combine the rice, salt, sugar, and milk in top of a double boiler. Heat to boiling, stirring constantly. Cook over boiling water 30 to 35 minutes, stirring several times, until the milk is absorbed and the rice is tender.
2. Add the nuts, rind, and raisins to the rice mixture.
3. Spoon into serving dishes and sprinkle with cinnamon.

Yield: 4 servings

—————————— Main-Dish Rice Salad ——————————

	Standard	Metric
Salad oil	3 Tbsp.	45 mL
Vinegar	1 Tbsp.	15 mL
Dry mustard	1 tsp.	5 mL
Sugar	1/2 tsp.	2 mL
Cooked warm rice	2 cups	500 mL
Diced cooked ham	1 cup	250 mL
Cooked green peas	1/2 cup	125 mL
Chopped green onion	2 Tbsp.	30 mL
Sliced cooked carrot	1/2 cup	125 mL
Chopped green pepper	1/2 cup	125 mL
Chopped parsley	1 Tbsp.	15 mL

1. Combine the salad oil, vinegar, dry mustard, and sugar in a jar with a lid. Shake vigorously to blend the ingredients.
2. Stir the salad dressing lightly into the cooked warm rice. Place in the refrigerator to cool.
3. When the rice mixture is chilled thoroughly, add the diced ham, green peas, carrot, and green pepper to the rice.
4. Serve on salad greens and sprinkle with chopped parsley.

Yield: 4 servings

—————————— Baked Rice and Cheese ——————————

	Standard	Metric
Diced American cheese	2 cups	500 mL
Cooked rice	3 cups	750 mL
Eggs, slightly beaten	2	2
Milk	1-1/4 cup	310 mL
Salt	1 tsp.	5 mL
Cayenne pepper	1/8 tsp.	0.5 mL
Dehydrated minced onion	1 tsp.	5 mL
Buttered bread crumbs	1/4 cup	60 mL

1. Preheat the oven to 350° F (175° C).
2. Arrange alternate layers of cheese and rice in a greased baking dish.
3. Combine the beaten eggs, milk, salt, pepper, and

onion. Pour over the cheese and rice mixture. Sprinkle the top with bread crumbs.

4. Bake for approximately 45 minutes or until the mixture is set and the top is lightly browned.

Yield: 4 to 6 servings

——————— Peanut Butter Pudding ———————

	Standard	Metric
Peanut butter	1/2 cup	125 mL
Milk	2 cups	500 mL
Instant vanilla pudding	1 pkg. (3-1/4 oz.)	92 grams

1. Beat the peanut butter until it is very creamy. Gradually add the milk, a little at a time, and beat until thoroughly blended.
2. Add the pudding mix and beat until creamy.
3. Pour into serving dishes and chill.

Yield: 4 to 6 servings

——————— Peanut Butter Soup ———————

	Standard	Metric
Butter or margarine	2 Tbsp.	30 mL
Flour	2 Tbsp.	30 mL
Chopped onion	2 Tbsp.	30 mL
Chopped celery	2 Tbsp.	30 mL
Milk	2 cups	500 mL
Peanut butter (may need adjustment to suit taste)	3/4 cup	175 mL

1. Melt the butter in a heavy saucepan. Sauté the celery and onion until translucent. Stir in the flour.
2. Gradually stir in the milk and cook until thickened, stirring constantly.
3. Stir in the peanut butter and adjust the proportion to suit taste.

Yield: 4 to 6 servings

——————— Almond Nut Butter ———————

	Standard	Metric
Chopped almonds	1-1/2 cup	375 mL
Salad oil	2 Tbsp. plus 2 tsp.	40 mL

1. Whirl small amounts of the almonds with all the salad oil in a food blender or pass the nuts through the fine blade of a food grinder as often as is necessary to make a smooth paste and then blend with the salad oil.
2. Store in a covered jar in the refrigerator or freeze.
3. This may be used as a topping for vegetables or as a sandwich spread. It may also be extended by whipping in 1/2 cup butter.

Yield: approximately 1 cup

——————— Peanut-Rice Fiesta ———————

	Standard	Metric
Cooked rice	3-1/2 cups	875 mL
Peanut butter	1 cup	250 mL
Milk	2 cups	500 mL
Green chilis, drained, seeded, and chopped	1 (4 oz.) can	1 (113 gm)
Chili powder	2 tsp.	10 mL
Salt	1/2 tsp.	2 mL
Ginger	1/4 tsp.	1 mL
Garlic cloves, crushed	2	2
Shredded cheddar cheese	1 cup	250 mL
Chopped parsley	3 Tbsp.	45 mL

1. Preheat the oven to 375° F (190° C).
2. Gradually blend the milk in small amounts into the peanut butter until smooth.
3. Stir in the chilis, chili powder, salt, ginger, and garlic.
4. Toss together the cheese and parsley.
5. Put half the rice in a buttered 2-quart casserole. Pour over half the peanut butter mixture.
6. Sprinkle over half the cheese and parsley.
7. Repeat the layers, omitting the cheese and parsley.

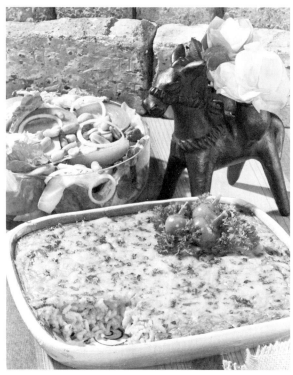

Figure 10-11.
Peanut butter, cheese, and rice combine to make a complete protein dish. (Oklahoma Peanut Commission)

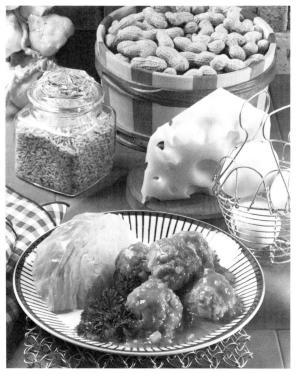

Figure 10-12.
Meatless meatballs are served with a tangy sauce. (Oklahoma Peanut Commission)

8. Bake for 35 to 40 minutes. Sprinkle over the remaining cheese and parsley. Let stand until the cheese melts. Garnish with parsley and peppers.

Yield: 6 to 8 servings

Recipe: Courtesy of Oklahoma Peanut Commission and shown in Figure 10-11.

_____ Meatless Meatballs _____

	Standard	Metric
Cooked brown rice	1 cup	250 mL
Ground cocktail peanuts	1 cup	250 mL
Shredded Swiss cheese	1 cup	250 mL
Minced onion	1/4 cup	60 mL

	Standard	Metric
Egg, beaten	1	1
Crushed Rosemary leaves	1/4 tsp.	1 mL
Thyme	1/4 tsp.	1 mL
Cayenne pepper	1/8 tsp.	0.5 mL
Sauce:		
Oil	1 Tbsp.	15 mL
Minced onion	1/4 cup	60 mL
Garlic clove, crushed	1	1
Stewed tomatoes	1 (1 lb.) can	1 (454 gm)
Chopped dill pickle	1/4 cup	60 mL
Salt	1/2 tsp.	2 mL
Cornstarch	1 tsp.	5 mL
Water	2 tsp.	10 mL

1. Preheat the oven to 350° F (175° C).

2. In a bowl combine the rice, peanuts, cheese, onion, egg, rosemary, thyme, and cayenne. Moisten hands and shape the mixture into 20 balls, using a rounded Tbsp. for each ball.

3. Place the meatless balls in a lightly-greased 2-quart rectangular baking dish; cover while preparing the sauce.

4. In a saucepan sauté the onion and garlic in oil until tender. Stir in the tomatoes, dill pickle, and salt.

5. Blend together the cornstarch and water until smooth and stir into the tomato mixture.

6. Heat the sauce to boiling while stirring constantly; boil 2 minutes. Pour the sauce over the meatless balls; cover and bake for 20 to 25 minutes.

Yield: 20 meatless meatballs

Recipe: Courtesy of Oklahoma Peanut Commission and shown in Figure 10-12.

LEARNING ACTIVITIES

1. At the grocery store see how many food products can be found that contain textured vegetable protein. Report your findings to the class.

2. Make a list of the foods you normally eat that could be classified as meat alternates.

3. Compare the cost of making macaroni and cheese from basic ingredients and preparing it from a canned and dehydrated form.

4. Investigate the varieties of legumes that can be bought at the market. As a class, prepare 1/2 cup uncooked portions of each of the legume varieties and sample each for flavor and texture.

5. Develop a recipe or find a recipe, that uses one of the legumes prepared in number 4. Prepare the recipe and figure its cost per serving.

6. Compare the cost of two varieties of cooked canned legumes with the uncooked varieties of the legumes. Base the comparison on 1/2 cup servings.

7. Plan a breakfast menu using a meat alternate as the entrée. Evaluate the nutrient composition of the meat alternate food dish.

8. Plan a week's dinner menus using meat alternates as the main entrée for 4 of the 7 days.

9. Investigate the different kinds of pastas that are available at the local market. Prepare a dish from a pasta that you have not eaten before.

10. Cook a long-grain rice in boiling, salted water and in water that is not heated before the rice is added. Compare the difference in the textures of the finished products.

11. Cook an uncooked rice and a precooked rice. Note the differences in time preparation and in the texture of the cooked rices. Decide which rice would be the better buy for a given situation.

12. Cook 1/2 cup of rice in three different liquids. Taste the product and plan a menu around each of the different rices.

13. Cook a meat analog and serve it to a group of your friends, family, or classmates. Note their approval or disapproval of the product.

14. Prepare a report on why it is difficult for some people to accept meat alternates in place of meat.

15. If soy flour can be purchased in your area, prepare a white sauce using soy flour rather than regular flour and note the difference in taste.

16. Prepare chili using a soybean meat extender as the substitute for meat. Note the difference in flavor and compare the cost.

17. Compare the cost difference for a nut that is available in whole, half, and broken form.

18. Compare the cost difference between the same nut that is available in both blanched and unblanched form.

REVIEW QUESTIONS

1. Define a meat alternate.
2. What are some foods that make suitable meat alternates?
3. What are two reasons for using meat alternates in meal planning?
4. What meat alternate has a high fat content?
5. Why are meat alternates incomplete proteins?
6. How is the protein value of a meat alternate raised?
7. Which food is the most complete protein of the plant group?
8. Which food is the most complete protein of the cereal group?
9. Which nut is the most complete protein of the nut group?
10. What is the characteristic flavor of meat alternates?
11. Why are pasta and rice products usually good for people who are on special diets?
12. How can a busy time schedule affect the form in which legumes are purchased?
13. What foods are members of the legume family?
14. What is pasta made from?
15. What is the difference between noodles and macaroni besides their shape?
16. What is the textural difference between cooked long-grain rice and cooked short- and medium-grain rice?
17. What is the difference between brown, parboiled, regular-milled, and precooked rice?
18. What is wild rice?
19. What is a meat analog?
20. What are three factors to look for when purchasing legumes?
21. Which is the most economical form in which to purchase nuts?
22. How should legumes, pasta, and rice be stored?
23. Why are some legumes soaked?
24. Which legumes should not be soaked before they are cooked?
25. What is the quick way to soak legumes?
26. How are dried beans cooked in a saucepan?
27. How can pasta and rice be prevented from sticking to the bottom of the pan?
28. Why should rice be started to cook in boiling water?
29. What are four methods that may be used in cooking rice?
30. How can the flavor of rice be varied by adding liquid, herbs, spices, and other ingredients? Name five flavor ingredients that can be used.
31. What is the procedure for blanching nuts?

11

Fruits

Fruit, one of the most colorful and flavorful foods, comes from the flowering portion of the plant. A ripened fruit has a delectable aroma.

There are many kinds of fruit, and many fruits have several varieties. Fruit is eaten both in its raw form and as a cooked food. The color, flavor, and texture of fruits make them a major ingredient in many salads, pies, puddings, and other desserts.

In the United States fruits are widely available in both the fresh and processed forms. Some fruits grow only in certain geographic locations and during certain seasons of the year, but modern transportation and storage now make many fruits available the year around.

Nutritional Factors to Consider

Fruits are as variable in some of their nutrient composition as they are in their flavor and color. Therefore, if fruit is to provide a specific nutrient at a meal, the nutritive composition of the fruit must be carefully studied.

Carbohydrate

Most of the carbohydrate found in fruits is in the form of sugar or cellulose. Some fruits contain carbohydrate in the form of starch that is changed to sugar as the fruit ripens. For example, an apple that is eaten before it has ripened has a starchlike flavor, whereas a ripe apple tastes sugar-sweet.

The cell walls of fruit are composed of cellulose, which is an indigestible form of carbohydrate for the human body, but cellulose is important in the diet because it serves to keep food moving through the digestive system. Pectic substances are another form of carbohydrate found in fruits. Under proper conditions they contribute to the gelling quality of fruits.

151

Fat and Protein

With the exception of avocados, olives, and coconuts, most fruits contain only a trace of fat.

A very small amount of protein is found in fruits, mainly in the form of enzymes that cause certain reactions to take place. Enzymes are responsible for the ripening action in fruits.

Vitamins and Minerals

Citrus fruits, such as oranges and grapefruits, are excellent sources of ascorbic acid. Strawberries and cantaloupes are also rich in ascorbic acid. Since citrus fruits are commonly available the year around, their ascorbic acid contribution to the human diet is of special importance.

Yellow fruits, such as peaches and apricots, are good sources of vitamin A, and dried fruits, such as peaches, apricots, raisins, and prunes, are good sources of iron. Fair sources of calcium are found in citrus and dried fruits. Fruits contain varying amounts of other vitamins and minerals.

Calories

Fruits are basically water and carbohydrate with the average water content of fruit being 85 per cent, so that fruits are relatively low in calorie content. However, the calorie content of the diet can rapidly be increased by consuming an overabundance of dried fruits, which, when processed, have most of the water removed from them.

Menu-Planning Points

Inherent Factors

Balance. Fruits can provide balance to a menu in many ways. They can give the right color,
the needed shape, the sweet or tart flavor, or the texture that may be needed to balance a meal. Figure 11-1 shows fruit as part of a breakfast meal.

Color. Pleasant color combinations can be achieved by including fruits in menu planning. Color in a breakfast menu is most often achieved by the addition of fruit. For example, a wedge of cantaloupe, a dish of strawberries, or a glass of orange juice will brighten up a breakfast planned around cereal and milk. The sack lunch looks more appetizing if it includes a brightly colored fruit, such as an apple or an orange. Fruits, such as spiced apricots, cranberry relish, or green grapes, are colorful and nutritious garnishes to accompany dinner meals.

Shape. Fruits grow in a variety of shapes. Small fruits, such as berries and grapes, add interest to a meal, and larger fruits, such as melons, can be cut into wedges or scooped into balls. Most fruits can be sliced or cut into chunks to add more design to a meal. A variety of fruit shapes is shown in Figure 11-2.

Flavor. In planning menus with fruit it is important to consider the flavor of the fruit. Most fruits have a slightly sweet flavor with a tart overtone. Some fruits, such as pears and bananas, have a delicate flavor, and other fruits, such as grapefruits and lemons have a more robust flavor. A meal featuring a meat with a tangy barbecue sauce would be complemented with a lightly flavored fruit, such as peaches.

Texture. Most ripened fruits have a soft and pulplike texture, but fruits, such as ripe apples, are firm and crisp; overripe apples will be mushy. The texture of fruits can be made more tender by cooking. Dried fruits, such as apricots, are chewy, whereas dried apples slices are crisp.

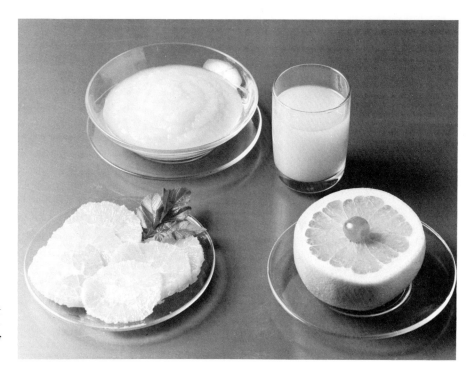

Figure 11-1.
Orange slices, grapefruit half, fruit sauces, or juice are nutritious parts of breakfast.

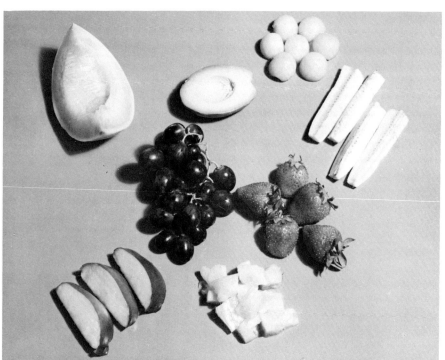

Figure 11-2.
Preparing fruits in a variety of shapes adds variety and interest to a meal.

External Factors

Age and Culture. There is no age limit to the enjoyment of fruit, and its nutrient composition and ease in preparation make fruit an excellent food to serve as a snack.

Certain fruits may be related to a given culture because they grow best in given geographical areas. For example, mangoes, papayas, and guava, are accepted fruits of peoples who live in the tropical areas where these fruits grow.

Economics. Modern methods of cultivating, processing, storing, and transporting fruit have contributed greatly to making fruit an economical purchase. When certain fruits are not available in fresh form, they are usually available in a processed form. The biggest changes in the availability and price of fruit are affected by unseasonal climatic changes. For example, an unexpected freeze in the citrus-growing areas of the country can lead to a rapid change in the price and availability of oranges and grapefruit.

Space, Equipment, and Time Scheduling. Since most fresh fruits need to be refrigerated, it is important to purchase only an amount that can be stored and consumed within a short time. Canned and dried fruits are best stored on the kitchen shelf.

Fruits are a great time-saver in scheduling meal preparation because they can often be eaten in raw form. Canned, dried, and frozen forms of fruit can be used with a minimum of preparation.

Grading

Quality grading standards for fresh and processed fruits have been established by the USDA. The inspection service offered is voluntary and is paid for by the user.

Fresh fruits are graded according to the following standards. US Extra Fancy applies only to apples and means that the fruit is of extremely high quality and shows no defects; US Fancy implies that the fruit is of good color and shape; and US No. 1 means that the fruit is of good shape and appearance but may have some defects. The grades are widely used at the wholesale level but are not commonly seen on fruits that the consumer purchases.

Processed fruits have three quality grading standards. US Grade A or US Grade Fancy is given to fruits of extremely high quality; US Grade B or Choice is for fruit that is not quite as perfect but still highly acceptable; and US Grade C or Choice applies to fruit that does not have the color, flavor, and appearance of the other grades. However, Grade C is still an acceptable product for eating. These grades may be seen on the label of some processed fruits.

Fruit Forms

In the past, fresh fruit was available only during its growing season and much effort was put toward the home preservation of fruits for the winter months. Although fruits are still preserved in many homes, a wide variety of fruit is available on the market in fresh, frozen, canned, and dried forms; of these, fresh and canned forms are the most numerous.

Fresh

The fruits that are most commonly available throughout the year include apples, bananas, cantaloupes, grapefruits, lemons, limes, oranges, and pineapples. Seasonal fresh fruits include apricots, avocados, berries, cherries, grapes, guava, melons, mandarin oranges, nectarines, papayas, peaches, pears, plums, and rhubarb.

Frozen

Several kinds of fruit are available in frozen form, whole, in slices, or as a varied mixture.

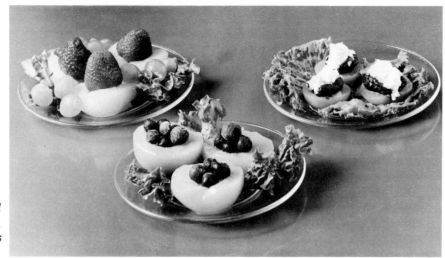

Figure 11-3.
Pear, peach, and apricot halves can hold other small fruits such as strawberries, grapes, blueberries or dates stuffed with cream cheese.

These fruits may be frozen without sugar, with sugar, or in a sugar syrup. Frozen fruits have a high retention of fresh flavor but may exhibit textural changes when they are thawed. The most common frozen fruits available on the market include blueberries, strawberries, and raspberries. However, many other fruits can be satisfactorily frozen for home use.

Frozen fruit juice concentrates have become increasingly popular. Orange, grapefruit, cranberry, grape, and lemonade juices are available in concentrated frozen form.

Canned

The many kinds and varieties of canned fruits are available for purchase. These are cooked fruits, packed either in water, natural juices, or in a light, medium, or heavy syrup. Variety is offered by the form in which these fruits are canned, such as whole, halves, slices or sections, chunks, and crushed fruit. Canned sauce, combinations of mixed fruits, and fruit juice are other varieties. Many canned fruits are available in various can sizes that enable the consumer to select the fruit for a specific need. As shown in Figure 11-3, canned fruit halves are attractive holders for other fruits.

Dried

Fruits are dried either by the sun or by mechanical methods. A fruit that is dried by mechanical methods is often called a dehydrated fruit. Dried or dehydrated fruits have had more than 50 per cent of the water removed from them. One mechanical method called "vacuum drying" removes 96 per cent or more of the water. Most dried fruit contains an average of 25 per cent water. All dried fruits are a concentrated source of sugar.

Apricots, peaches, pears, raisins, figs, prunes, currants, and dates are fruits that are marketed in dried form. When dried fruits are eaten they have a chewy consistency. Some dried fruits are partially rehydrated before they are packaged to give the fruit a higher moisture content and to make it more tender, these are sometimes called "tenderized."

Purchasing

Fresh

The best time to buy fresh fruits is at the peak of their season. Although some fruits are available the year around, the price is higher during the off-season months. Crop losses resulting from climatic conditions also will cause the price of the fruit to be higher. It is important to purchase fruit of high quality; just because the price is low does not mean that the fruit is a good buy. Since fruit may decay faster than it can be used, a familiarity with the quality characteristics of a fruit is an asset and can prove to be a money-saver. It is also important to purchase only the amount of fruit that can be used within a short period of time. Most fruits do not store well over an extended period of time.

Before fruit is purchased, a decision should be made on how quickly it is to be eaten. For example, bananas that will not be eaten for 2 or 3 days are best purchased when they are more green than yellow. Avocados should feel firm to the touch if they are not to be eaten for 3 or 4 days. Fruits, such as berries and cherries, are picked ripe and need to be eaten quickly. A very ripe fruit is sometimes desirable for cooking and often can be purchased at a lower price. The best banana bread is made when the bananas are very ripe, and a fruit puree calls for a riper fruit than that which would be eaten fresh.

The size of fruit that is purchased is also an important factor. For example, if apples are being purchased for a young child's brown-bag lunch, the better buy to eliminate waste is the smaller size. No fruit is a good buy if it spoils and is thrown out before it can be used.

When selecting fruits, it is important to handle them gently. When a fruit is squeezed with too much force, it is bruised and this leads to more rapid decay of the fruit.

Some fruits have different varieties that are suitable for different purposes. Certain varieties of apples are better for cooking and others are best for eating.

If the use of the fruit is not dependent on its being fresh, the price of a fresh fruit should be compared with the same fruit in another form.

For example, frozen fruit juice is usually a better buy than freshly squeezed juice.

Some fruits are sold by weight and other fruits are sold as a unit package. For example, apples may be sold at $.49 a pound or they may be sold as a unit package of six apples for $.89. The following section discusses the quality characteristics to look for when selecting fresh fruits.

Apples. There are many varieties of apples for eating, but some varieties are common only to certain geographical areas and others are available nationwide. Apples that are suitable for fresh eating include Delicious, Golden Delicious, Jonathan, McIntosh, and Winesap. Apples that are more tart and excellent for pies and sauces include Gravenstein, Grimes Golden, Jonathan, and Newton. Good apples for baking include Rome Beauty and Winesap.

Apples should be selected that are firm to the touch and do not show soft spots or a shriveled skin. The color should be representative of the variety.

Apricots. Apricots should have a golden orange color and a skin that does not look withered. A greenish tinge is a sign that an apricot is not fully ripe.

Avocados. Avocados should be selected on the basis of when they are to be used. Avocados with a dark green or black color and a firm feeling will ripen at room temperature in a few days. Those with a soft feeling are ready for immediate use.

Bananas. Bananas are usually green when they are harvested. Bananas ripen readily at room temperature and are ready to eat when they are a bright yellow with brown flecks in the skin. Unless bananas are to be eaten immediately, it is best to select those that are just changing to a yellow color. Bananas ripen at room temperature.

Berries. The selection of berries with a uniform color characteristic of the variety, and a lack of soft spots or mold, is most important. Strawberries should be selected, if possible, with the stem attached, whereas other berries, such as blackberries, blueberries, and raspberries, should not have the stem attached.

Cherries. Cherries should be selected, if possible, with the stem on, although many times the stems are lost in shipping. Cherries should be free of mold growth and cracks in the skin. Light red cherries have a very tart flavor and are called "pie" or sour cherries. Queen Anne cherries are a light-cream colored, sweet variety. Dark red cherries are sweet and good for fresh eating. Dark varieties include Bing, Black Tartarian, and Chapman.

Citrus Fruits. The two most common varieties of oranges are the thin-skinned Valencia and the thick-skinned navel. Navel oranges are easiest to peel and eat fresh, whereas Valencias yield the most juice and are best for slicing. Oranges should feel heavy for their size, and have good color and a skin that is relatively smooth without soft spots or signs of decay. Oranges are also sold as California and Florida varieties. Coloring is added to the skin of some oranges.

Grapefruits have either a pink or white flesh and a thick or thin skin. Thin-skinned varieties yield the most juice and have a firmer texture. Like oranges, grapefruits should feel heavy in relation to their size.

Lemons are chosen on the basis of a bright yellow color, a smooth skin that is not shriveled or spotted with decay, and a weight in relation to size. Limes should have a shiny skin appearance.

Cranberries. Cranberries should be firm with a rich-red to a deep-red color.

Grapes. Grapes should not show signs of leak-

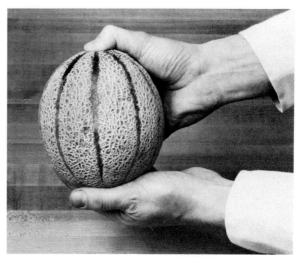

Figure 11-4.
One sign of a ripe cantaloupe is when the blossom end yields to thumb pressure.

age or decay and should be firmly attached to the stem. Thompson grapes are a yellowish green and contain no seeds. Tokay and Emperor grapes are a deep red to purple and contain seeds as do the black grapes Ribier and Concord.

Melons. Cantaloupe should have no stem and the skin color segmented between the rough surfaces should be a yellowish color. The blossom end of the cantaloupe should yield to light pressure when touched with the thumb, as shown in Figure 11-4. A ripe cantaloupe has a cantaloupe smell when it is held to the nose.

Casaba and crenshaw melons should have a golden yellow rind color and should yield to light pressure at the blossom end.

Honeydew and honeyball melons should have a yellowish, creamy skin color and be slightly soft at the blossom end.

Watermelons, if cut, should have a good red color. Whole watermelons should have a creamy underside and ends that are rounded and filled out.

Peaches. Peaches that are ready to eat have a yellow skin with tinges of red. The freestone peach has a seed that is easily freed from the flesh, and the clingstone peach has a seed which adheres to the flesh. Because clingstone peaches have a firmer flesh, they are generally preferred for canning.

Pears. Pears should be selected with a slightly green skin if they are not to be eaten immediately. They will ripen at room temperature. Pears that do not feel firm, particularly at the stem end, and which have a shriveled skin, are of poor quality.

Pineapple. A ripened pineapple has a yellowed skin and fresh-appearing green leaves. As many pineapples are picked green for shipment, the leaves may have shriveled and turned brown. Good pineapples should have a rich, sweet odor and have no decayed or bruised spots.

Plums. Depending on the variety, plums may be red, green, or yellow. Freestone plums are called prunes. Plums that are shriveled and hard, or very soft plums that show signs of decay, should not be selected.

Rhubarb. Rhubarb, unlike other fruits, is the stem part of the plant. Stalks that are narrow in diameter should be selected since larger stalks are likely to be more fibrous.

Canned

Canned fruits are sold under national brands, and most large grocery chains have one or two qualities of fruits under their own brand label. Many times, the only difference between labels is the price of the fruit. The brand and kind of fruit that should be bought is determined by its intended use, the amount of money available, and the time available for preparation.

The most expensive brands are most often the fruits of highest quality, and they are usually packed in a heavy syrup. Less expensive fruits are usually pieces of fruit that are often of irregular sizes and packed in a medium or light sugar syrup. Although the flavor and appearance of lower-priced fruits may not be of as high a quality as the more expensive varieties, they are equally as nutritious and good for eating.

The label of canned fruit will provide the information as to the form of the fruit, the type of syrup in which it is packed, and the amount of fruit in the container. The number of ounces of fruit that a can contains will serve as a guide to the number of servings; some labels will give suggested servings. An easy guide to adjust ounces to number of servings is this: 8 ounces of fruit equal 1 cup, 16 ounces equal 2 cups, and 32 ounces equal 4 cups. One-half cup is an average serving of fruit.

Many varieties of canned fruit juices and drinks are available in the market. When purchasing fruit drinks the common labeling terminology used must be understood.

1. Juice is the pure, strained liquid of a fruit or vegetable.
2. Fruit juice drink is composed of 50 per cent fruit juice and 50 per cent water. Additional sweeteners are usually added.
3. Fruit drink is the same as a fruit juice drink except that it contains less fruit juice.
4. Nectar is a fruit juice containing some of the pulp of the fruit.
5. Fruit concentrate is a fruit juice that is processed to four times its original strength.

Cans with bulging ends or signs of leakage should never be purchased. Jars of fruit with twist-off lids should always be checked to make sure that the lid has not been loosened.

Frozen

Frozen fruits are sold in plastic-coated cartons, plastic bags, and plastic containers. When purchasing frozen fruits, signs of defrosting should be checked for. If the carton is not hard, or if signs of leakage appear on the container, the fruit may be partially thawed or may have defrosted and been frozen again.

The label on the frozen-fruit container will most often tell the style of the contents and provide directions for thawing and serving the fruit.

Dried

Dried fruits should be purchased according to the way they will be used. Some dried fruits require cooking before they are used in other kinds of food preparation, and some dried fruits come in varieties for special uses.

Dark raisins are used for snacking and cooking. Small boxes of dark raisins are good additions for snacks and lunches but are more expensive. Light-colored raisins are used the same way as dark raisins but are preferred for their color in fruitcakes and some other baked products. Dates and prunes may be pitted or unpitted, and come in low- and high-moisture varieties. The drier, low-moisture varieties of dates and prunes usually require some cooking before they are eaten. Prunes are also sold according to size—extra-large, large, medium, and small.

Storage

Fresh

Most fruits are refrigerated to control the ripening process. Another reason for refrigerating fruit is that chilled fresh fruit is more enjoyable to eat. Fruits that can be further ripened by being left at room temperature include bananas, avocados, and pears. As fruits ripen, the skin color changes, the flesh becomes softer, the flavor becomes sweeter, and the true aroma of the fruit develops.

Fruits that should be washed, dried, and stored in the refrigerator include apples, grapefruits, oranges, pears, plums, and rhubarb. Fruits that should be refrigerated but not washed until they are ready to use include apricots, berries, cherries, grapes, and peaches. The stem, if it is present, should be left on strawberries, cherries, and grapes to lessen the danger of spoilage. Berries and cherries will keep best if they are spread out on a tray in the refrigerator.

Fruit may be stored in plastic bags or in the hydrator drawers of the refrigerator.

Canned and Frozen

Canned fruits are stored in a cool, dry, well-ventilated place. Frozen fruits are stored at 0° F (–18° C) or below.

Dried

Dried fruits are stored in a cool, dry place or they may be refrigerated or frozen. It is important that the dried fruit container be properly closed at all times to preserve the fruit's quality.

Basic Methods of Preparation

Fruits are prepared and served in either the raw or cooked form. Almost everybody enjoys eating raw fresh fruit. Fruits may be cooked and served alone or they may be cooked as a part of another dish to add variety to meals.

Raw

Fruits should always be thoroughly washed with water before they are prepared. Washing fruit helps to eliminate microorganisms or any

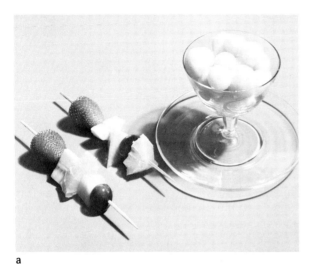

a

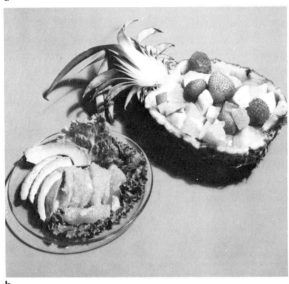

b

Figure 11-5.

(a) Small pieces of fruit put on skewers make attractive appetizers or small pieces of fruit such as melon balls may serve as an appetizer or a dessert. (b) Avocado and grapefruit slices provide an interesting taste combination for a salad and a pineapple half can be an attractive container for fruit pieces.

chemical residue that may be left on the fruit.

Fresh fruits are served whole, or they may be sliced, diced, sectioned, crushed, or pureed to be served alone or in combination with other fruits as a salad, appetizer, garnish, or dessert. Figure 11-5 shows a variety of ways to prepare fruits. Chapter 13, "Salads," gives more information on the preparation of raw fruits.

Certain fruits, such as apples, bananas, avocados, and peaches, discolor or turn brown when their flesh is exposed to air. This discoloration is caused by an enzymatic reaction of the fruit with the oxygen of the air. Coating the fruit with lemon juice, pineapple juice, or a commercial preparation containing ascorbic acid (vitamin C) helps to prevent its discoloration.

Cooked

When fruit is cooked, the flesh becomes more tender and translucent. The cooking of fruit is particularly advantageous when the fruit is underripe, and cooking or canning overripe fruit helps to preserve them. The addition of sugar to the cooking water also helps to preserve the fruit.

Many fruits lose much of their flavor, sugar, and nutrients to the water in which they are cooked. If the juice of canned fruit is not consumed with the fruit when it is served, the juice may be used in other food preparation but it will have a high sugar content. For example, the juice may be used as the liquid for a food dish made with a gelatin base, or it may be used as part of the liquid for a fruit drink.

Baked. Fruits may be baked whole or as pieces of fruit in a casserole. Fruits cooked in the skin retain more flavor than those that are pared before cooking. The most commonly baked fruit is apple, as shown in Figure 11-6. To bake apples, the cores are removed and the apples are placed in a casserole dish. Water is added to the dish to come up to 1/4 inch from the base of the apple. The apples are baked at 350° F (177° C) for 60 minutes, or until they are tender. The center of the apples may be

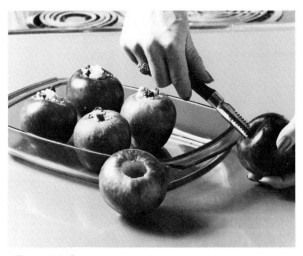

Figure 11-6.
Baked apples are cored and stuffed before being baked.

filled with 1 tablespoon of brown or white sugar and/or raisins or dates. The apples should be basted several times with the liquid in the dish during baking.

Sauces. Fruits that are cooked to a sauce are cooked in a slight amount of water over low heat until the fruit is tender. After the fruit is removed from the heat but is still warm, the sugar is added and stirred into the mixture until it is dissolved. Sugar tends to dilute cooked fruit mixtures, so it is important to cook the mixture with a small amount of liquid and add the sugar after cooking. Fruit, such as cranberries, rhubarb, and apples, are often served as fruit sauces.

Stewed Fruits. Stewed fruits are cooked in a sugar syrup over low heat with care being taken to retain the shape of the fruit while it is being cooked. Fruits will best retain their shape when they are cooked in a proportion of two parts water to one part sugar. Excess sugar can cause the fruit to shrink and become hard. Fruits such as berries and apricots are prepared by the stewing method, and mixtures of fruits, called

fruit compotes, may also be cooked by this method. Stewed fruits in combination are shown in Figure 11-7.

Dried Fruits. Dried fruits are cooked in water at a low boil or simmer until the fruit is tender. Sugar is added, if needed, near the end of the cooking time. If the fruit has a low-moisture content, it may be necessary to cover the fruit with boiling water and allow it to stand for a short time before it is cooked in the same water. It is best to read the directions on the package to determine the cooking process to be followed and the correct cooking time.

Other Methods. Fruits may be broiled for an additional variety in serving. Common fruits that are broiled include grapefruit halves, banana halves, and pineapple slices. Canned fruits may also be heated under the broiler. Fruits to be broiled are usually coated with sugar or a sugar syrup to give them a glazed effect. Different ways to serve fruits are illustrated in Figures 11-8 and 11-9.

Figure 11-7.
Stewed fruits are good served as a breakfast fruit or as a meat accompaniment.

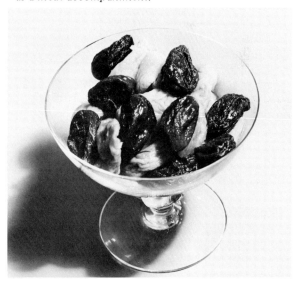

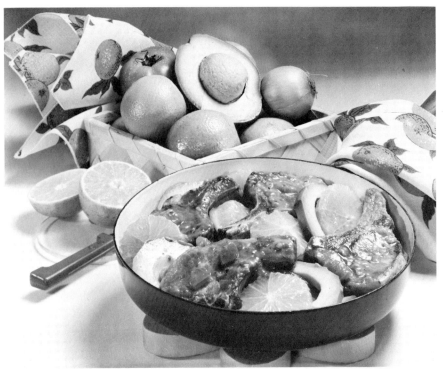

Figure 11-8.

Pork chops cooked in an orange juice sauce and served with avocado and orange slices give special flavor to a meal. (Florida Citrus Commission)

Figure 11-9.

Orange and pineapple chunks provide a light fruit flavor to chicken dishes. (Florida Citrus Commission)

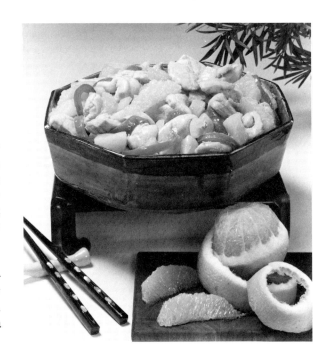

Fruits such as apples may also be lightly fried in a small amount of fat. The fruit may be dipped in a coating before being cooked in such a manner. This is often the preliminary preparation for an exotic flaming dessert such as bananas flambé. Sugar is usually sprinkled over the cooked fruit.

Microwave. Fruits such as apples and cranberries maintain their shape and are quickly tenderized when cooked in a microwave oven. Defrosting of fruits in a microwave oven is a quick process.

RECIPES

Rhubarb Sauce

	Standard	Metric
Chopped Rhubarb	2 cups	500 mL
Sugar	1/2 cup	125 mL
Water	2 Tbsp.	30 mL

1. Wash and chop the rhubarb into 1-inch pieces.
2. Combine the rhubarb and water in a saucepan.
3. Cover and cook over low heat until tender, approximately 20 minutes.
4. Stir in sugar.

Yield: 3 to 4 servings

Apple Sauce

	Standard	Metric
Apples, medium-sized	4	4
Sugar	1/4 cup	60 mL
Water	1/4 cup	60 mL

1. Wash the apples; pare, quarter, and core the apples and cut each quarter section into four slices.
2. Add the apples and water to a saucepan.
3. Cover and cook over low heat until the apples are tender, approximately 15 minutes.
4. Remove from the heat and stir in the sugar until it dissolves.
5. After being cooked, the apple sauce may be put through a sieve for a finer consistency.

Variations
1. Apples may be cooked unpeeled. One tsp. of cinnamon may be added with the sugar.

Yield: 3 to 4 servings

Spicy Dried Fruit Compote

	Standard	Metric
Dried prunes	1 cup	250 mL
Dried apricots	1 cup	250 mL
Raisins	1/2 cup	125 mL
Water	2 cups	500 mL
Sugar	1-1/2 cup	375 mL
Cider vinegar	3/4 cup	175 mL
Whole cloves	24	24
Cinnamon sticks	2	2

1. Place the fruit in a saucepan with water. Cover and cook over low heat for 10 minutes.
2. Add the remaining ingredients, cover, and cook over low heat for 10 minutes.
3. Carefully remove the fruit to a bowl; remove cloves and cinnamon sticks; add liquid; cover and refrigerate. Serve as an accompaniment to meat or poultry.

Yield: 3 cups

Hot Fresh Fruit Compote

	Standard	Metric
Sugar	1 cup	250 mL
Water	2 cups	500 mL
Vanilla extract	1 tsp.	5 mL
Diced fresh peaches	1 cup	250 mL
Fresh pineapple chunks	1 cup	250 mL
Fresh pear chunks	1 cup	250 mL

1. Add the sugar to water in a saucepan and boil for 5 minutes.
2. Add the fruit and vanilla extract to the sugar syrup and cook over low heat until tender, approximately 10 minutes. Serve warm.

Yield: 3 cups

Cranberry Relish

	Standard	Metric
Fresh or frozen cranberries	2 cups	500 mL
Orange, medium	1	1
Sugar	1 cup	250 mL

1. Wash the cranberries and discard any decayed ones.
2. Peel the orange, saving enough peel to make 2 tsp. Cut the orange flesh into sections.
3. Force the cranberries, orange, and orange peel through a food grinder.
4. Mix the ground fruit with the sugar.
5. Place in a covered container and refrigerate several hours before serving.

Yield: 2 cups

Spicy Orange Relish

	Standard	Metric
Oranges, medium, whole, unpeeled	4	4
Sugar	2-1/2 cups	625 mL
Water	1-1/2 cups	375 mL
Vinegar	2/3 cups	150 mL
Cloves, whole	12	12
Stick cinnamon	1	1

1. Simmer the whole oranges in water to cover for 20 minutes. Drain, cool, and slice into 1/8-inch-thick slices.
2. Combine the sugar, water, vinegar, cloves, and cinnamon. Bring to a boil and add the oranges. Simmer for 20 minutes.
3. Remove the cinnamon and cloves and pour the fruit into a covered dish. Refrigerate. Use as a garnish for many dishes.

Yield: 2 pints

Fried Apple Rings

	Standard	Metric
Apples	2	2
Cinnamon	1 tsp.	5 mL
Sugar	1 tsp.	5 mL
Egg, beaten	1	1
Fat	2 Tbsp.	30 mL

1. Wash and core the apples. Cut into 1/4-inch slices.
2. Combine the sugar and cinnamon.
3. Dip the apple slices in the egg and sprinkle with the cinnamon-sugar mixture.
4. Melt the fat in a heavy skillet.
5. Fry the apple slices slowly over moderate heat until tender.

Yield: 2 to 3 servings

Glazed Apples

	Standard	Metric
Butter	4 Tbsp.	45 mL
Apples	4	4
Vanilla	1 tsp.	5 mL
Sugar	1/4 cup	60 mL

1. Wash the apples. Peel, core, and cut the apples into 1/8-inch-thick slices.
2. Melt the butter in a saucepan. Add the sliced apples and vanilla. Cover and cook over low heat for approximately 6 minutes or until tender.
3. Add the sugar; serve immediately.

Yield: 4 servings

Broiled Peach Halves

	Standard	Metric
Peach halves, canned	4	4
Brown sugar	4 tsp.	20 mL
Crushed pineapple, drained	1/4 cup	60 mL

1. Turn the broiler on to preheat.
2. Fill each peach half with 1 Tbsp. of crushed pineapple and sprinkle with 1 tsp. of brown sugar.
3. Place on a broiler pan and broil 3 inches from heat until heated through. Serve immediately.

Yield: 4 servings

————————— Fresh Peach Whip —————————

	Standard	Metric
Pureed peaches	1 cup	250 mL
Salt	1/8 tsp.	0.5 mL
Sugar	1/2 cup	125 mL
Egg whites, stiffly beaten	2	2
Lemon juice	1 Tbsp.	15 mL

1. Combine the peaches, salt, and sugar in a saucepan. Heat until the sugar is dissolved and the mixture is of a syruplike consistency.
2. Pour the hot syrup mixture slowly over stiffly beaten egg whites, beating constantly.
3. Add the lemon juice.
4. Spoon into serving dishes and serve immediately.

Yield: 4 servings

Variations
1. Substitute any fresh fruit or cooked dried fruit for the peaches.

————————— Apple Crisp —————————

	Standard	Metric
Apples	6	6
Water	1/4 cup	60 mL
Sugar	3/4 cup	175 mL
Flour	1/2 cup	125 mL
Cinnamon	1 tsp.	5 mL
Butter	6 Tbsp.	90 mL

1. Preheat the oven to 375° F (190° C).
2. Wash, core, and slice the apples to a thickness of 1/8-inch.

3. Place the sliced apples in a buttered baking dish and add water.
4. Combine the sugar, flour, and cinnamon. Blend in the butter until the mixture is of a crumbly consistency.
5. Pour the mixture over the sliced apples. Bake uncovered for 1 hour.
6. Serve warm or cold.

Yield: 4 to 6 servings

————————— Baked Orange Fluff —————————

	Standard	Metric
Eggs, separated	4	4
Sugar	1 cup	250 mL
Orange juice	1/2 cup	125 mL
Almond extract	1/2 tsp.	2 mL
Grated orange rind	2 tsp.	10 mL

1. Preheat the oven to 350° F (175° C).
2. Beat the egg yolks until they are light. Gradually add the sugar and continue beating.
3. Combine the orange juice, rind, and almond flavoring; add to egg yolk mixture and mix until well-blended.
4. Beat egg whites until stiff peaks form.
5. Fold the mixture into the stiffly beaten egg whites.
6. Pour the mixture into a greased baking dish. Place the baking dish in another pan and add hot water to come up to 1 inch on the sides of the casserole dish. Bake 35 minutes or until firm. Serve immediately.

Yield: 6 servings

Lemon Pudding

	Standard	Metric
Eggs, separated	4	4
Butter	4 Tbsp.	45 mL
Lemon juice	1/4 cup	60 mL
Lemon rind	1/2 lemon	1/2 lemon
Sugar	1/2 cup	125 mL
Sugar	1/2 cup	125 mL
Bread crumbs	1/2 cup	125 mL

1. Preheat the oven to 350° F (175° C).
2. Melt the butter.
3. Combine the butter, egg yolks, lemon juice (reserving 1 tsp.), lemon rind, and 1/2 cup sugar. Beat until the mixture is smooth.
4. Beat the egg whites until they are foamy. Add 1 teaspoon of lemon juice and gradually add the sugar; continue beating until shiny, stiff peaks form.
5. Fold the mixture into the stiffly beaten egg whites.
6. Pour the mixture into a greased 9-inch × 2-inch square casserole dish. Sprinkle with the bread crumbs. Bake for 25 to 30 minutes.

Yield: 4 servings

Orange Apricot Cooler

	Standard	Metric
Orange juice	2 cups	500 mL
Lemon juice	2 Tbsp.	30 mL
Cooked dried apricots	1/2 cup	125 mL

1. Cook the apricots according to the package directions.
2. Blend until smooth in a food blender or put through a food grinder.
3. Combine with the orange juice and lemon juice. Serve over ice.

Yield: 2 servings

LEARNING ACTIVITIES

1. Plan breakfast, lunch, and dinner menus in which a fruit fulfills the daily need for ascorbic acid.
2. Prepare a list of the different ways that citrus fruits can be served for breakfast.
3. Consult a local newspaper and determine which fruits are the best buy for a given week. Plan and prepare a fruit dessert from one of these fruits.
4. Compare the price of fresh oranges and canned and frozen orange juice at a local market. Determine how much an 8-ounce glass of orange juice would cost from the three forms. Assume that it would take three oranges to make an 8-ounce glass of juice.
5. If possible, compare the price of a fruit other than a citrus in fresh, frozen, and canned form. Determine how much it would cost for a half-cup serving of the three forms.
6. Study the quality characteristics of fresh fruits that are available in a local market and describe to the class what is important to look for.
7. Slice an apple. Dip one half of the slice in a lemon solution. Place the dipped and undipped slices on a plate and note the changes that take place on the apple surface over several hours.
8. Cook one sliced apple in 2 tablespoons of water until tender. Add 1 tablespoon of sugar. Cook a second sliced apple in 2 tablespoons of water with 1 tablespoon of sugar added at the beginning of the cooking. Note the difference in the sauce consistency.
9. Compare the flavor, texture, and appear-

ance of the same fruit packed in a heavy, medium, and light syrup.
10. Prepare a list of five fruit recipes using the fruit analyzed in number 9. Determine which variety of the fruit should be used in each recipe.
11. Stew a fresh fruit and prepare a menu including it.
12. Prepare a fruit by broiling and note the flavor changes that occur.
13. Thaw a package of frozen berries and note the textural changes that take place. Develop a fruit drink recipe that uses the frozen fruit and prepare it.

REVIEW QUESTIONS

1. From what portion of the plant does fruit come?
2. What are the three main quality characteristics that make fruit such an enjoyable food?
3. What is the main form of carbohydrate found in an unripened fruit?
4. Why is cellulose important in the human diet?
5. What five fruits are an excellent source of ascorbic acid?
6. What is the average water content of fruit?
7. How does the water content of dried fruit relate to a higher caloric content?
8. What quality does the pectic substance in fruit give?
9. Why is the use of fruits in menu planning a timesaving factor?
10. Why does the consumer not often see US grade standards on fresh fruits?
11. In what two forms are fruits most widely available?
12. What quality characteristics should be looked for when purchasing apples, berries, and citrus fruits?
13. What is one method that helps to determine when a melon is ripe?
14. How are frozen fruits sold in relation to size and added sugar?
15. What are four common variety forms of canned fruits?
16. What are two ways in which fruit is dried?
17. What is the difference between a vacuum-dried fruit and other dried fruits?
18. When are fresh fruits the best buy?
19. What three decisions need to be made before purchasing fresh fruits?
20. What is the major difference between buying expensive and less costly canned fruits?
21. What is the difference in content of a fruit juice labeled "juice" and one labeled "fruit juice drink"?
22. What changes occur as fruit ripens?
23. How are berries best stored in the refrigerator?
24. What is the purpose of washing fruits before they are used?
25. How can the discoloration of some fruits be reduced?
26. What changes occur when fruit is cooked?
27. Why is sugar most often added after a fruit sauce is cooked?
28. What kind of care needs to be taken when fruits are cooked in a sugar syrup?
29. What are four methods that may be used to cook fruits?

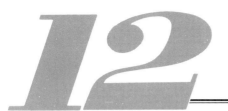

Vegetables

Vegetables are plants that are used as food. Several different parts of the plant are eaten, including the root (carrots), the leaf (spinach), the fruit of the plant (tomatoes), the bud and stem (broccoli), the seed (peas), and the underground stem or tuber (potatoes). Legumes are considered part of the seed family, but because of their high protein content they were discussed in Chapter 10. Each vegetable makes an important nutritive contribution to the daily diet and vegetables are high contributors of flavor, color, and texture to any meal.

A wide variety of vegetables in several different forms can be purchased today. Many vegetables are homegrown, and children acquire a fondness for vegetables they help to grow and prepare for eating. Even city dwellers can grow a few vegetables in containers and enjoy the foliage as the plant matures.

Vegetables can become a taste adventure when previously unfamiliar vegetables are tried. Vegetables are one of the most economical foods and can be prepared in many different ways to add variety to meals. Figure 12-1 illustrates a variety of vegetables that can be homegrown in most geographical areas of the United States.

Nutritional Factors to Consider

Carbohydrate and Fat

All vegetables are a good source of carbohydrate. Carbohydrate, mainly in the form of starch, is found chiefly in vegetables whose edible portion comes from the ground, as in potatoes. Root vegetables, like carrots, parsnips, and beets, also contain a small amount of

168

sugar. As vegetables mature, the sugar in them is converted to starch. The fruits of vegetables, such as winter squash and pumpkin, are also good sources of carbohydrate.

Vegetable leaves and stems contain cellulose, which is a nondigestible form of carbohydrate for the human body. Cellulose is important because the bulk it contributes allows food to pass through the digestive system more readily.

Vegetables as a group contain only a trace of fat.

Protein

The protein in vegetables is incomplete, meaning that vegetables do not contain the nine essential amino acids necessary for the body's proper utilization of protein. However, the protein quality is increased when vegetables are served in a sauce made with milk products.

Vitamins and Minerals

Vegetables are excellent sources of both vitamins and minerals. Dark-green vegetables like broccoli and spinach and deep-orange vegetables like winter squash and carrots are excellent sources of vitamin A. Tomatoes, green peppers, cabbage, potatoes, and broccoli are good sources of ascorbic acid. Vegetables contain varying amounts of the B vitamins.

Dark-green leafy vegetables such as spinach or kale are one of the best sources of iron. Mustard greens, collards, and broccoli are good sources of calcium. Although calcium is present in spinach and beet greens, the presence of

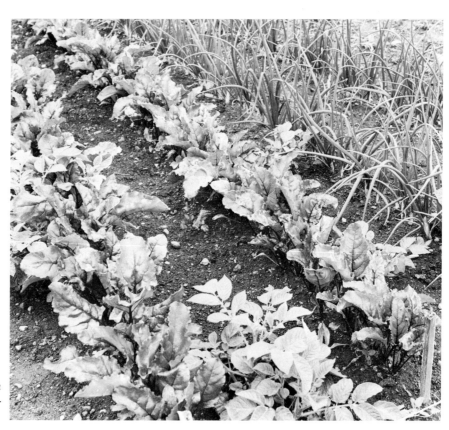

Figure 12-1.
Beets, potatoes, and green onions adapt well to home-growing as pictured here.

Table 12-1
Calorie, Carbohydrate, Vitamin, and Mineral Content of Some Vegetables

Food	Food Energy Calories	Carbo-hydrate gm	Cal-cium mg	Iron mg	Vit-amin A I.U.	Thi-amine mg	Ribo-flavin mg	Niacin mg	Ascor-bic Acid mg
Asparagus, 1/2 cup cooked	18	3.3	19	0.6	810	0.5	0.16	1.	24
Broccoli, 1/2 cup cooked	20	3.5	68	.6	1940	0.7	0.15	.6	70
Cabbage, 1/2 cup shredded, raw	11	2.5	22	0.2	60	0.02	0.02	0.1	21
Carrots, 1 whole, raw	30	7	14	0.5	7930	.04	0.04	.3	6
Potatoes, 1, baked	145	33	14	1.1	Trace	.15	0.07	2.7	20
Spinach, 1/2 cup, fresh cooked	21	3	84	2	7290	.7	.13	.5	25

Nutritive Value of American Foods, Agriculture Handbook No. 456, USDA, 1975.

oxalic acid in these vegetables does not allow the body to properly absorb the calcium.

Calories

Vegetables are low in calories. An average one-half cup serving of vegetables contains between 25 and 50 calories. Many individuals avoid the more starchy vegetables such as potatoes if they are counting calories. However, one medium-sized baked potato contains only 95 calories as compared to a 1-ounce serving of plain fudge that contains 115 calories. It is not the vegetable, but how the vegetable is prepared that accounts for the additional calories. Table 12-1 gives the calorie, carbohydrate, vitamin, and mineral content of some vegetables.

Menu-Planning Points

Inherent Factors

Balance. Vegetables balance a meal by providing the necessary nutrients, such as vitamins A and C, that may not be present in other foods being served. Properly prepared, vege-

tables add the color, texture, and flavor that balance a meal and give additional enjoyment to eating.

Color. A pleasing contrast in color can be achieved in a meal through the proper selection of vegetables. For example, a menu with white fish as the entrée is made more colorful by a healthy serving of green beans; the rosy entrée of baked ham can be balanced in color by using cauliflower as the vegetable.

Shape. The shape of the vegetable plant offers an interesting contrast to other foods served for a meal. Vegetables grow in globular shapes, as in Brussels sprouts and beets, and in length-wise form, as in asparagus, green beans, and carrots. Shape can also be created by cutting vegetables lengthwise, as with zucchini; cutting chunks, as with eggplant; or cutting the vegetable in half for serving, as with acorn squash.

Flavor. The flavor of vegetables varies widely. In planning menus the proper flavor of a vegetable is an important consideration. Strongly flavored vegetables such as onions and cabbage should be served with a mildly flavored entrée like veal cutlets. A sweetly flavored vegetable such as parsnips would not be a good choice to serve with a dish like sweet and sour pork.

Texture. Some vegetables are crisp and some have a softer texture in raw form. Raw, young vegetables are more tender than the older, mature ones. For example, fresh young carrots are tender to the bite, whereas the older, more mature carrot can have a tough, stringy texture. Cooking to the proper stage of doneness also affects the texture of vegetables.

External Factors

Age. As children grow older, they often develop a dislike for certain vegetables. This dislike probably originates from the preferences of other family members, the forced-feeding concept that "you must eat the vegetables," or from having to eat vegetables that are unappetizing because of the way they are prepared.

Culture and Economics. Few vegetables are not eaten by all cultures, although some vegetables are more readily available in certain geographical areas and are more acceptable to a group.

Modern food technology has greatly increased the availability and quality of vegetables, many of which are now on the market the entire year at an affordable cost.

Space, Equipment, and Time Scheduling. The form in which a vegetable is purchased is directly related to the amount of space available for storage and the type of equipment available. For example, frozen foods cannot be stored if a freezer is not available. Fresh vegetables have to be purchased in quantities relative to the amount of refrigerator storage space.

Special tools that are necessary for vegetable preparation include a parer and a vegetable scrub brush. Special cooking containers that can be used in vegetable preparation include a wok, a steamer, and a deep-fat fryer.

Vegetables are usually the last food to be cooked before serving, and time schedules need to be carefully planned to allow for it. The flavor of a cooked, lukewarm vegetable is not appealing. If serving is delayed, the vegetable can be quickly cooled by setting the pan in cold water and then reheating.

Vegetable Grading

The U.S. Department of Agriculture has set standards of quality for most of the fresh and processed vegetables marketed in the United States. A standard of quality is based on the taste, texture, and appearance of the vegetable. The use of these standards and the federal inspection of vegetables is a voluntary service that is paid for by the food industry using the service.

The consumer who purchases vegetables usually does not see the U.S. grade standards on the product, but the standards were probably used by wholesalers involved in the processing of vegetables. If the vegetable was packed and processed under continuous inspection, it may carry the U.S. grade mark and the inspection shield, the statement "USDA Inspected" or "Packed under Continuous Inspection of the U.S. Department of Agriculture," as shown in Figure 12-2.

U.S. No. 1 is the most common grade mark used for fresh vegetables. This designates that the vegetable has few blemishes and is of good quality. The top grade for canned and frozen vegetables is US Grade A or US Fancy. Vegetables that are of high quality but are not as tender or of as good a color as the top grade are marked US Grade B or US Extra Standard.

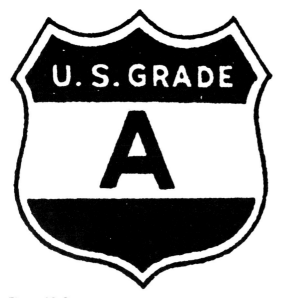

Figure 12-2.
U.S. grade A name may appear on the label and denotes a vegetable of excellent appearance and texture.

US Grade C is used for vegetables that do not have the flavor, texture, and appearance of the other two grades.

Vegetable Forms

Vegetables are available in fresh, frozen, canned, and dehydrated forms. Improved methods of growing, harvesting, processing, storing, and transporting have made available a large variety of vegetables in each of these forms.

Fresh

Fresh vegetables may either be vegetables from a local harvest or they may have been shipped from many hundreds of miles away. Vegetables commonly available during the entire year include cabbage, carrots, celery, potatoes, and squash.

Frozen

As homes have increased their freezer storage, more frozen vegetables have become available to the consumer. Many vegetables are also home-frozen. Frozen vegetables should be picked at their peak of desired maturity and immediately processed. The nutrient content of frozen vegetables is near that of fresh vegetables. Vegetables with a high water content such as lettuce, cabbage, celery, and tomatoes do not freeze well.

Canned

The greatest array of vegetables on the market is found in canned form and many vegetables are also home-canned.

Dehydrated

The smallest variety of vegetables available is the dehydrated form, in which the water is removed from the vegetables. Small-scale food dehydrators can be purchased for the home, and many individuals are now using dehydration as a method of food preservation.

Purchasing

The form in which a vegetable is purchased is dependent on many factors including how the vegetable is to be used, the amount of storage space available, and the vegetable's availability at the market. Portions of fresh vegetables often have to be discarded because of bruises, decay, or wilted leaves, whereas vegetables in canned or frozen form do not have these waste factors. In this situation the choice of vegetable is based on personal preference and cost.

Fresh

Fresh vegetables should always be purchased in an amount that can be used while they are still fresh. Most vegetables will not keep longer than 2 to 5 days, with the exception of root vegetables, such as carrots and turnips. Fresh vegetables that do not show signs of bruising, decay, and wilt are the best to purchase. These factors cause the vegetable to deteriorate more rapidly and lessen the amount of the vegetable that is edible. The following discussion describes what to look for in purchasing some fresh vegetables.

Artichokes. There are two kinds of artichokes. Good-quality French artichokes have a globe or cone shape with green petals or scales that do not show a brownish discoloration. The artichoke should feel heavy in relation to its size. The Jerusalem artichoke resembles a thick, tuberlike potato.

Asparagus. The asparagus spears should be green and smoothly rounded, the tips tightly closed, and the stalk about 1/2 inch in diameter.

Beans. The pods of beans should feel firm to the touch. Green beans should be bright in color, and wax or yellow beans should have a good yellow color.

Beets. Fresh, high-quality beets are a deep red color and have a round root that feels smooth without scaly areas on the surface.

Broccoli. The buds should be compact and a rich green, not a yellowish color that reflects a sign of overmaturity.

Brussels Sprouts. The leaves of the sprout should be tight fitting around a firm head. Worm injury can be detected by small holes or jagged leaves.

Cabbage. The head of both green and red cabbages should be firm and the outer leaves should not show signs of wilting. Yellowed leaves of green cabbage are a sign that the cabbage has been stored too long. Savoy cabbage has green, crinkly leaves and Chinese cabbage has a more elongated firm head with crinkly leaves.

Carrots. The root should be smooth and firm with a deep-orange color. Carrots that are excessively rough or cracked are a sign of poor quality.

Cauliflower. The white portion of the cauliflower should be firm and compact with no sign of discoloration. Any green leaves still attached should have good color.

Celery. The celery stalks should feel firm and the upper leaves should be of good green color.

Corn. The husks should have a good green color and the ears should be filled out with bright yellow kernels. The corn tassel should be dark brown.

Cucumbers. The skin of a cucumber should be a smooth green and should have a firm feel.

Eggplant. The color of high-quality eggplant is a rich, deep purple. The vegetable should feel firm and heavy and the skin should be free from defects.

Leafy Greens. Greens should have a healthy color, be free from blemishes and insects, and not look wilted or dried out.

Mushrooms. The cap of the mushroom should be tightly closed around the stem and be of a white to creamy color.

Okra. The pods of okra should be small to medium-sized, be green in color, and have a fleshy feel.

Onions. The dry onion bulb should feel firm

and the neck should be small. The outer covering should have a papery texture with no sign of mold. Green onions should have tops that are crisp and of good green color.

Peas. The pods should be bright green and contain peas that are of medium size. Pods that are flat contain immature peas, and pods of a dull green or yellowish color contain overly mature peas.

Parsnips. A fresh parsnip is small to medium in size and has a firm feel.

Peppers. Peppers vary in shape from small to large bell-shaped and are red or green in color. The surface should be free of decay and bright in color.

Potatoes. New potatoes are harvested early and may show a slight amount of skin discoloration; however, those with large areas of skin defect should not be purchased. More mature potatoes should be firm and free of skin defects. Potatoes with green discoloration and sprouts protruding from the skin should be avoided. Sweet potatoes should have a smooth skin and not show signs of decay.

Squash. Summer squash should be firm with a shiny, blemish-free, and tender skin. Varieties of summer squash include the yellow crookneck, patty pan, and zucchini. Winter squash, which should have a heavy feel with a tough rind, include acorn, butternut, and hubbard.

Tomatoes. Tomatoes should have a smooth skin that is free from blemishes. They should not be purchased if there are signs of cracks, bruising, and decay. Fully ripe tomatoes have a rich, red color, whereas tomatoes that are less than ripe will be light red and feel more firm.

Frozen

Frozen vegetables are available in many different forms including whole, sliced, julienne, or chopped. Some vegetables are frozen in combination with other vegetables, whereas others are available as specially prepared dishes like a soufflé. Special seasonings and sauces are also sold with frozen vegetables. These special additions add to the cost and may result in a decreased amount of nutrients in a serving.

Packages that show signs of excessive frost or which are soft in feel should not be purchased because the package was either partially thawed and refrozen or was not being held at a proper storage temperature. Frozen vegetables sold under a national brand are usually of high quality because of standards set by the industry. Sometimes large chain stores carry two qualities under their own label, but there is little difference in quality between brand names of frozen vegetables except for their price.

Large packages of frozen vegetables are now available in free-pour bags that allow the cooking of just the right amount of vegetables. It is important to immediately return the unused portion to the freezer. These large bags are usually a good buy.

Canned

The ease in storing canned vegetables and their economical price make canned vegetables a good purchase. Many kinds of vegetables are available whole, chopped, sliced, and in several combinations. Some vegetables are available in a marinade, have special seasonings added, or have part of an additional cooking process completed, such as creamed corn.

As with the frozen form, vegetables are sold under national brand labels; some large stores have their own brand labeling. The choice of which brand to buy is very much dependent on how the vegetable is to be used. If the vegetable is to be served in its existing form, then top quality is important. If the vegetable is to be used in combination with other ingredients, such as in a casserole, a lower quality is acceptable. There is no difference in nutrients between brands, but there can be a difference in flavor and texture. It is wise to sample different brands to determine which brand is desirable for one's needs.

Many brands of vegetables offer nutritional labeling that is helpful to the consumer in planning meals with needed nutrients. Cans of vegetables that show bulging ends, or leakage or which are deeply dented should always be avoided in purchase.

Dehydrated

The most common dehydrated vegetables available on the market are onions, garlic, parsley, mushrooms, and potatoes. Other forms of dehydrated vegetables are available on a limited basis in specialty stores that offer services to hikers and campers. Aside from the vegetables mentioned, dehydrated foods are quite expensive, but they can be economical purchases for the individual who uses small amounts because they are easy to store and do not spoil.

Storage

Fresh vegetables are stored in the refrigerator with the exception of potatoes, winter squash, unripe tomatoes, and dry onions. Potatoes, squash, and onions can be stored in a cool dry area. Unripe tomatoes may be left at room temperature to ripen fully and then be refrigerated.

Other vegetables are washed, dried, placed in plastic bags or plastic covered containers, and refrigerated. Some refrigerators have special drawers called hydrators that are used for storing vegetables. The use of a vegetable brush helps to remove the dirt from hard-surfaced vegetables, such as potatoes and carrots. A colander helps to remove the excess water from leafy green vegetables.

The green tops of vegetables such as carrots and radishes should be trimmed to within 1 inch of the top of the vegetable and the stem root cut off. The woody stalk of corn can be stored in the husk, or the husk and silk may be removed and the corn stored in plastic bags. Green peas should be left in the pod until they are ready to use. Instructions for the proper care of leafy greens are discussed in Chapter 13, "Salads."

Frozen vegetables are stored at 0° F (-18° C) or below. Canned and dehydrated vegetables are stored in a dry, well-ventilated area. Vegetables that are home-dried can be stored in plastic bags, covered jars, or other containers.

Basic Preparation

Vegetables can be prepared in many ways to make them delectable companions to be served with other foods or to be served alone as a tasty snack or appetizer. Some vegetables are eaten raw, some are cooked before eating, and some are eaten either raw or cooked, as shown in Figure 12-3. Vegetables can be cooked whole, or diced, sliced, shredded, chopped, or cut into strips. Some vegetables are mashed after they are cooked. Vegetables like tomatoes, zucchini, or acorn squash can be hollowed out and used as a cooking container for other food ingredients. Stuffed acorn squash is shown in Figure 12-4. Vegetables such as potatoes, carrots, and beets can be cooked in their skins and eaten or they may be peeled before they are eaten. If vegetables are to be pared before they are cooked, a vegetable peeler should be used in place of a knife. Many nutrients are close to the skin of vegetables and

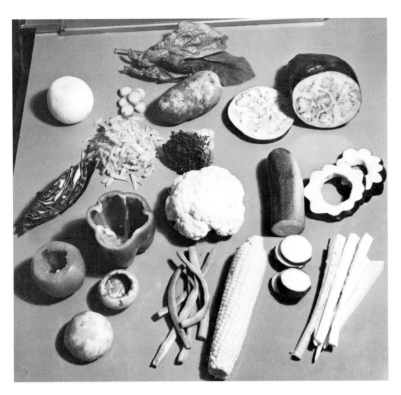

Figure 12-3.
Vegetables can be cooked whole, shredded, cut into strips or chunks or hollowed out and stuffed before being cooked.

Figure 12-4.
Acorn squash can be filled and baked with a variety of ingredients for a nutritious and flavorful vegetable entree. (The R. T. French Co.)

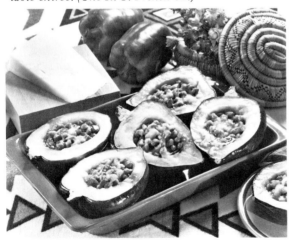

it is desirable to remove only a thin layer of skin.

The length of time a vegetable is cooked is somewhat a matter of personal preference. Some people like cooked vegetables with a crisp texture, whereas others may prefer a softer texture. Nutrients, fresh flavors, and bright green color are best retained when vegetables are cooked for a short period of time. The woody stems of such vegetables as broccoli and asparagus will not become more tender with prolonged cooking and so are usually discarded.

The flavor of vegetables such as broccoli, Brussels sprouts, cabbage, cauliflower, kale, and turnips becomes stronger with prolonged cooking. Green vegetables will retain a better color if they are stirred several times during the cooking process and are not overcooked. Although the addition of baking soda to green vegetables helps to retain their color, it destroys the ascorbic acid and causes the vegetable to have a mushy texture. Baking soda should thus not be used in cooking vegetables.

Red cabbage and beets may develop color problems during their preparation. The red color of cabbage can be maintained by adding a small amount of vinegar, lemon juice, or apple to the cabbage while it is being cooked. Beets peeled before they are cooked tend to lose their color in the cooking water. Beets will retain their color if they are cooked unpeeled and skinned after being cooked.

Peeled white and sweet potatoes will turn brown if they are allowed to stand because of enzymatic reactions. This discoloration can be eliminated by placing the potatoes in salted water.

Raw

Cleaned, raw vegetables should be served chilled. Vegetables with a high water content such as zucchini or cucumber should be chilled in the refrigerator for a short period, and firmer vegetables like carrots and radishes should be chilled in ice water before they are served. Chapter 13, "Salads," gives more details on the preparation of raw vegetables.

Baked

Thick-skinned vegetables such as squash and mature potatoes are often baked in the skin. Potatoes may be wrapped in foil and steam baked or directly baked in the skin in the oven. Potatoes wrapped in foil need no special pretreatment. However, potatoes without a covering may be very lightly coated with fat to prevent a hard crust from forming, and should be pricked in several places with a fork to allow the steam to escape during the baking process. Potatoes that are not pricked may explode in the oven.

The oven temperature for baking potatoes is dependent on the length of time desired for

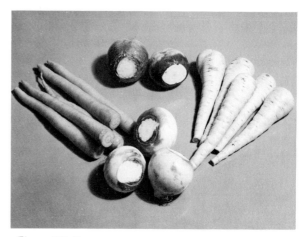

Figure 12-5.
Popular root vegetables include carrots, rhutabagas, parsnips, and turnips.

cooking. For example, medium-sized potatoes baked at 400° F (205° C) take approximately 45 to 60 minutes to cook. At times it may be desirable to cook potatoes in the oven with other foods at a lower temperature, such as meat dishes cooked at 325° F (165° C). The time for cooking the potatoes would then be approximately 90 minutes.

Root vegetables such as carrots, beets, potatoes, parsnips, or turnips may also be baked in the oven. The cleaned vegetable is first shredded and then placed in a lightly greased casserole dish with a tight-fitting lid. Root vegetables are baked at 375° F (190° C) for 45 to 60 minutes. The length of cooking time is dependent on the amount of vegetables being cooked, and the size and kind of the casserole. Root vegetables are pictured in Figure 12-5.

Broiled

Vegetables that can be broiled satisfactorily include root vegetables, potatoes, onions, and tomatoes. Root vegetables need to be partially cooked first by boiling. They may be marinated for several hours to add additional flavor. If root vegetables are being broiled, they need to be turned frequently to permit even cooking. Vegetables such as tomato halves and onion slices are usually topped with some type of seasoning such as cheese or bread crumbs. Vegetables should be broiled about 3 inches from the broiler unit for approximately 5 to 8 minutes. A variety of vegetables are often alternated on skewers and broiled. Barbecuing over coals is another method for broiling vegetables.

Boiled

Many vegetables are boiled. The basic rule with this method of vegetable preparation is to boil the vegetables in a minimum amount of water for the shortest time possible to assure doneness. The proper way to boil vegetables is to bring the water to a boil, add the vegetables, cover, bring the water back to a boil, turn the heat to simmer, and cook until fork tender. The length of cooking time will vary with the type of pan, how tight the lid fits on the pan, the quantity of vegetables being cooked and personal preference. Green vegetables will have a better color if cooked without a lid. The water in which vegetables are boiled contains many of the water-soluble minerals and vitamins and is a flavorful and nutritious addition to gravies, sauces, soups, stews, and casseroles. Vegetables with a high water content, such as leafy greens, are cooked with a minimum of water; if there is moisture clinging to the leaves, no additional water may be needed. Firmer vegetables like carrots will require 1/4 to 1/2 cup of water, but the amount varies with the quantity being cooked. Strong-flavored vegetables may be cooked in a large amount of water uncovered.

The stalk vegetables like asparagus and broccoli cook more slowly than the buds. It is advisable to cook these vegetables with the stalks in the water and the buds above the water. Figure 12-6 shows asparagus tied to-

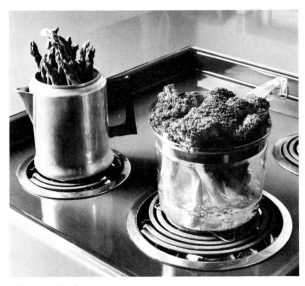

Figure 12-6.
Vegetables with a heavy stalk are best cooked with the stalk in water. The buds are cooked by steam from the simmering water. The bottom of a double boiler or a coffee pot make good cooking containers.

gether and being cooked in the bottom of a coffee pot and broccoli cooked in the bottom of a double boiler. Brussels sprouts will cook more quickly if a deep cross is cut in the stem end, and artichokes will cook faster if a one-half inch cross is made on the top.

Frozen vegetables are boiled in the same manner as fresh ones. They need a minimal amount of water and should not be thawed before they are cooked. The stems of vegetables such as asparagus will cook more evenly if they are gently pried apart during the cooking process. Frozen vegetables cook more quickly than fresh ones because they have been partially cooked prior to being frozen.

Most canned vegetables are cooked by boiling. The liquid from the vegetable is poured into a pan, brought to a boil, and heated to evaporate some of it. The vegetable is then added and heated to the correct temperature for serving. If the vegetables were home-canned, the process as described in Chapter 3 must be followed.

Fried

Pan Frying. Vegetable greens such as chard or spinach can be quickly cooked by pan frying. One to 2 tablespoons of fat is melted in a heavy pan, which has a tight-fitting lid. The greens, which should have a small amount of moisture still clinging to the leaves, are then added. The vegetables are brought to a simmer, stirred, and covered. If the stems are being cooked, they should be added first and cooked for a few minutes before the greens are put in the pan. To assure even cooking the greens should be stirred several times while they are being cooked. Greens that are pan fried cook very quickly and will be tender and cooked in 1 to 2 minutes, depending upon the amount being prepared. Pan frying is illustrated in Figure 12-7.

Deep Frying. A different way to prepare vegetables is to deep fry them. This process is discussed in Chapter 5, "Fats."

Stir Frying. Stir frying is similar to pan frying except that the food is not covered during the cooking and the food is continuously stirred. Because cooking is done over a high heat, a fat with a high smoking point is used. A heavy fry pan, an electric skillet, or a wok can be used. A small amount of fat is heated in the pan. The proper temperature has been reached when it will light toast a cube of bread. The vegetables are added and stirred continuously over moderate to high heat until they are just tender.

Vegetables should be cut into small uniform pieces to assure even cooking, as shown in Figure 12-8. If a mixture of vegetables is being

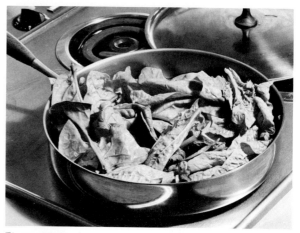

Figure 12-7.
Pan frying is a quick and easy way to prepare vegetable greens such as spinach.

used, the firmer vegetables such as carrots and cauliflower should be cooked a few minutes before the vegetables higher in water content like celery, onions, and green pepper are added. Vegetables cooked in a wok are shown in Figure 12-9.

Microwave Oven

Vegetables cooked in a microwave oven retain most of their fresh flavor, color, texture, and nutrients because of the minimum amount of water used in microwave cooking. The biggest problem encountered in cooking vegetables in a microwave oven is the tendency to overcook. A 5-minute, carry-over cooking time should be allotted for vegetables being cooked in a microwave oven. The following basic rules describe some of the procedures to remember when cooking vegetables in a microwave oven.

1. Frozen and fresh vegetables cooked in a casserole dish need a minimum of water. Usually 2 to 3 tablespoons are ample for vegetables for four people. The vegetable

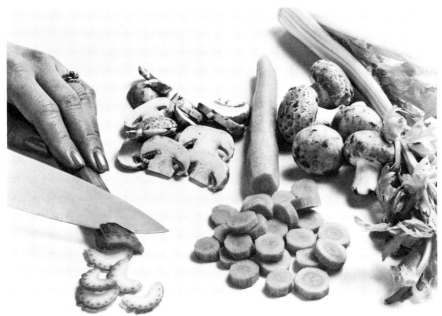

Figure 12-9.
Many vegetables are stir-fried in a special pan, the wok. They are cooked until barely tender, retaining their crunchy texture and good flavor. (Mazola Corn Oil)

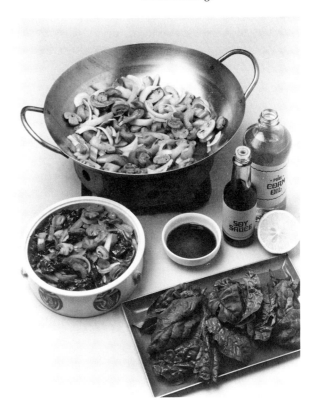

is cooked covered, and if a lid is not available, waxed paper is suitable. Plastic wrap tends to melt in a microwave oven.

2. Frozen vegetables may be cooked in the carton if one end of the carton is removed. Frozen vegetables in a plastic pouch may be cooked in that container if the pouch is slit to allow the steam to escape.

3. Potatoes and squash may be cooked in their skins if the skin is pierced with a fork before cooking to prevent a buildup of steam and an explosion in the oven. Corn can be cooked in the husk or wrapped in waxed paper for cooking.

4. When cooking more than one vegetable

180 *Vegetables*

such as potatoes or corn, the vegetables should be evenly spaced and turned during the cooking time.

5. Salt may be stirred into the cooking water before adding the vegetables, or it may be added after cooking. Other seasonings can be cooked with the vegetables.

Pressure Cooked

This method is usually used for the firmer vegetables like those from the root and tuber groups. It is best to follow the recommended water, temperature, and cooking time of the pressure cooker instructions to assure that the vegetable will be properly cooked.

Steamed

A steamed vegetable is one that has not come in contact with the water in which it is cooked.

Young, tender vegetables cook quickly by steaming. Firm, mature vegetables are more quickly cooked by boiling. Vegetables may be steamed in a specially purchased steamer, on the rack of a pressure cooker, or in a container such as a colander that keeps the vegetables out of the water in the pan.

Additional Ingredients

Many spices, herbs, sauces, and other foods can be added to vegetables before cooking or just after cooking to enhance their flavor and appearance. Figure 12-10 shows an appetizing dish of broccoli with a cheese sauce. Additional ingredients should not mask the flavor of the vegetable being served. Table 12-2 provides some suggested variations for certain cooked vegetables. Table 12-3 is a list of terms and their definitions that are commonly associated with vegetable cookery.

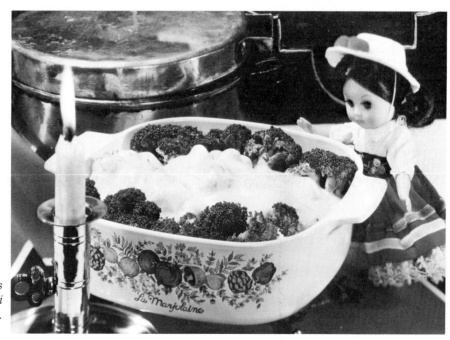

Figure 12-10.
Sauces are flavorful additions to vegetables such as broccoli served with cheese sauce. (Corning)

Table 12-2
Vegetable Variations

Vegetable	Variations
Artichokes	Fresh; boiled in water with a peeled clove of garlic; with a bay leaf and 2 Tbsp. oil; canned; in a white sauce.
Asparagus	In a cheese sauce or hollandaise sauce; topped with sieved egg yolk; topped with buttered crumbs.
Green beans	Flavored with herbs such as basil, marjoram, thyme, or savory; served with a mushroom sauce; cooked with onion and tomato.
Beets	Served with butter or with sour cream and horseradish; served with orange or Harvard sauce.
Broccoli	Served with a cheese sauce, lemon butter, or hollandaise sauce.
Brussels sprouts	Served with butter; cooked lyonnaise; in a cheese sauce; cooked in bouillon; served with sour cream.
Cabbage	Served with a cheese sauce; cooked with celery or apple.
Carrots	Served with butter; glazed; in a white sauce with peas.
Celery	Cooked in bouillon; broiled with Parmesan cheese.
Corn	Cooked with tomato and green pepper; cooked as a pudding.
Eggplant	Breaded and fried; cooked in combination with other vegetables; cooked with onion or celery juice.
Green peppers	Stuffed and cooked in combination with other vegetables.
Mushrooms	Sautéed; creamed; stuffed.
Okra	Stewed; lyonnaise; fried.
Onions	Buttered; creamed; French fried; broiled.
Peas	Buttered; creamed; combined with water chestnuts; cooked with mint leaves.
White potatoes	Baked; stuffed; scalloped; shredded and fried; with cheese sauce.
Sweet potatoes	Baked; candied; in casserole with pineapple or oranges.
Squash	Buttered; baked; mashed.
Tomatoes	Stewed; baked; broiled; in combination with other vegetables.
Turnips	Served with butter; glazed; mashed.

Table 12-3
Terms Used in Vegetable Cookery

Term	Definition
Au beurre	Cooked or sautéed in butter
Au beurre noir	Served with a brown butter
Au gratin	Cooked with a grated cheese and bread crumbs; baked in the oven
Creamed	Served with milk or cream, usually in the form of a white sauce
Creole	Combined with rice
Glazed	Cooked in a sugar-butter sauce
Lyonnaise	Fried sliced onion
Maitre d'hotel butter	Served with sauce that is prepared with butter or butter and oil that has lemon juice or dry white wine added
Sauce Provençal	Served with sauce made by simmering a garlic clove in butter
Scalloped	Cooked in a milk sauce
Stewed	Cooked at a simmering temperature

RECIPES

―――――――――― **Baked Stuffed Tomatoes** ――――――――――

	Standard	Metric
Tomatoes, medium-sized	4	4
Bacon	3 slices	3
Onion, medium-sized, finely chopped	1	1
Chopped green pepper	1/4 cup	60 mL
Minced parsley	2 Tbsp.	30 mL
Basil	1 tsp.	5 mL
Monosodium glutamate	1/4 tsp.	1 mL
Salt	to taste	to taste
Pepper	to taste	to taste
Grated sharp cheddar cheese	1/2 cup	125 mL
Dry bread crumbs	1/4 cup	60 mL

1. Preheat the oven to 350° F (175° C).
2. Cut a small slice from the tops of the tomatoes and scoop out the pulp. Save the centers for the stuffing.
3. Fry the bacon until it is crisp. Drain and crumble.
4. Sauté the onion, green pepper, parsley, and tomato pulp in the bacon fat until tender.
5. Season the sautéed mixture with the basil, monosodium glutamate, and salt and pepper.
6. Remove the pan from the heat and stir in the crumbled bacon and grated cheese.
7. Place the tomato shells in a shallow baking dish; fill with the stuffing mixture. Sprinkle the tops with bread crumbs.
8. Bake for 30 minutes. Garnish with parsley sprigs. For microwave cooking, place the tomatoes in a glass pie pan, cover with waxpaper and cook for 8 minutes, rotating dish 1/4 turn 4 minutes through cooking time. Let stand 5 minutes before serving.

Yield: 4 servings

French Fried Onion Rings

	Standard	Metric
Sweet onions, large	2	2
Milk	2 cups	500 mL
Salt	1/2 tsp.	2 mL
Flour	1/2 cup	125 mL

1. Slice the onion crosswise into 3/8 inch slices. Press out to make rings.
2. Combine the milk and salt and add the onion rings. Allow to soak for 30 minutes.
3. Remove the onions from the milk and lightly coat in the flour.
4. Fry in deep fat heated to a temperature of 380° F (194° C). Brown on both sides. Drain on absorbent paper.

Yield: 4 servings

Deep Fried Vegetables

	Standard	Metric
Flour	1 cup	250 mL
Egg	1	1
Water	3/4 cup	175 mL
Fresh green beans	1/4 pound	113 gm
Whole mushroom caps	8	8
Asparagus stalks	8	8

1. Combine the flour, egg, and water to make batter.
2. Heat the fat in a deep fryer to 350° F (175° C).
3. Dip the vegetables into the batter and lower gently into the hot fat. When the vegetables are cooked, drain on absorbent paper. Remove the free-floating pieces of the batter with a slotted spoon as needed.

Yield: 4 servings

Brussels Sprouts in Chicken Bouillon

	Standard	Metric
Fresh Brussels sprouts	2 cups	500 mL
Minced onion	2 Tbsp.	30 mL
Butter	2 Tbsp.	30 mL
Chicken bouillon	1 cube	1
Boiling water	1 cup	250 mL

1. Wash the Brussels sprouts and remove any damaged outer leaves. Cut a cross in the stem end.
2. Sauté the onion in butter over low heat until it is soft.
3. Dissolve the bouillon in boiling water in a saucepan.
4. Add the cooked onion and Brussels sprouts.
5. Cook over low heat until the sprouts are tender, approximately 15 minutes.

Yield: 4 servings

Variations

1. One 10-oz. package of frozen Brussels sprouts may be substituted for the fresh sprouts.
2. One beef bouillon cube may be substituted for the chicken.

Glazed Carrots

	Standard	Metric
Carrots, medium-sized	8	8
Butter or margarine	4 Tbsp.	60 mL
Brown sugar	4 Tbsp.	60 mL

1. Preheat the oven to 325° F (165° C).
2. Scrape the carrots and cook in a small amount of boiling salted water for 10 minutes, covered. Drain.
3. Melt the butter in the oven in a shallow baking dish. Stir in the brown sugar. Add the carrots and coat with the sugar-butter mixture. Bake uncovered for 10 minutes or until tender.

Yield: 4 to 6 servings

Dilled Green Beans

	Standard	Metric
Green beans	1 (16 oz.) can	1 (454 gm)
Dill weed	1-1/2 tsp.	7 mL

1. Drain the liquid from the beans into a saucepan and boil until 1/2 of the liquid remains in the pan.
2. Add the green beans and dill weed; stir to mix in the dill weed. Cook covered at a low temperature until the green beans are heated; approximately 5 minutes. For microwave cooking, combine the beans, 1/4 cup liquid, and the dill weed in a casserole dish. Cover and heat for 3 minutes.

Yield: 4 servings

Red Cabbage with Apple

	Standard	Metric
Bacon	6 slices	6
Red cabbage	1 head	1
Apple, chopped and peeled	1	1
Sugar	1 Tbsp.	15 mL
Vinegar	1 Tbsp.	15 mL
Salt	To taste	To taste
Pepper	To taste	To taste

1. In a heavy saucepan fry the bacon until it is crisp.
2. Cut the cabbage into quarters; rinse with water.
3. Add the cabbage to the bacon and bacon fat in the pan. Cook covered over low heat for 1 hour, stirring several times.
4. Add the chopped apple, sugar, vinegar, and salt and pepper to taste; stir to blend the ingredients into the cabbage mixture.
5. Let cook over low heat until the apple is soft, approximately 15 minutes.

Yield: 4 servings

Pan Fried Spinach Parmesan

	Standard	Metric
Butter or margarine	3 Tbsp.	45 mL
Garlic clove, peeled	1	1
Spinach, washed and drained	1-1/2 pounds	680 gm
Grated Parmesan cheese	1/2 cup	125 mL

1. Melt the butter or margarine in a heavy fry pan with a tight fitting lid. Add the garlic and sauté 1 to 2 minutes. Remove.
2. Add the spinach and bring to a simmer. Stir and cover. Stir several times while cooking. Drain off any excess cooking liquid.
3. Remove the spinach to a serving bowl and sprinkle with the Parmesan cheese.

Yield: 4 servings

Glazed Parsnips

	Standard	Metric
Parsnips	4	4
Water	3/4 cup	175 mL
Salt	1/2 tsp.	2 mL
Butter	3 Tbsp.	45 mL
Brown sugar	1 Tbsp.	15 mL

1. Wash and scrape the parsnips. Slice lengthwise into quarters.
2. In a shallow pan with a lid, combine the parsnips, water, and salt. Cover and cook 8 minutes or until tender; drain.
3. Add the butter and sprinkle with brown sugar. Cook uncovered over medium high heat, turning the parsnips in butter until they are well glazed.

Yield: 4 servings

Stir-Fried Vegetables

	Standard	Metric
Fat	3 Tbsp.	45 mL
Shredded cabbage	1 cup	250 mL
Chopped celery	1 cup	250 mL
Chopped green pepper	1/2 cup	125 mL
Chopped green onions	3	3
Zucchini, medium, sliced	1	1
Salt	1/2 tsp.	2 mL

1. Heat the fat in a heavy skillet or wok.
2. Add the vegetables to fat and stir constantly while cooking over high heat.
3. Sprinkle with salt. Serve immediately.

Yield: 4 servings

Sweet Potatoes in Orange Sauce

	Standard	Metric
Sweet potatoes, medium	4	4
Cornstarch	1 Tbsp.	15 mL
Sugar	2 Tbsp.	30 mL
Orange juice	1 cup	250 mL

1. Scrub the sweet potatoes. Do not peel.
2. Place in a pressure pan with 1/2 cup water for a 4-quart cooker. Cook according to pressure cooker directions for 10 minutes.
3. Remove the skin from the potatoes; slice and place in a serving dish.
4. In a small saucepan combine the sugar and cornstarch. Stir in the orange juice and cook, stirring constantly, until the sauce is thick.
5. Pour the sauce over the sweet potatoes and serve immediately.

Yield: 4 to 6 servings

Broccoli in Cheese Sauce

	Standard	Metric
Frozen broccoli spears	1 (10 oz.) pkg.	1 (284 gm)
Medium white sauce	1 cup	250 mL
Grated cheddar cheese	1 cup	250 mL

1. Cook the broccoli in 1/2 cup (125 ml) of boiling, salted water until tender. Drain.
2. Add the cheese to the white sauce and stir over warm heat until the cheese is melted.
3. Place the broccoli on serving platter and pour cheese sauce over. Serve immediately.

Yield: 4 servings

Broccoli Soufflé

	Standard	Metric
Butter or margarine	3 Tbsp.	45 mL
Flour	3 Tbsp.	45 mL
Milk	1 cup	250 mL
Salt	1/2 tsp.	2 mL
Grated American cheese	2-1/2 cups	625 mL
Frozen chopped broccoli, partially thawed	1 (10 oz.) pkg.	1 (284 gm)
Dehydrated onion flakes	1 tsp.	5 mL
Eggs, separated	3	3

1. Preheat the oven to 350° F (175° C).
2. Melt the butter or margarine in a saucepan; stir in flour; cook 1 minute. Gradually stir in the milk and salt. Cook 5 minutes, stirring constantly.
3. Add the cheese; stir until melted. Fold in the partially thawed broccoli and onion flakes. Set the pan off the burner.
4. Beat the egg whites until they are stiff, but not dry.
5. Beat the egg yolks well and stir into the broccoli sauce mixture. Fold in the beaten egg whites.
6. Pour into a 2-quart baking dish with straight

sides. Set the dish in a pan filled with 1/2-inch of hot water. Bake for 45 minutes or until a table knife when inserted comes out clean. Serve immediately.

Yield: 6 servings

——————— Tomato Pudding ———————

	Standard	Metric
Butter	4 Tbsp.	20 mL
Thinly sliced onions	2 cups	500 mL
Sugar	1 Tbsp.	15 mL
Salt	1 tsp.	5 mL
Cooked tomatoes	2-1/2 cups	625 mL
Butter	3 Tbsp.	45 mL
Soft bread crumbs	1 cup	250 mL
Pepper	dash	dash
Grated cheddar cheese	1/2 cup	125 mL

1. Preheat oven to 350° F (175° C).
2. Melt 4 tablespoons butter in saucepan; add the onions and sprinkle the onions with the sugar and salt. Cover and cook the mixture for 25 minutes over low heat. Do not allow the onions to brown.
3. Brown 1/2 cup of the bread crumbs in 3 tablespoons of butter. Set aside.
4. Arrange onions in a 9″ × 9″ baking dish. Add tomatoes, 1/2 cup of bread crumbs, and pepper. Sprinkle the top with the remaining browned bread crumbs and the grated cheese.
5. Bake for 20 minutes.

Yield: 4 servings

——————— Potatoes Lyonnaise ———————

	Standard	Metric
Boiled potatoes, large	2	2
Fat	2 Tbsp.	30 mL
Minced onion	2 tsp.	10 mL
Salt	to taste	to taste
pepper	to taste	to taste
Chopped parsley	1 Tbsp.	15 mL

1. Dice the potatoes.
2. In a heavy fry pan melt the fat. Add the onion and cook until tender.
3. Add the potatoes to the fry pan and season to taste with salt and pepper. Cook the potatoes over medium heat until tender, stirring lightly, to evenly brown the potatoes. Sprinkle with parsley before serving.

Yield: 4 servings

LEARNING ACTIVITIES

1. Investigate a local food store to determine whether the store carries its own brand label on vegetables. If it does, compare the cost between the store brand label and a national brand label. Read the information on the labels to determine the label that is most informative and discuss with the class how this information might affect your choice of purchase.
2. Compare the contents of a national-brand container and two store-label containers of the same vegetable. Check the appearance, color, flavor, and texture of the vegetables to determine if there is any difference. Present the results of your findings to the class.
3. Select a vegetable that is available in fresh, frozen, and canned form. Do a cost comparison of the various forms of the vegetable to determine which would be the best buy. Make a list of other factors that might influence which form you would purchase.

4. Prepare the vegetable selected in number 3 by boiling each form of the vegetable. Compare the differences in flavor and texture between the different forms.

5. Bake one potato in its skin and another steamed in foil to determine if there is a difference in the texture and flavor between the two.

6. Compare the cost of a serving of fresh potatoes against the cost of a serving of dehydrated potatoes and determine which is more costly.

7. Cook and mash a fresh potato and prepare a serving of dehydrated potato flakes and compare the flavor and texture of the two products.

8. Plan a menu in which most of the daily need of ascorbic acid is contributed by a vegetable.

9. Plan a menu in which the daily need for calcium is met by a vegetable. Do not include spinach as a source of calcium.

10. Plan a day's menu in which vegetables account for one half of the female's daily need for iron.

11. Select a vegetable and prepare it by boiling and by steaming. Note the difference in cooking time, flavor, color, and appearance between the two.

12. Prepare a frozen vegetable in a white sauce that you have made, and then prepare a frozen vegetable packed in a white sauce. Summarize the difference in time preparation and in cost between the two.

13. Prepare a variety of vegetables in a deep fryer, practicing the rules of safety.

14. If available, cook one whole carrot in a microwave oven and cook another by boiling. Compare the time of preparation and flavor of the two products.

15. Interview 20 people to determine which vegetables they dislike the most and the reasons for their choices. Make a chart displaying your results.

16. Select a vegetable green that is unfamiliar to you and pan fry it. Note your reactions to preparing and tasting an unfamiliar food.

17. Plan and prepare an oven meal around a baked root vegetable.

18. Develop a pleasing combination of vegetables to be stir-fried. Determine which vegetables, if any, should be cooked first. Prepare and serve the dish.

19. Prepare a vegetable using an additional ingredient with which you are unfamiliar, such as an herb.

20. Prepare a root vegetable by broiling. Partially cook and marinate the vegetable first.

REVIEW QUESTIONS

1. What different parts of the plant are eaten?

2. What is the advantage of eating a vegetable that is high in carbohydrate?

3. What two major nutrients are lacking in vegetables?

4. How can one tell from the color of a vegetable that it is high in vitamin A?

5. Which vegetables are major sources of ascorbic acid?

6. Why are spinach and beet greens not considered good sources of calcium?

7. Why is the potato not a "fattening" food?

8. How can a vegetable give a meal a pleasing appearance?

9. What are some reasons that people develop a dislike for certain vegetables?
10. What is the difference in the nutrient content of fresh, frozen, and canned vegetables?
11. What is the major advantage in purchasing canned or frozen vegetables over fresh vegetables?
12. What are some factors that may influence the purchase of a fresh vegetable?
13. What are some signs that a fresh vegetable is deteriorating?
14. How can one determine if a national brand or a store brand is the better buy?
15. Why are dehydrated onions considered a good buy?
16. How should perishable vegetables be cared for and stored?
17. Why should a green vegetable be stirred several times during the cooking process?
18. How is the color of red cabbage retained?
19. Why are beets cooked in the skin?
20. How can the enzymatic reaction of peeled potatoes be retarded?
21. Why is a thick-skinned vegetable pricked before it is baked in an oven or cooked in a microwave oven?
22. What factors affect the length of time a vegetable is boiled?
23. What is the proper way to cook asparagus?
24. For what types of vegetables is the pressure cooker most suited?

13

Salads

The versatility of the salad in planning nutritious and aesthetically appealing meals comes from the many different foods that can be used in a salad. Salads are important components of brunch, lunch, and dinner menus. They may be part of an afternoon or late evening snack or the featured food for a festive occasion, such as a bridal shower.

Some salads are served hot but most salads are served cold. Most salads are served on a base of greens or the greens are used as the main ingredient. Salads are usually served in medium-sized portions and the pieces are small enough in size to be eaten with a fork.

Nutritional Factors to Consider

Carbohydrate

Salads are high in carbohydrate when the main ingredient of the salad is a food such as potatoes, apples, macaroni, rice, or various legumes. Fruits that have been prepared in a heavy sugar syrup are also a concentrated source of carbohydrate.

Fat

The fat content of a salad comes mainly from the dressings and coatings used to mix the salad. Vegetable oils, mayonnaise, and cream are major ingredients in salad dressings and all have a high fat content.

Protein

Complete protein foods such as meat, seafood, poultry, cheese, and eggs are commonly used in entrée salads. Incomplete protein foods from the pasta, grain, and legume families are combined with a lesser amount of a complete protein food in a salad to provide part of the daily protein requirement.

Vitamins and Minerals

Most fruits and vegetables are excellent sources of vitamins and minerals. The daily need for ascorbic acid might be filled by a serving of cole slaw or by an orange and grapefruit salad. Other important food sources of ascorbic acid that are commonly used in salads include cantaloupe, green peppers, raw green leaves, strawberries, and tomatoes. A salad green used as a base for other salad ingredients would not constitute an adequate daily serving of ascorbic acid, but a generous serving of assorted salad greens could. Deep green vegetables such as asparagus and broccoli and yellow vegetables such as carrots are good sources of vitamin A, whereas leafy green vegetables provide thiamine, riboflavin, calcium, and iron.

Calories

Salads whose chief ingredients are fruits and vegetables are relatively low in calories, but salads in which the chief ingredients are potatoes or starchy foods from the pasta, grain, or legume families are relatively high in calories. Dressings with a high content of salad oil or cream, such as mayonnaise or French dressing, have much higher calorie values than are dressings made from a fruit or vegetable base, such as lemon or tomato juice.

Menu-Planning Points

Inherent Factors

Color. The use of brightly colored fruits, vegetables, and salad greens is an excellent way to add color variety to a meal. Meat, potato, macaroni, and bean salads that have less colorful main ingredients can be brightened by adding garnishes made from carrots, tomatoes, parsley, or green pepper.

Shape. A wide variety of interesting shapes can be achieved in salad preparation. For example, if the tomatoes are sliced, the green pepper can be cut into strips, or if the orange is sectioned, the banana can be cut crosswise. Small fruits such as berries and grapes have a more interesting shape when they are left whole. Large fruits such as pears and peaches are more pleasing when they are cut in half, sliced in small wedges, or cut into chunks.

Texture. Salads can provide the balance in texture that is needed in most meals. For example, meals in which soups or chowders are the entrée and that are served with a crisp vegetable relish tray have a balance in texture. A meal featuring salmon loaf as the entrée would be enhanced with a cole slaw. Salads made from soft fruits like pears and strawberries or a molded tomato aspic complement entrées such as fried chicken, roast beef, or baked pork chops.

Flavor. A meal that is strongly flavored and highly spiced will benefit from an accompanying salad that is mild in flavor. For example, lamb curry goes well with the refreshing flavor of a combination of cantaloupe and watermelon balls. Spaghetti served with a meat sauce is complemented in flavor with a cold, crisp green salad. A mildly flavored entrée like creamed chicken suggests the serving of a tartly flavored salad combination of onion rings and sliced pickled beets.

External Factors

Temperature. Meals are more acceptable if they include a balance of hot and cold foods. A salad most often serves as the cold part of the meal, although the season of the year also dictates the temperatures at which food is served. A variety of chilled salads on a hot summer day could serve as the complete meal for a summer luncheon or dinner.

Preparation Time. A meal preparation schedule should allot time for certain salad ingredients such as greens to be cleaned, dried, and chilled before they are used. When this is done, many fresh salads can be prepared in a short period of time. Quick-to-prepare salads can also be made from canned foods. For example, some canned vegetables and legumes are available in a marinade and some fruits come already mixed. Molded salads take longer to prepare and require a longer setting time before they are ready to serve.

Availability of Ingredients. Since many fresh foods called for in salad recipes are not available in certain geographic locations, or are available only at certain times of the year, substitution of ingredients may have to be made. Some fresh fruits and vegetables are available 12 months of the year but the price of such fruits and vegetables during certain months may necessitate the selection of alternate ingredients. For example, soft fruits such as peaches, melons, and berries and vegetables such as tomatoes may either not be available or may be available only during the summer months.

Tools and Equipment. Kitchen tools such as a sharp paring knife, kitchen shears, a melon-ball scoop, and a set of different-sized graters are assets to creating salads. A colander for draining greens and a cutting board are also important pieces of equipment to have. Many types of food slicers and food blenders can be used to prepare various salad ingredients.

The amount of storage space in the refrigerator is a decisive factor in the type of salads that can be prepared. For example, if the refrigerator is small and has space to store only the basic perishable foods, then it would be unwise to attempt to prepare a large molded salad. The choice of greens may also be restricted because of limited storage space.

Types of Salads

Appetizer Salads

The appetizer salad is served as the first course of the meal and is intended only to whet the appetite. The serving portions of these salads are small but menu planning factors are still important. The appetizer salad is offered as an individual serving or as a tray of selections from which people may help themselves. Appetizer salads may include greens mixed with an oil and vinegar dressing; a fruit cup composed of pears, oranges, and pineapple; or a platter composed of cherry tomatoes, fresh mushrooms, celery sticks, and green pepper wedges served on a plate of greens to which people may help themselves. Figure 13–1 shows a pleasing array of vegetables in a bowl that can serve as an appetizer salad.

Accompaniment Salads

Designed to go with the entrée, the accompaniment salad complements the other foods being served. Fruits, vegetables, and salad greens are the usual ingredients, although the choice of the salad ingredients will depend on the entrée. For example, a casserole of meat and vegetables calls for a salad without multiple ingredients; an appropriate choice would be a tossed salad of greens. A plain fish entrée

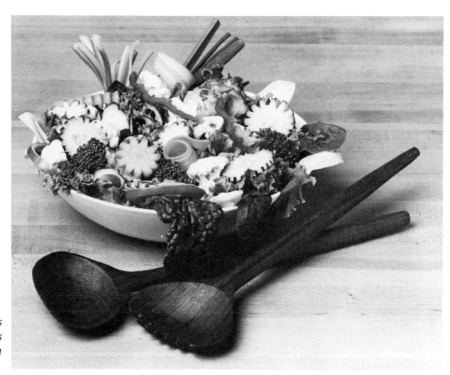

suggests the use of more ingredients in the accompanying salad.

Entrée Salads

The entrée salad, which is the central theme of the meal, is served in larger portions. Entrée salads may be hot or cold. The major ingredient of the entrée salad is either a complete protein food such as chicken, an incomplete protein food such as a pasta that is high in carbohydrate, a starchy vegetable such as potato, or a combination of drained canned fruits which were packed in a heavy syrup.

Dessert Salads

The main ingredient of the dessert salad is canned, frozen, or fresh fruit. Dessert salads, such as a fresh fruit ambrosia, may be served as the refreshing finale to a heavy meal. A molded fruit salad is often served as the entrée for a late evening snack or as the featured food at a party. A dessert salad for a festive occasion is shown in Figure 13-2.

Ingredients

The basic salad ingredients are used in either their fresh, frozen, or canned form. The classic green salad has become a standard part of every American menu in restaurants and in the home. Green salads are used in menu planning for their crisp texture, color, flavor of greens, and nutritional contribution. Green salads also adapt well to many different and flavorful dressings.

Depending on the geographical location and the season of the year, several kinds of salad

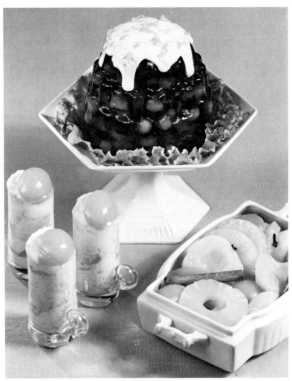

Figure 13-2.
Salads are decorative when served as a dessert. (Libby, McNeil & Libby)

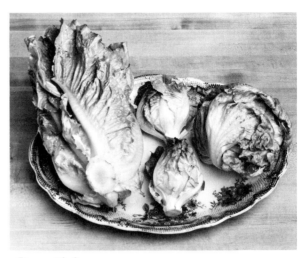

Figure 13-3.
From the left: romaine, leaf, and iceberg—commonly used salad greens.

greens will be available at most local markets. Figure 13-3 shows a variety of salad greens that are usually available.

Greens

Lettuce. Iceberg lettuce, sometimes referred to as "head" lettuce is crisp and compact. Red or green leaf lettuces have a loose-leaf unheaded structure and are mild in flavor. Bibb lettuce is a softly compacted head with a delicate texture and flavor and a light-green color.

Romaine. The outer leaves of romaine, which are dark green in color, contrast with the pale green of the heart. The leaves are rectangular in shape and have a stronger flavor than that of iceberg lettuce.

Curly Endive. This green grows as a spreading plant with branchy leaves that have curly edges. The dark-green leaves are slightly bitter in flavor.

Escarole. This green is a loose-leaf head similar to endive but is characterized by a jagged-edge leaf and a strong flavor.

Spinach. This green, which is normally served as a cooked vegetable, is equally good when served raw in a salad.

Cabbage. The head of a cabbage is tightly compact, light-green or bluish-red in color, and crunchy in texture. Finely shredded cabbage mixed with a dressing is called cole slaw. Figure 13-4 shows cole slaw garnished with a tomato rose.

Other Vegetables

When mixed with greens or served on greens, vegetables provide flavor, color, texture, shape, and nutrition to a salad. Vegetables found in the produce section of a supermarket or a

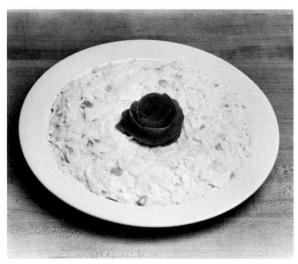

Figure 13–4.
Coleslaw is a nutritious accompaniment to many meals.

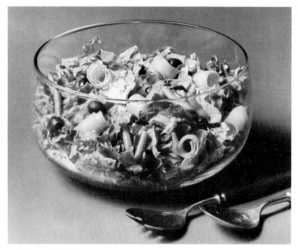

Figure 13–5.
Winter salads use both fresh and canned foods as shown in the salad of greens, carrot curls, canned green beans, and olives.

food store that are acceptable for salads include cabbage, carrots, cauliflower, celery, cucumbers, green onions, green or mild flavored red peppers, lettuce, mushrooms, radishes, and whole or cherry tomatoes. Other vegetables that can be used in salads are Bermuda onions, potatoes, spinach, turnips, and zucchini. Although these vegetables are usually available throughout the year, their price will vary according to the season. Fresh vegetables that are available only at certain times of the year include artichokes, asparagus, and several greens.

Vegetable salads are planned according to the foods that can be economically purchased or for which substitutions can be made. Figure 13–5 shows a winter accompaniment salad using greens, carrot curls, and canned green beans that have been marinated. If tomatoes are too expensive, carrots may be substituted to provide color, flavor, and nutrition. When certain fresh vegetables are not available, canned or frozen varieties, well-drained such as canned or frozen asparagus for fresh may readily be used.

Fruits

Geographical location and the season of the year will dictate the fruits that are available in local areas. However, modern transportation and storage provide a wide array of choices of fruit. Citrus fruits and apples are in plentiful supply all year, whereas soft fruits like apricots, bananas, avocados, berries, cherries, grapes, peaches, pears, plums, and melons vary in their availability.

Fruit salads should be planned according to the season of the year or canned fruits may be substituted. For example, canned peaches and pears are satisfactory substitutes for the fresh fruits. Some fruits such as strawberries and blueberries are available frozen. Frozen fruits are best used in a molded salad because they tend to lose their shape and texture when they are thawed and the gel helps to maintain their shape and texture when they are thawed and the gel helps to maintain their shape. The section of this chapter on molded salads discusses precautions that should be followed in using frozen pineapple.

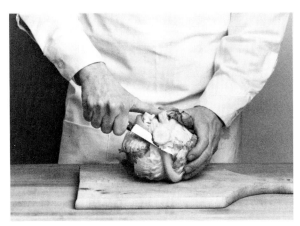

Figure 13-6.

The core of iceberg lettuce is removed with a sharp knife.

Preparation of Ingredients

Greens

The improper care of greens can result in a loss to the food budget, but the proper care and storage of greens will eliminate the need to discard greens because of spoilage. The following steps are the best way to care for greens.

1. Leafy greens are rinsed under cold water to clean off dirt, insects, microorganisms, and chemical residues. Crinkly leaves will open out more if they are rinsed under warm water. Since vitamins and minerals are found in greatest abundance in the outer leaves, only those leaves that show damage should be discarded.

2. The core of iceberg lettuce is removed with a sharp knife. The proper method for removing the core is illustrated in Figure 13-6. The cored side is held under running water to clean and remove the leaves easily. The separated leaves can be used as lettuce cups.

3. Excess water is drained from the leaves by laying them on paper or on cloth towels; water may also be removed by draining the greens in a colander or a wire basket. Water that is left on leaves causes brown spots called rust to form and hastens spoilage.

4. Salad greens may be stored in the drawers of a refrigerator in plastic bags. If the greens are not completely dry before they are stored, they may be wrapped in paper or cloth towels to absorb the excess moisture. Towels should be removed in 1 or 2 days as they draw moisture from the leaves. In turn, the towels become a wet surface that causes rust to develop on the greens.

5. Parsley keeps best when it is placed in a glass of water with a loose-fitting cover in the refrigerator.

A crisp, well-chilled green salad is best when the greens are torn shortly before the salad is served. Depending upon the type of greens and the salad being prepared, it is also proper to cut the greens. For example, cabbage is sliced or shredded. Cut or torn, the greens should be bite-size. Since the crispness of greens may be lost after 3 or 4 hours, greens that are prepared in advance should be stored in a plastic bag or in an airtight container.

Other Vegetables

Vegetables may be sliced, diced, shredded, cubed, sectioned, or left whole depending on which are used in the salad. When possible, the skin should be left on vegetables as the greatest quantity of vitamins and minerals is near the surface. Another determining factor is the size and shape that is desired in relation to the other ingredients. At times it is desirable to cook the raw vegetables before adding them to a salad.

Celery. Celery is cut on the diagonal, diced, cut in julienne strips, made into celery fans

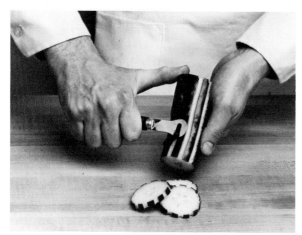

Figure 13-7.

A scored cucumber produces an attractive design on the outer edges when sliced. A zester is the implement used here.

(see garnishes), or left whole for stuffing. Julienne means to cut in thin, matchlike strips. Celery may also be cooked and marinated in an oil and vinegar dressing.

Carrots. Carrots are cut in julienne strips, diced, cut crosswise in a coin shape, shredded, or made into carrot curls (see garnishes). Carrots can be cooked and marinated.

Peppers. Peppers are cut in julienne strips, diced, or cut crosswise for rings. The seeds can be removed from the interior and the whole shell can be used as a container for a salad dressing.

Cucumbers and Zucchini. These two vegetables are cut in strips or sliced crosswise, or the skin can be scored and the vegetable cut crosswise. To score a vegetable means to cut the skin lightly to make lines. The tines of a fork or a zester are best for scoring vegetables. Figure 13-7 demonstrates the scoring of a cucumber and the effect achieved when the cucumber is sliced.

Fruits

Whole Fruits. Smaller fruits like berries and grapes are most often left whole. Not only are they more attractive when they are served in this manner but they also retain more ascorbic acid.

Fruit Sections. Apples and melons are cut into wedges or diced. The peel of an apple that is left on adds more color but melons are most often served with the skin removed. Bananas and avocados are peeled and sliced lengthwise or crosswise. An attractive way to prepare melons is with a utensil that scoops out small melon balls, and avocado balls are made in the same manner. Citrus fruits are sliced crosswise or sectioned. Oranges and grapefruit are more attractive in a salad if the following steps are taken in paring and sectioning them.

1. Skin and white membrane are cut through with a paring knife to expose the fleshy surface. A circular motion is used to remove all of the skin and membrane.
2. The knife should be inserted between the fruit section and the membrane to expose a section of fruit, and sections of fruit are removed without the membrane covering.

Figures 13-8a through 13-9 illustrate the paring of an orange, the removal of a fruit section, the cutting of fruit sections, and decorative touches added to the fruit shell.

Fruits should be prepared just before they are served to aid in vitamin retention. Cutting fruit into pieces and bruising, peeling, and exposing them to air decreases the retention of ascorbic acid. Citrus fruits retain ascorbic acid more readily than other fruits.

Fruits that have a low acid content, such as bananas, apples, avocados, peaches, and pears, will darken after they are cut and exposed to air because of oxidative enzymes that cause a chemical reaction in the fruit. These fruits

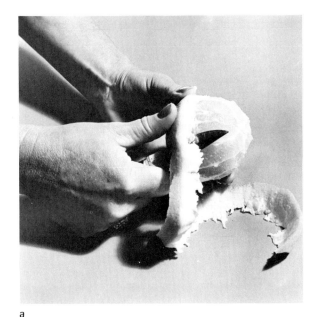

a

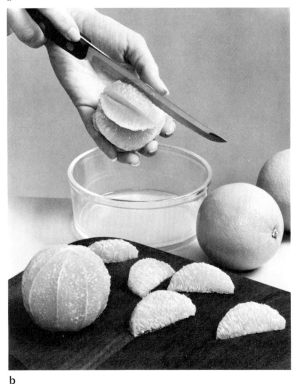

b

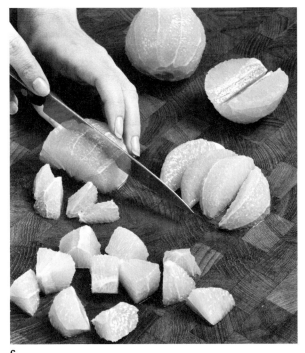

c

Figure 13-8.

(a) To prepare a citrus fruit for sectioning, the skin is removed with a sharp knife, making sure that all of the white membrane is removed. (b) Fruit sections are removed by cutting along the membrane to expose and cut out a fruit section. (c) Citrus can then be cut up into bite-size pieces. ((b) and (c) Sunkist Growers, Inc.)

must be coated with an ascorbic acid solution such as lemon, orange, or pineapple juice or a commercial product to inhibit the darkening process.

Canned and Frozen Fruits and Vegetables

A suitable fruit or vegetable is often not available in fresh form and a canned fruit or vegetable is sometimes selected both for its variety and to save time. Although it is more expensive, a top grade fruit or vegetable is purchased for use because of its size uniformity, freedom from blemishes, and degree of ripeness.

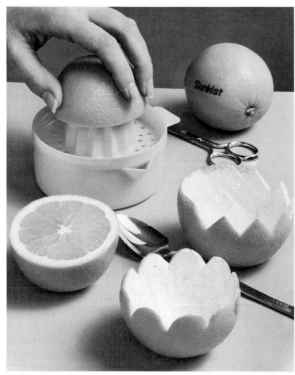

Figure 13-9.
Hollowed out shells can be made decorative containers by cutting the edges with scissors or a sharp knife. (Sunkist Growers, Inc.)

Preparation of Canned Fruits and Vegetables. Canned fruits and vegetables will be best if they are chilled before being used in a salad. To use canned fruits and vegetables in a salad the liquid must first be drained from the food.

Preparation of Frozen Fruits and Vegetables. Frozen fruits are best used in a molded salad, and are usually partially thawed before they are used. Care needs to be taken that the fruits are used immediately after partial thawing so that they do not develop a mushy texture. Fruits frozen in a syrup need to be drained before being used. Frozen vegetables are first cooked and then chilled before being used in a salad.

Marinating. To marinate means to allow foods to stand for an hour or longer, depending upon the flavor preference, in a dressing. Before the food is used in a salad the marinade is drained off. Canned, freshly cooked, or raw vegetables are often marinated. Fresh greens are not marinated because of their tendency to wilt. Suitable fresh vegetables for marinating include cabbage, cucumber, green peppers, onions, and tomatoes. Examples of cooked vegetables that can be marinated include artichokes, carrots, potatoes, beets, cauliflower, asparagus, broccoli, and green beans. Members of the legume family, including kidney beans, garbanzo beans, chick peas, and soybeans, have an appreciable flavor after being cooked and then marinated. Figure 13-10 (a) shows vegetables being cooked in the marinade and 13-10(b) shows marinated vegetables on a platter.

Molded Salads

A molded salad is one whose ingredients are held together by gelatin or another congealing base, such as a cooked starch paste or an egg. These salads can be served as an appetizer, accompaniment, entrée, or dessert salad and are always an attractive highlight.

Gelatin

Gelatin is made from collagen, a protein found in the connective tissue of animals. Collagen is, however, the one animal protein that is incomplete because tryptophan, one of the nine essential amino acids, is lacking. Therefore, gelatin used alone does not make a significant nutritional contribution to the salad. The addition of other ingredients is the determining factor for the salad's nutrient contribution to a meal.

Unflavored Gelatin. Unflavored gelatin is sold in individual packets that contain 1 tablespoon.

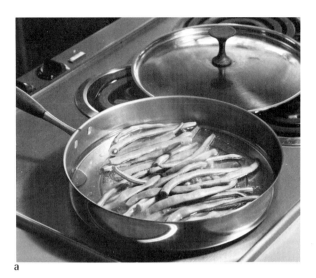

a

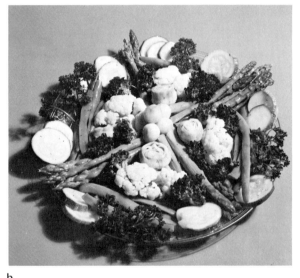

b

Figure 13-10.

(a) Raw vegetables for a marinated salad may first be cooked in the marinade for additional flavor. They are then chilled in the marinade until the salad is prepared. (b). Marinated vegetables are attractive, flavorful and nutritious.

A recipe will often call for 1 tablespoon or one packet of gelatin. To form a gel, the proportions are usually 1 tablespoon of gelatin to 2 cups of liquid. The type of liquid used to dissolve the gelatin and the other ingredients used in the salad will determine the flavor of the salad. The following are the steps to follow to attain a gel from unflavored gelatin.

1. The gelatin granules are mixed with a small amount of cold liquid and allowed to stand a few minutes. Although this technique allows for a better dispersion of the gelatin granules before the hot liquid is added for dissolving, it is not always included in directions.

2. The swelled granules are placed over hot water and the required hot liquid is added and stirred to dissolve. This solution will gel in 2 to 4 hours under refrigeration.

3. If the process must be hastened, part of the liquid can be added in a chilled or frozen form. The more rapidly the solution is cooled, such as by placing the solution in the freezer or in a bowl of ice cubes, the quicker it will gel. However, the resulting gel will break down more quickly when it is exposed to warm air.

4. A recipe that contains more than 2 tablespoons of an acid ingredient such as vinegar or lemon juice per 1 cup of liquid may need an increase of 1–1/2 teaspoons more gelatin per 1 cup of liquid. The reason for this is that acidic ingredients tend to reduce the strength of the gel.

Commercially Flavored Gelatin. The commercially flavored product contains gelatin, sugar, artificial color, and flavoring. It is available in many different flavors and is sold in 3- and 6-ounce packages. A 3-ounce package contains 1 tablespoon of gelatin. Because of the flavoring included, the liquid used for dissolving commercially flavored gelatin is usually water. Preflavored and sweetened gelatin should not be substituted for unflavored gelatin in a recipe. Commercially flavored gelatin mixes are prepared by the following steps:

1. One cup of boiling water is added to the gelatin mix and stirred to dissolve.
2. One cup of cold water is added, and the mixture is then chilled.

Ingredients

To add ingredients to a gelatin base, the gelatin is allowed to chill until it has the consistency of unbeaten egg whites. If ingredients are added before this point they will rise to the surface or sink to the bottom and will not be evenly dispersed throughout the mixture. If the gel is allowed to become too thick, it will become chunky and coarse, which results in a less acceptable product.

Fresh or frozen pineapple contains the enzyme bromelin, which will prevent gel formation. However, if these two types of pineapple are boiled for 2 minutes before they are added to the gelatin mixture, the gelation process will not be affected. Canned pineapple is completely acceptable for use in a gelatin mixture without boiling.

Fruits and vegetables are added to a molded salad to provide color, shape, texture, flavor, and nutritional value. Bits, pieces, chunks, and whole fruits and vegetables are all acceptable for a molded salad and either fresh or canned foods may be selected. Meats, seafood, poultry, and cheeses can be used for the entrée salads, and nuts and pickles are added to add flavor and texture. Many fruits and vegetables can serve as containers for other fruits and vegetables in a molded salad. For example, peach halves can hold blueberries and be molded in a lemon gelatin base, or pear halves can hold cream cheese balls and be molded in a raspberry gelatin base.

Layering different flavors of gelatin and ingredients creates an attractive molded salad. The first gelatin mixture is poured into a mold and chilled until it is just firm. The second layer is prepared and chilled until it is partially thickened, and is then poured over the first layer. This process is repeated until the salad layers are complete. Figure 13-11 shows a layered salad.

Molds

Salads are molded in individual molds or large molds that hold more than one serving. The shape of an individual mold should be a com-

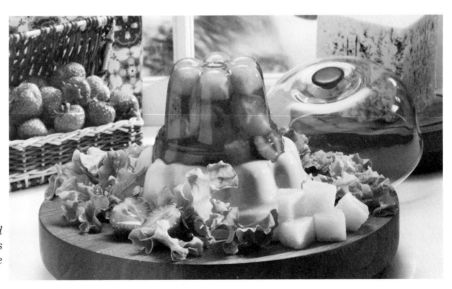

Figure 13-11.
Layering molded salads and adding decorative garnishes make attractive salads. (Castle & Cooke Foods; Dole)

plementary shape for the meal. Ideas for individual molds include custard cups, Mary Ann molds, paper baking cup liners for firmer gelatin mixtures such as salads with a cream cheese base, or fruits and vegetables with firm exterior shells such as green peppers or oranges. Other containers that can be used to mold salads are seashells, small cans, muffin tins, and ice-cube trays.

Square, rectangular, and oval-shaped dishes serve as satisfactory molds for large salads. Other molds include a heart-shaped cake pan for Valentine's day, a fish mold for a seafood salad, a loaf pan, a tube cake pan, or a coffee tin. Mixing bowls of various sizes and shapes are also suitable molds. The size and shape of the mold will affect the length of time required for the gelatin to set.

Prior to putting the ingredients into the mold, it should be sprayed with one of the nonstick products that are available on today's market. The spray prevents ingredients from sticking to the pan when unmolding.

To unmold the salad, the serving plate is rinsed with cold water to help the molded salad to slide easily into position. The mold is then set into warm water for just a few seconds and then removed. The plate is then inverted over the mold and both are turned over. The salad should slide out easily. If it does not, a knife may be run around the edge to allow air under the salad, and the process is repeated. The salad must be refrigerated if it is not to be served immediately and the greens added as garnish just before serving.

Additional Ingredients

Additional ingredients in a salad can provide more texture, flavor, color, shape, and nutrition. Bean or alfalfa sprouts and nuts, either chopped or left whole, may be added to salads, and coconut is a tasteful addition to a fruit salad. A frozen ring of ice with flowers or sea-

shells may become a creative table piece to hold a molded salad. Flavorful herbs add a dash of aroma and spice to many salads. Herbs such as basil, mint, oregano, tarragon, thyme, dill-weed, fresh from the garden or sprinkled from a jar, or combinations of these and other herbs are also good additions to salads.

Toasted cubes of bread, called croutons, are crunchy additions to serve with a green salad. To make 1 cup of croutons, 3 slices of bread are first cut into 1/2-inch cubes, and one-fourth cup of butter is melted in a heavy skillet. The cubed bread is added and stirred to coat the cubes in the butter, and is then toasted slowly over low heat, turning frequently. Croutons can burn easily so they need to be carefully watched. If desired, the croutons can be lightly sprinkled with an herb as soon as they are removed from the pan.

Salad Dressings

The three basic types of salad dressings are French dressing, mayonnaise, and salad dressing. Each has a standard of identity established by the FDA. These dressings can be purchased or they can be prepared at home. All three types of dressing have many variations.

French Dressing

French dressing is composed of a vegetable oil, vinegar or lemon juice, and seasonings like salt, pepper, herbs, sugar, honey, or paprika. The standard proportions for a French dressing are three to four parts oil to one part vinegar. When the dressing is made at home, the basic procedure is to shake the ingredients together in a jar and immediately toss with the salad just prior to serving.

Mayonnaise

Mayonnaise is made from a vegetable oil, vinegar and/or lemon juice, and whole egg or egg yolk. Additional seasoning such as mustard, paprika, and salt are usually added. The whole egg or the egg yolk used in mayonnaise creates a permanent emulsion, which is a dispersion of one liquid in a second liquid in which it does not dissolve. The egg or egg yolk contains an emulsifying agent which keeps the vegetable oil dispersed in the vinegar or lemon juice.

Mayonnaise that is sold commercially must meet the FDA's standard of identity and contain by weight no less than 65 per cent vegetable oil. Since mayonnaise is readily available in the supermarket, most people purchase commercially prepared mayonnaise. The recipe section of this chapter gives ideas for additions to mayonnaise.

Salad Dressing

Salad dressing resembles mayonnaise in appearance but differs in some of the ingredients used and in the method of preparation. The basic ingredients of salad dressing include a vegetable oil, vinegar or lemon juice, whole egg or egg yolk, milk or water, and a cooked starch paste. Some recipes for salad dressing call for the egg to be used as the single thickening agent, but better results are achieved by using a starch agent for thickening.

A commercial salad dressing labeled as such must meet the standard of identity of the FDA and contain by weight no less than 30 per cent vegetable oil and by weight no less than 4 per cent liquid egg yolk or the equivalent. Many flavorful salad dressings can be prepared with ease at home.

Ingredients

Vinegar. A good vinegar is essential to a good salad dressing. Vinegars available on the market include cider, white and red wine, and fruit vinegar. Tarragon- and garlic-flavored vinegar are also popular. Personal choice dictates which vinegar is to be used in the dressing.

Oil. The oil chosen for a salad dressing is a matter of personal preference. Olive oil is expensive, and if it is not used within a short period of time it will develop an off-flavor. Some of the oils sold today in the market are combinations of several different vegetable oils, such as soybean, cottonseed and safflower oil.

Eggs. Eggs are used in making mayonnaise and salad dressing.

Spices and Flavorings. The herbs most commonly used in making salad dressings include basil, oregano, tarragon, thyme, and dillweed, or mixtures of these. Other condiments from the spice shelf used in salad dressings include paprika, cayenne pepper, dry or prepared mustard, Worcestershire sauce, celery and poppy seeds, freshly ground pepper, celery and garlic salt, parsley, onion, and garlic.

Cheeses such as Roquefort and blue add flavor to a salad dressing. The flavor of these two cheeses is similar and they can be used interchangeably. Parmesan or Romano cheese, which can be purchased in bulk or grated form, is sometimes mixed in with the dressing, but most often these cheeses are sprinkled over the salad in grated form just before the dressing is added. Sour cream or plain cream can be used for both thinning the consistency of a salad dressing or as a main ingredient, but they will increase the number of calories in the dressing.

Choice of Dressing

The choice of dressing for a salad will be dependent upon the ingredients of the salad. Salad dressings should complement the flavor of the salad ingredients, and be of a suitable consistency for them. Thick, rich dressings such as Roquefort, blue cheese, and thousand island are suitable for leafy-green salads but are not suitable for most other salads.

A green salad is mixed with the dressing just before the salad is served. A dressing should lightly coat the salad greens but not completely mask them. Potato salad and salads made from pastas and grains are enhanced in flavor by being mixed with the dressing a few hours before the salad is served and is then refrigerated until serving time. Although many molded salads are served with no dressing, some are enhanced by an accompanying dressing.

Garnishes

A garnish is an added decoration or an ornament added to a food to make it more attractive and colorful. Garnishes are the final touch to any food being served. Some garnishes are simple and quick to prepare, whereas others are time-consuming in preparation. Garnishes are most often edible. The following are examples of garnishes that use foods which are commonly thought of as salad ingredients.

Carrot Curls

The carrot is pared to make lengthwise strips, rolled into a circle, and held together with a toothpick as shown in Figure 13-12(a). The curls are thoroughly chilled in ice water. The toothpick is removed and the carrot curl is used as part of a relish tray or as a green salad ingredient.

Carrot and Cucumber Flowers

The carrot is pared first. One-sixteenth gashes are made lengthwise around the carrot or cucumber with a knife or zester. The tongs of a fork may also be used for slashing the cucumber skin. One-eighth inch slices are made crosswise; a toothpick is used for the stem. Carrot and cucumber flowers make attractive vegetable platter garnishes. Carrot flowers are shown in Figure 13-12(b).

Cucumber Slices

The seedy portion of the cucumber is scooped out with a small spoon. The shell is stuffed with a soft-spread filling such as softened cream cheese and chilled. The cucumber is sliced crosswise and served as part of a relish tray or appetizer salad.

Radish Roses

Large, well-rounded radishes are used to make the roses shown in Figure 13-12(c). They are chilled in ice water until they bloom.

Celery Fans

Gashes are made on a 2-inch stalk of celery, on either end to the center with care being taken to not cut through to the other end. The celery is placed in ice water until fans form.

Tomato Roses

With a sharp paring knife the tomato skin is peeled from the pulp in a continuous thin strip. The strip is then coiled to form a rose. Figure 13-12(d) shows the making of a tomato rose.

Turnip Lilies

The same procedure is used as in making carrot curls, but the pared strips of the turnip are rolled in the shape of a cornucopia.

Additional Ideas

Pimiento or cream cheese or a flavorful gelatin base provides a medium for small cutouts to garnish a salad. Green pimiento-stuffed olives cut in slices are an attractive garnish for a salad. Pitted olives provide a holder for julienne strips of carrot and celery. Cheese that has been softened can be molded into petite balls and rolled in parsley.

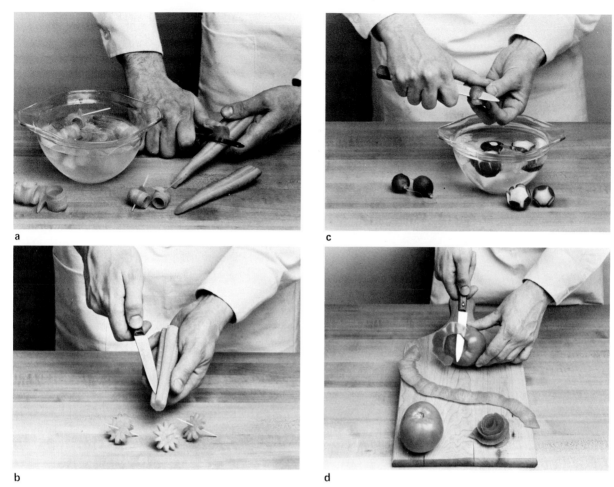

a

b

c

d

Figure 13-12.
Carrot curls, carrot flowers, radish roses, and tomato roses are edible and decorative garnishes.

Serving

Meal Pattern

The appetizer salad is served as the first course of a meal. Accompaniment salads may be served prior to or with the entrée. It is also proper to serve a salad, especially a green salad, after the entrée has been eaten and the entrée dishes cleared from the table.

Serving Dishes or Plates

Many types of dishware make attractive serving dishes for salads. Wooden ware has long been a favorite as a salad serving dish. Some individuals prefer to let their wooden salad bowl season with use and wipe it out after each use. However, wooden salad bowls are attractive for many kinds of salads. Washing the bowl with a mild soap or detergent, rinsing,

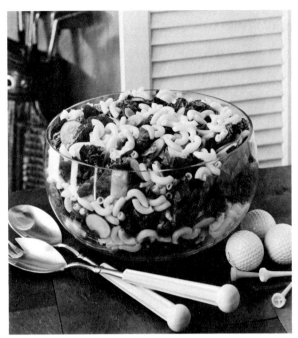

Figure 13-13.
Glass makes an attractive dish for serving, as shown in this combination, leafy green and pasta salad. (National Macaroni Institute)

and thoroughly drying it prevents strong flavors such as garlic from becoming impregnated in the wood. Repeated washing with a detergent can cause a wooden bowl to dry out and crack.

Salads are attractive when served in glassware, and glass platters are particularly pleasing for a large molded salad. A large glass bowl or individual bowls or salad plates are appropriate choices for both green salads and fruit salads. A green salad is attractively served in a glass bowl as shown in Figure 13-13. Ovenproof stoneware and pottery are appropriate choices for hot salads and some cold salads.

Relish Trays

A relish tray is a substitute for a salad and can be served as the appetizer portion of the meal or in place of the accompaniment salad. Vegetable garnishes, marinated vegetables, fruit slices and sections, seafoods, deviled eggs, and cheese cubes or slices can be used alone or in combination to create attractive relish trays. A dip or spread is often included and some type of bread or cracker may accompany the relish tray. Colors are alternated for eye appeal, and the shapes and textures of foods help to create a pleasant appetizing array.

The choices of the serving dish or tray and of the salad green used as a base need to be considered. If a dip or spread is being served as an addition to the tray, a container should be chosen that will not slip when the tray is being passed. If the relish is to be served at the table, it is sometimes better to use several small relish dishes rather than one large tray.

Convenience Salad Food Products

In addition to the various canned fruits and vegetables that are available for salads, some markets may have available precut or shredded vegetables for salads. Many bottled salad dressings and dry, instant forms of salad dressings are also available in a variety of flavors.

———————— French Dressing ————————

	Standard	Metric
Mild vinegar	1/4 cup	60 mL
Vegetable oil	1 cup	250 mL
Sugar (optional)	1/2 tsp.	2 mL
Salt	to taste	to taste
Pepper	to taste	to taste

1. Combine the ingredients in a container with a lid and shake just prior to tossing with the salad ingredients.

Variations

1. To use the French dressing as a marinade for cooked vegetables, increase the vinegar to 1/2 cup and the sugar to 1/4 cup. Let the vegetables stand in the marinade for an hour or longer.
2. The addition of paprika and dry mustard to the basic ingredients gives French dressing a tangy flavor. Herbs such as basil, thyme, or tarragon give a different flavor variation. The type of vinegar used will increase or decrease the dressing's pungency.
3. A sweeter flavor and a thicker consistency is developed by using honey as the sweetening agent. Celery or poppy seeds are flavorful additions to a sweet French dressing. Fruit salads and some vegetable combinations adapt well to this sweeter version.
4. Lemon or lime juice can be used for all or part of the vinegar.
5. The addition of catsup, Worcestershire sauce, and fresh onion, garlic, or horseradish to the basic recipe create a tangy dressing that is also suitable for a meat marinade.

Yield: 1-1/4 cup

———————— Hot French Dressing ————————

	Standard	Metric
Diced bacon	3/4 cup	175 mL
Vinegar	1/4 cup	60 mL
Sugar	1 tsp.	5 mL
Diced green onion	3/4 cup	175 mL
Salt	to taste	to taste
Pepper	to taste	to taste

1. Fry the bacon until it is crisp. Drain on a paper towel.
2. To the bacon fat in the skillet add the sugar and vinegar and bring to a boil.
3. Add the bacon bits and the diced green onion to the salad greens and toss with the hot dressing. Serve immediately.

Yield: dressing for 4 cups greens

The hot French dressing is used to coat fresh garden lettuce or endive. The basic difference from a French dressing is that bacon fat is used in place of the vegetable oil and the dressing is heated before being tossed with the salad greens to create a "wilted lettuce" salad.

———————— Mayonnaise ————————

	Standard	Metric
Egg yolk	1	1
Salt	1 tsp.	5 mL
Dry mustard	1/4 tsp.	1 mL
Olive oil or other salad oil	1 cup	250 mL
Lemon juice or wine vinegar	2 Tbsp.	30 mL

1. Beat the egg yolk, salt, and mustard together.
2. Add the oil a few drops at a time and beat after each addition at the start. Gradually add more oil

and continue beating until the mixture is thick and stiff.

3. Thin with the vinegar or lemon juice.

The ingredients for a mayonnaise should be at room temperature before mixing. It is important that mayonnaise be refrigerated after being prepared as it contains egg and is susceptible to bacterial growth.

Yield: 1 cup mayonnaise

Variations

1. Many flavorful dressings can be made from mayonnaise by adding such ingredients as chili sauce, horseradish, chopped pickles, Worcestershire sauce, or blue or Roquefort cheese.

2. Sour cream combined with mayonnaise makes a creamier dressing for such salads as cole slaw or potato salad.

3. The addition of parsley, onion, anchovies, and a small amount of tarragon-flavored vinegar to mayonnaise makes the dressing known as green goddess.

———————— **Cooked Salad Dressing** ————————

	Standard	Metric
Sugar	1/4 cup	60 mL
Flour	1-1/2 Tbsp.	22 mL
Salt	1/2 tsp.	2 mL
Pineapple juice	3/4 cup	175 mL
Egg, slightly beaten	1	1

1. Mix the sugar, flour, and salt together in a saucepan.

2. Slowly stir in the pineapple juice and cook over low heat until thickened.

3. Add to the slightly beaten egg and return to heat and cook 2 minutes longer.

4. Remove from the heat and add the vinegar. Chill before serving.

Yield: 1 cup

Many molded, frozen, or fresh fruit salads are enhanced with a cooked dressing. Because cooked

dressings contain egg and sometimes milk or cream, it is important that they be stored in the refrigerator until use to prevent the growth of harmful microorganisms.

———————— **Macaroni Salad** ————————

	Standard	Metric
Macaroni, cooked	2 cups	500 mL
Diced celery	1/2 cup	125 mL
Minced onion	1 Tbsp.	15 mL
Diced sweet pickle	2 Tbsp.	30 mL
Eggs, hard cooked	2	2
Lettuce leaves	4	4
Green pepper strips	12	12
Mayonnaise	3/4 cup	175 mL

1. Combine all ingredients except the lettuce and green pepper. Chill.

2. Spoon onto the lettuce cups and garnish with the green pepper strips.

Yield: 4 servings

Variations

1. Add 1 cup diced cheese, 1 cup cooked seafood, 1 cup chopped ham or luncheon meat, or 1 cup cooked meat.

2. Garnish with pimiento strips or tomato wedges.

3. Serve in green pepper cups.

———————— **Rice Salad** ————————

	Standard	Metric
Rice, cooked	2 cups	500 mL
Chopped onion	2 Tbsp.	30 mL
Minced green pepper	1/2 cup	125 mL
Shredded carrot	1/2 cup	125 mL
Diced pineapple	1/2 cup	125 mL
French dressing	3/4 cup	175 mL
Curry powder	1/2 tsp.	2 mL

1. Combine all the ingredients except for the French dressing and curry powder. Chill.

2. Just before serving toss with dressing to which curry powder has been added.

Yield: 3 to 4 servings

———————— Hot Kidney Bean Salad ————————

	Standard	Metric
Canned kidney beans, drained	2 cups	500 mL
Thinly sliced celery	3/4 cup	175 mL
Cubed sharp cheddar cheese	3/4 cup	175 mL
Minced onion	2 Tbsp.	30 mL
Sweet pickle relish	2 Tbsp.	30 mL
Mayonnaise	1/2 cup	125 mL
Dry bread crumbs	1/4 cup	60 mL

1. Combine all the ingredients except the bread crumbs and spoon into four 8-ounce custard cups.
2. Sprinkle with the bread crumbs.
3. Bake at 450° F (230° C) for 10 minutes.

Yield: 4 servings

———————— Seafood Salad ————————

	Standard	Metric
Canned tuna, shrimp or salmon, drained	1 cup	250 mL
Diced celery	1/2 cup	125 mL
Mandarin oranges	1 cup	250 mL
Chopped and unpeeled apple	1 cup	250 mL
Ground walnuts	1/2 cup	125 mL

1. Combine all the ingredients except for the walnuts.
2. Mound on lettuce leaves and garnish with walnuts.
3. May be served with cooked pineapple dressing.

Yield: 3 to 4 servings

———————— Cole Slaw ————————

	Standard	Metric
Mayonnaise	1/2 cup	125 mL
Sour cream	1/4 cup	60 mL
Sugar	2 tsp.	10 mL
Cider vinegar	1 tsp.	5 mL
Shredded cabbage	2 cups	500 mL
Diced cucumber	1/2 cup	125 mL
Minced parsley	2 Tbsp.	30 mL
Salt	to taste	to taste
Pepper	to taste	to taste

1. Combine the mayonnaise, sour cream, sugar, and vinegar.
2. Toss the dressing with the cabbage, cucumber, and parsley. Season to taste.

Yield: 4 servings

Variations
1. Substitute red cabbage for green cabbage or use a mixture of the two.
2. Vary the cole slaw by adding shredded carrot, diced apple, diced green pepper, or thinly sliced cauliflower.
3. The dressing may be changed to a French dressing and changed in flavor by adding celery or poppy seeds.

———————— Garden Salad ————————

	Standard	Metric
Greens, torn in bite-size pieces	2 cups	500 mL
Cucumber, scored and thinly sliced	1/2 cucumber	1/2
Tomatoes, cut in wedges	2	2
Avocado balls	1/2 cup	125 mL
French dressing	1/2 cup approx.	125 mL
Blue cheese, crumbled	2 Tbsp.	30 mL
Croutons	1 cup	250 mL

1. Combine the greens and cucumber slices.

2. Sprinkle crumbled Blue cheese over and lightly toss with the French dressing.
3. Garnish with the tomato wedges and avocado balls.
4. Serve croutons as a salad accompaniment.

Yield: 4 to 6 servings

Marinated Vegetable Platter

	Standard	Metric
Whole green beans, drained, and freshly cooked or canned	2 cups	500 mL
Carrots, sliced crosswise, cooked and drained	2 cups	500 mL
Peas, frozen, cooked and drained	2 cups	500 mL
Asparagus, cooked and drained	2 cups	500 mL
Tomatoes, sliced	2	2
Onion, sliced	1	1
French dressing	1-1/2 cups	375 mL
Carrot curls	8 to 10	8 to 10
Radish roses	6	6
Pimiento strips	4	4
Salad greens	4 to 6	4 to 6

1. In separate dishes marinate the green beans, carrots, peas, asparagus, tomatoes, and onion in the French dressing for 2 hours in the refrigerator.
2. Vegetables may need to be carefully rotated during the marinating time to assure complete coverage.
3. Drain the marinade from the vegetables.
4. Arrange the vegetables in separate lettuce cups on a platter.
5. Garnish the asparagus with the pimiento strips. Garnish the entire platter with the carrot curls and radish roses.

Yield: 4 to 6 servings

Fruit Ambrosia in Orange Cups

	Standard	Metric
Oranges	4	4
Seedless grapes	1/2 cup	125 mL
Miniature marshmallows	1/2 cup	125 mL
Pineapple tidbits, drained	1 cup	250 mL
Flaked coconut	1/2 cup	125 mL
Sour cream	1/2 cup	125 mL

1. Slice 1/2 inch from the top of the four oranges. Carefully remove the orange pulp from the shell of the orange. Remove the seeds and membrane from the orange pulp and dice.
2. Combine the diced orange, grapes, marshmallows, pineapple, and flaked coconut with the sour cream.
3. Chill the mixture and the orange shells for several hours or overnight.
4. Spoon the fruit ambrosia into the orange shells and serve.

Yield: 4 servings

Variation
1. Mandarin oranges may be substituted for the fresh oranges and the chilled ambrosia may be served in lettuce cups.

Tomato Aspic

	Standard	Metric
Tomato juice	2 cups	500 mL
Chopped onion	2 Tbsp.	30 mL
Chopped celery leaves	2 Tbsp.	30 mL
Brown sugar	1 Tbsp.	15 mL
Salt	1/2 tsp.	2 mL
Bay leaf	1	1
Whole cloves	2	2
Unflavored gelatin	1 envelope	1
Water, cold	2 Tbsp.	30 mL
Lemon juice	1-1/2 Tbsp.	22 mL
Finely diced celery	1/2 cup	125 mL

1. Combine the tomato juice, onion, celery leaves, brown sugar, salt, bay leaf, and cloves in a saucepan. Simmer 5 minutes.
2. Strain the mixture in a sieve.
3. Soften the gelatin in 2 Tbsp. cold water and dissolve in the hot tomato mixture.
4. Add the lemon juice and chill until partially set.
5. Add the celery and pour into a 3-cup mold or four individual molds.
6. Chill until set.

Yield: 4 servings

──────── **Layered Fruit Salad** ────────

	Standard	Metric
First layer		
Strawberry gelatin	1 (3 oz.) pkg.	1 (85 gm)
Water, hot	1-1/2 cup	375 mL
Raw cranberries, ground	3/4 cup	175 mL
Ground orange	1/2 cup	125 mL

1. Dissolve the gelatin in hot water. Add the cranberries and orange.
2. Pour into a 2-quart ring mold or a 10 × 5 × 3-inch loaf pan and chill until just firm.

Second layer		
Lemon gelatin	1 (3 oz.) pkg.	1 (85 gm)
Cream cheese	2 (2 oz.) pkg.	1 (170 gm)
Water, hot	2 cups	500 mL

1. Dissolve the lemon gelatin in hot water.
2. Beat in cream cheese until smooth.
3. Let the mixture cool.
4. Pour over the first layer and chill until just firm.

Third layer		
Lime gelatin	1 (3 oz.) pkg.	1 (85 gm)
Water, hot	1 cup	250 mL
Pineapple juice	1 cup	250 mL
Pineapple tidbits, drained	1 (9 oz.) can	1 (255 gm)

1. Dissolve the gelatin in hot water and stir in pineapple juice.
2. Add the pineapple and let cool.
3. Pour over the second layer and chill until firm.

Yield: 6 to 8 servings

──────── **Molded Vegetable Medley** ────────

	Standard	Metric
Unflavored gelatin	1 envelope	1
Water, cold	2 Tbsp.	30 mL
Water, hot	1-1/2 cups	375 mL
Sugar	1/4 cup	60 mL
Salt	1/2 tsp.	2 mL
Lemon juice	1/4 cup	60 mL
Grated carrot	1-1/2 cup	375 mL
Grated cabbage	1/2 cup	125 mL
Diced green pepper	1/2 cup	125 mL

1. Soak the gelatin in cold water.
2. Combine the hot water, sugar and salt, and gelatin in a saucepan and stir constantly over low heat until the gelatin is dissolved.
3. Remove from the heat and stir in the lemon juice.
4. Chill until partially set.
5. Fold in the remaining ingredients and pour into individual molds or a 3-cup mold. Chill until set.

Yield: 4 to 6 servings

LEARNING ACTIVITIES

1. Plan menus for brunch, lunch, dinner, late evening snack, and a festive occasion that include either an appetizer, accompaniment, main entrée, or dessert salad.
2. Analyze and report on the major nutrient contribution that each salad in number 1 makes to the complete meal.
3. Investigate the fresh salad ingredients available at a local market. Determine

which might be considered staple produce items and which might be considered seasonal foods.

4. Prepare a fresh salad from locally available fruits and vegetables. Determine the cost per serving.
5. Prepare a salad from canned vegetables. Determine the cost per serving.
6. Make a marinade and prepare a salad composed of marinated ingredients.
7. Make a list of all the different combinations of fresh fruits and vegetables that can be used in a salad.
8. Plan and prepare a salad that meets a substantial portion of the daily ascorbic acid recommendations.
9. Prepare a tray of vegetable garnishes.
10. Make two gelatin salads, one with an unflavored gelatin and the other with a commercially flavored gelatin with the same flavor in the unflavored gelatin base as the flavoring that is present in the commercial base. Do a flavor and a cost comparison.
11. Prepare three gelatin bases. Chill one in the refrigerator, one in the freezer, and one in a bowl of ice cubes. Compare the time required for gelling and the texture and holding characteristics of the three products.
12. Make up an original combination for a layered gelatin salad. Plan a menu for the salad, and prepare the salad.
13. Plan a summer menu for dinner featuring salads. Include an accompaniment, entrée, and dessert salad.
14. Investigate the availability and cost of special salad-making equipment.
15. Compare the cost and flavor difference between a low-priced and a high-priced commercial mayonnaise.
16. Prepare a French dressing. Add different ingredients and try on different salad combinations. Evaluate the flavors.
17. Prepare a French dressing that has ingredients similar to a commercially prepared French dressing. Compare the flavors and costs.
18. Prepare an entrée salad from the legume family and plan a balancing menu to accompany it.
19. Prepare an individual fruit salad and a cooked dressing to accompany the salad.
20. Prepare a bulletin board demonstrating the proper care of salad greens.
21. Investigate available convenience foods that can be used in salad preparation.

REVIEW QUESTIONS

1. What are the main factors to be considered in planning a salad for a meal?
2. What are some basic characteristics of all salads?
3. What is the difference between an appetizer salad and an accompaniment salad?
4. What are the main nutrient(s) found in the following salads:

Orange and grapefruit salad

Hot macaroni and tuna fish salad

Marinated carrot, green bean, and tomato salad

Molded egg and cheese salad

5. What is wrong with letting moisture remain on greens?
6. When is it wiser to use canned vege-

tables in place of fresh vegetables for use in a salad?

7. What procedure should be used to make a gel from an unflavored gelatin?

8. What steps should be taken to create the proper consistency of a gel before adding the other ingredients? Why is this necessary?

9. What is an emulsion? How does the term *emulsion* apply to mayonnaise?

10. What proportion of oil to vinegar should be used when making a French dressing?

11. For what salads are cooked dressings most suitable?

12. How should mayonnaise and cooked salad dressings be stored? Why?

13. What kinds of major ingredients are used in entrée salads?

14. What are the proper steps to follow in removing a salad from its mold?

15. What types of vegetables make suitable garnishes?

16. What is the difference between a relish tray and a salad?

17. What are four herbs that can be used in a salad dressing?

18. Why does a green salad have fewer calories than a potato salad?

19. What could greatly increase the caloric value of the green salad?

14

Meats

Meat is the popular entrée for most dinners and is frequently eaten for lunch and breakfast and as a snack. There is much to learn about the purchasing, preparation, and storage of the major kinds of meat including beef, veal, lamb, and pork.

Modern technology has improved the breeding and feeding practices of animals so that meats now have less fat and more lean meat per pound, which is highly desirable for a healthy diet. The methods for cutting, packing, and storing meat have also improved, and fresh meat is now available the year around. Federal regulations assure us that the meat we purchase in the market is wholesome.

Meat is cut in a variety of ways, which provides a greater diversity in meat selection and preparation. When meat is cooked properly it is a flavorful and nutritious component of a meal.

Nutritional Factors to Consider

Carbohydrate

Meats contain little carbohydrate.

Fat

The fat content of meat is dependent on the kind of meat, its grade, and the cut. Beef and pork have a larger percentage of fat to lean than do veal and lamb. Prime and choice grades have more fat than meat that is graded *good*. Some less tender cuts of meat, such as short ribs or a blade cut pot roast, have a high percentage of fat, but top-graded tender cuts, such as a rib or porterhouse steak, also have a high percentage of fat. It is advisable to trim excess fat from meat before the meat is cooked.

Protein

Meat contains the nine essential amino acids and is a high-quality protein food. One 3-1/2-ounce serving of lean meat supplies an average of 30 grams of protein; the average man, 23 years of age or older, requires only 56 grams of protein per day. The average female, 19 years of age or older, requires 46 grams of protein per day. Thus, by consuming two servings from the meat group, one's daily need for protein is adequately met. However, most Americans consume more than this amount.

Meats are easily digested, with approximately 97 per cent of the protein being absorbed and utilized by the body, whereas plant sources of protein, such as legumes, are only about 78 per cent utilized. This means that smaller portions of meat will provide more and better quality protein to the diet and that small portions of meat added to plant protein sources improve the total protein.

Vitamins and Minerals

Meats are a rich source of most vitamins and minerals. Thiamine, riboflavin, and niacin are present in all meats, with liver being the best dietary source for riboflavin and niacin, and pork for thiamine. Meats are also good sources of the other B vitamins, and liver is an excellent source of vitamin A. Because the B vitamins are water-soluble, the juices left from cooking meats should be used, when possible, in other dishes.

All meats are excellent sources of iron, but the liver and heart are the richest. Other minerals present in meat include phosphorus, potassium, sodium in salted meats, and zinc.

Calories

Approximately 12 per cent of the daily calorie intake is derived from protein foods, and meats account for a good portion of this. As discussed in Chapter 1, protein is essential for certain major body functions, but meats are too expensive to be used as a major source of energy.

Meat cuts vary in calorie content, depending on the amount of fat present. For example, a 3-ounce ground beef patty with 10 per cent fat contains 186 calories, whereas, a 3-ounce patty with a 21 per cent fat content contains 235 calories.

Menu-Planning Points

Inherent Factors

Balance. Meat can balance any menu, nutritionally, because it is a complete protein and is high in both vitamins and minerals. For example, a menu containing a green salad, vegetable, and a bread is balanced with the addition of a meat.

Color. With the exception of some cured meats, most meat is of a grayish color after it is cooked, and other foods of a more colorful nature must be added to make the meal more appetizing. However, cured meats, such as smoked ham or corned beef, have a pinkish color and are complemented with other foods that are not as bright. For example, cauliflower or creamed onions would be good vegetables to serve with these meats.

Shape. A variety of shapes can be achieved by using different cuts of meat. Steaks and chops have a unique shape because of the bone, beef ribs or spareribs add a lengthy shape, and a slice of roast adds a circular shape. Other shape variations can be achieved by using small-sized chunks of beef for stews or kabobs, or in such meat dishes as beef Stroganoff or lamb curry. Meats can also be cut into strips for stir frying. Ground meats can be shaped into balls, patties, or individual or regular-sized loaves, or they can be baked in a ring mold or made into cone-shaped croquettes.

Flavor and Texture. Meat has its own distinctive "meaty" flavor that can be influenced by many factors, including the kind of animal, the grade of the meat, the cut, and the method of cooking. Beef has more flavor than veal because it comes from a mature animal, and mutton has a stronger flavor than lamb for the same reason. Top grades of meat and some less tender cuts contain more fat, which adds to the richer flavor of the meat. In menu planning, tender cuts of meat with a high fat content are complemented by other foods that are not heavy, such as crisp green salads, fresh fruits, and fresh vegetables. Veal, which contains less fat and is less flavorful than beef, can be served in a flavorful cream sauce or can be accompanied by vegetables with a more tangy flavor, such as Harvard beets.

Most veal, pork, and lamb cuts have a fine texture, but beef cuts will have a coarse or fine texture, depending on the grade and cut. Tender cuts of beef that are a prime, choice, or good grade have a fine texture, but less tender cuts, such as pot roasts or shank cuts, may be coarse. Because of the texture of meat, both fresh and cooked fruits and vegetables are good accompaniments for meat dishes.

The flavor and texture of all meats can be changed and sometimes improved by the length of time and the method of cooking, plus the use of additional seasonings. For example, a pot roast can be made more tender and flavorful by adding an ingredient such as onion or garlic during cooking, and by cooking for an extended period of time. The flavor of tender cuts, such as steaks or ground meat patties, is altered slightly by changing the heat source and cooking over a charcoal fire.

External Factors

Age and Culture. Meat is a highly digestible and high-quality protein that is needed for growth and body maintenance. Some cultures do not consume the amount of meat that most Americans do. In many cultures, meat is simply not available and many of these cultures are ravaged by disease and premature deaths because high-quality protein is not available. For others, eating meat is not part of their life-style.

Economics. Meat is expensive, the price of meat being determined largely by supply and demand. Over the past several years, meat prices have continued to rise as land for grazing has become more scarce and as feed and production costs have increased. Some believe that Americans need to reduce their meat consumption to allow more land for the growth of meat alternates to help feed the starving peoples of the world.

Food Availability. Meat is usually plentiful unless the demand overtakes the supply, or unless wholesale prices become so low that farmers do not sell their cattle. However, even when beef is available, the family's food budget may not allow meat purchases.

Space and Equipment. The amount of available refrigerator or freezer storage space is a prime factor to consider when purchasing meat, because fresh meat is a perishable food. The section in this chapter on storage explains this in detail.

A heavy fry pan with a lid, a broiler drip pan and rack, and a roasting rack are necessary pieces of equipment for meat cookery. The use of a meat thermometer allows meat to be roasted with greater accuracy. A pressure cooker and a slow cooker are useful pieces of equipment for the individual who is away from the home all day.

Time Scheduling. Cuts of meat must be cooked according to the time available. Less tender cuts may be a good buy, but they usually take anywhere from 1 to 3 hours of cooking time unless special equipment is available. Tender cuts of meat cook more rapidly, and the time schedule for this meal must be planned so that other foods are cooked when the meat is done.

Inspection and Grading

All meat sold in interstate and intrastate commerce must be federally inspected, or be inspected at standards equal to federal guidelines as set forth in the Federal Wholesome Meat Act of 1967; this is further discussed in the chapter on food safety. Wholesale meat cuts and meat food products that have been Federally inspected are stamped "U.S. Inspected and Passed," a guarantee of the meat's wholesomeness. Because of trimming, this stamp is usually not visible on retail cuts.

Federal grading standards have been established by the USDA, but are not mandatory, as is inspection. If meat is graded by a federal meat inspector, the carcass will bear the U.S. grade shield. Only carcasses or wholesale cuts, and not retail cuts, are graded, and this voluntary service is paid for by the meat packer.

Meat is graded on both its conformation and quality to give some indication as to its tenderness, juiciness, and flavor. Conformation refers to the general shape of the animal. The quality of meat is judged by the maturity of the animal, the amount of fat within the tissue, called *marbling*, and the color and texture of the meat. Federal meat grading is used for beef, veal, lamb, and mutton as a means of identifying differences to the consumer, but is not used with pork. Slight variations of these factors are used, depending on which kind of meat is being graded.

Meat is also graded on its cutability, which means the amount of usable meat a carcass will yield. Cutability is done on a USDA yield scale designated by the numbers 1 to 5. An animal that is graded Yield 1 has a minimum of fat and a high proportion of thick muscle, and thus will yield a high proportion of usable meat. Cutability grading is of particular interest

to the meat packer and to the consumer purchasing wholesale cuts of meat.

Some meat packers and retailers have their own grade-branding system, which may or may not conform in scale to the government grading system, but it is usually a good system for controlling the quality of their products.

The following is a discussion of the five USDA major grades used for beef; Figure 14-1 illustrates the major grades of beef with top loin steaks.

USDA Prime

Prime grade designates meat that is from young, mature animals and is tender, juicy, and flavorful, with a high proportion of marbling. It is most often high-priced and sold to commercial eating establishments.

USDA Choice

Meat graded choice is most often sold to the consumer. Although it contains less marbling than prime, it is still tender, flavorful, and juicy.

USDA Good

A good grade of beef has even less marbling, with a higher proportion of lean. It is slightly less tender, but is a highly nutritious selection.

USDA Standard

This grade has a minimum of fat, is less flavorful and juicy, but because it comes from young animals, it is still fairly tender.

USDA Commercial

A commercial grade of beef comes from a mature animal, and although its fat proportion is similar to prime and choice grades, it is less tender and requires moist heat cookery.

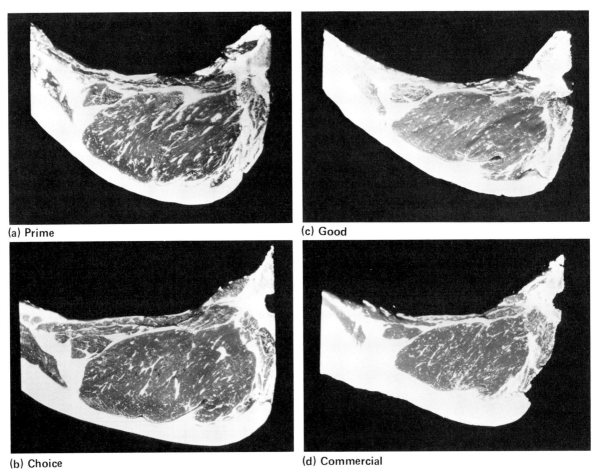

(a) Prime

(c) Good

(b) Choice

(d) Commercial

Figure 14-1.

The characteristics of beef grades are illustrated in these top loin steaks. (Photo: National Live Stock and Meat Board)

Kinds of Meat

Meats are composed of muscle, connective tissue, fat, and bone. Muscle, the lean part of meat, is made up of bundles of fibers; when these bundles are small, the meat has a smooth grain and texture. Connective tissue is the sheath, which holds the fibers together and attaches the muscle to the bone. The more connective tissue there is, the less tender is the meat. Muscles, such as those in the leg of an animal, do more work and contain more connective tissue and less fat; this accounts for these cuts of meat being less tender.

Connective tissue contains two proteins, elastin and collagen. When meat is cooked, the elastin does not change in composition. However, collagen, which is the substance from which gelatin is made, softens and hydrolyzes during cooking. This is the reason that less tender cuts of meat can be made more tender by long periods of cooking.

Fat in meat is either visible or invisible. The outer fat covering of meat and the marbling are visible fats; the fatty deposits within the muscle tissue are invisible.

The age of an animal can be somewhat judged by the bone. Mature animals have white and flinty bone, whereas a younger animal has bone that is porous and of a reddish color.

The color of meat is determined by the amount of the pigment myoglobin that is present. This color varies with both the species and the age of the animal. As animals age, the flesh color deepens from a light pink to a deeper red as seen in the difference between veal and beef.

Beef

Beef comes from mature cattle that are between 15 and 30 months of age. Most cattle are grass fed for 6 to 8 months and are then placed in a feed lot for another 3 to 5 months. However, some cattle are grass fed their entire growing time. Grass-fed animals have a lesser amount of fat than those that are fed in the feed lot.

Another type of beef that is sometimes available is called baby beef. This is grass-fed beef ranging from 7 to 10 months of age. Because there is only a small amount of fat in baby beef, baby beef is less flavorful and juicy than mature beef. The most acceptable forms of baby beef are the tender cuts and ground meat.

Veal

Veal is the name given to beef that is 3 months of age or younger. It is characterized by its grayish-pink color, lack of fat, and large amount of connective tissue.

Pork

Pork is the meat from young hogs, about 4 to 6 months of age; however, pork is usually sold by weight, not age. The color of pork is a light pink, and although the total fat content of pork may be higher than other meats, the amount of fat in the lean portion is about the same as for beef.

Lamb

The meat from young sheep less than a year old is called lamb. This meat is tender, flavorful, and juicy, with a pinkish-red flesh. Mutton is the meat from older sheep. Its stronger flavor and coarse grain make it less desirable than lamb.

Cured Meats

Fresh meats are cured to preserve them and to bring about desirable flavor changes. Curing methods include smoking, drying, or the use of a solution. Meat may be placed in a solution, the solution may be injected into the meat, or the solution may be spread on the surface of the meat. Ingredients used in curing solutions include sugar, salt, sodium nitrite, and spices. Special kinds of wood, such as hickory, are used for smoking.

Some meats are cooked or partially cooked during the curing process; some are cured in a solution and smoked. The label must be read to learn whether or not the cured meat has been cooked. Cured pork may be labeled "partially cooked," "fully cooked," or ready-to-serve." If the curing of pork results in an increase in water of 10 per cent or less, the product must be labeled "water added." If it is more than 10 per cent, the label must read "imitation."

An example of a cured, uncooked beef is "corned beef," which is the brisket cut. "Chipped beef" is cured and dried beef.

Luncheon meats and many sausages are cured and dried, or cured and cooked.

Sausages

A sausage is one or a combination of ground or finely chopped meats stuffed into a casing. Over 200 varieties of sausage are available and sold as fresh, fresh smoked, cooked or cooked smoked, and ready-to-serve. Some of the more popular varieties of sausage include pork sausage or links, bratwurst, frankfurters, pepperoni, and various luncheon meats.

Cuts of Meat

When learning about cuts of meat, it is helpful to think of the shape of the animal and the areas of the animal's body which get the most exercise. The heavily exercised areas have the most connective tissue and fibrous muscle and the least fat, and are the least tender cuts of meat. These areas include the shoulder, leg, and breast sections. The most tender cuts are located along the back section. The kind of animal also determines the amount of fat, connective tissue, and developed muscle. For example, veal is composed almost entirely of connective tissue with minimal fat deposits and, contrary to beef, most lamb cuts are tender because of their lack of connective tissue.

Understanding the wholesale cuts of meat and knowing from which wholesale section a retail cut comes can be a guide to the tenderness of meat and the method of cooking required. The wholesale and retail cuts for beef, veal, pork, and lamb are shown in Figures 14-2, 14-3, 14-4, and 14-5.

The shape of the bone found in retail cuts is similar in beef, veal, pork, and lamb and is an identifiable characteristic when selecting meat. The bone name is also used in the name of standardized retail cuts, such as a T-bone steak, a rib roast, or a blade pot roast. The seven major bones are illustrated in Figure 14-6.

Familiarity with meat cuts can still be confusing if the name of the cut is different in different stores. No federal regulation standardizes the names of various meat cuts throughout the country. However, the retail meat industry has established standard names for approximately 300 cuts of beef, veal, pork, and lamb, and these names have been adopted by many retail stores. The standardized meat label states the kind of meat, the wholesale cut from which it comes, and the retail cut.

Basically, the retail cuts of meat can be classified as ground meat, steaks or chops, ribs, roasts, and variety meats, although there are many variations to this generalization. The following discussion pertains to the most popular and commonly used cuts of meat.

Beef

One of the least expensive and most used forms of beef is ground beef, which is sold in several varying degrees of fat content. Under the standardized labeling system, ground beef can contain no less than 70 per cent lean meat, which is ground from the skeletal sections of the animal; no variety meats can be added. Ground beef may be labeled as "ground beef," "lean ground beef," or "extra lean ground beef." Variations may be labeled as "ground beef chuck" or "ground beef round," thus identifying the section from which the meat is ground.

Flavorful and juicy steaks are cut from the short loin, which contains the tender tender-

Figure 14-2.

[Opposite] Beef Chart, showing where the retail cuts of beef come from and how to cook them. (National Live Stock and Meat Board)

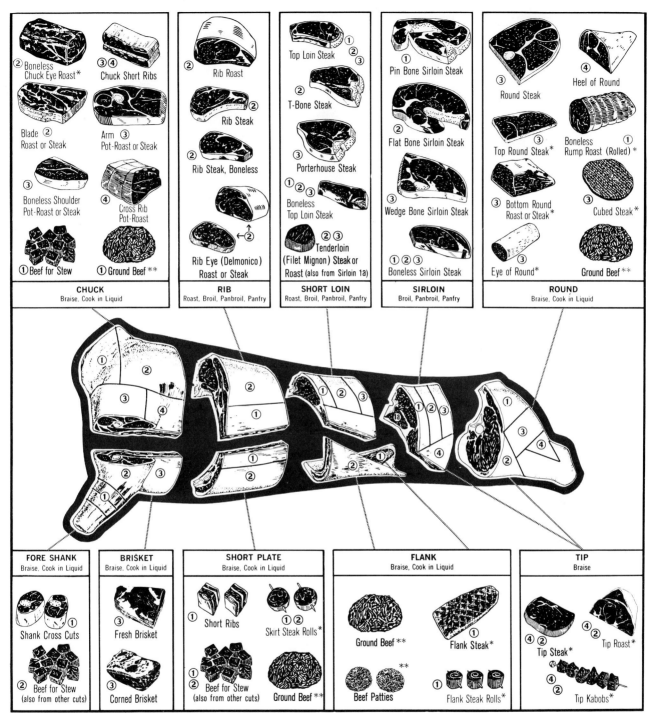

CHUCK
Braise, Cook in Liquid

② Boneless Chuck Eye Roast*
③④ Chuck Short Ribs
Blade ② Roast or Steak
Arm ③ Pot-Roast or Steak
③ Boneless Shoulder Pot-Roast or Steak
④ Cross Rib Pot-Roast
① Beef for Stew
① Ground Beef **

RIB
Roast, Broil, Panbroil, Panfry

Rib Roast
② Rib Steak
② Rib Steak, Boneless
② →
Rib Eye (Delmonico) Roast or Steak

SHORT LOIN
Roast, Broil, Panbroil, Panfry

① ② ③ Top Loin Steak
② T-Bone Steak
③ Porterhouse Steak
① ② ③ Boneless Top Loin Steak
② ③ Tenderloin (Filet Mignon) Steak or Roast (also from Sirloin 1a)

SIRLOIN
Broil, Panbroil, Panfry

① Pin Bone Sirloin Steak
① Flat Bone Sirloin Steak
③ Wedge Bone Sirloin Steak
① ② ③ Boneless Sirloin Steak

ROUND
Braise, Cook in Liquid

③ Round Steak
④ Heel of Round
③ Top Round Steak*
① Boneless Rump Roast (Rolled) *
③ Bottom Round Roast or Steak*
③ Cubed Steak *
③ Eye of Round*
③ Ground Beef **

FORE SHANK
Braise, Cook in Liquid

① Shank Cross Cuts
② Beef for Stew (also from other cuts)

BRISKET
Braise, Cook in Liquid

③ Fresh Brisket
③ Corned Brisket

SHORT PLATE
Braise, Cook in Liquid

① Short Ribs
① ② Skirt Steak Rolls*
① ② Beef for Stew (also from other cuts)
Ground Beef **

FLANK
Braise, Cook in Liquid

Ground Beef **
① Flank Steak*
Beef Patties **
① Flank Steak Rolls*

TIP
Braise

④ ② Tip Steak*
④ ② Tip Roast*
④ ② Tip Kabobs*

*May be Roasted, Broiled, Panbroiled or Panfried from high quality beef.   **May be Roasted, (Baked), Broiled, Panbroiled or Panfried.

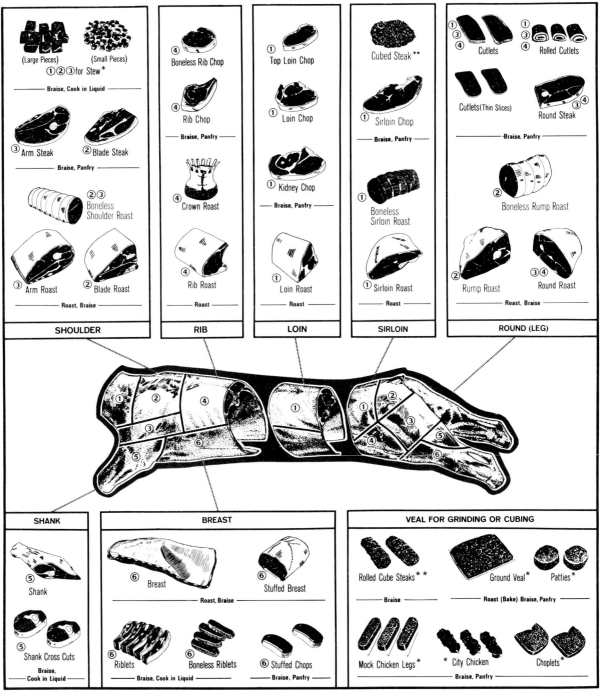

SHOULDER

(Large Pieces) (Small Pieces)
① ② ③ for Stew*
— Braise, Cook in Liquid —
③ Arm Steak   ② Blade Steak
— Braise, Panfry —
② ③ Boneless Shoulder Roast
③ Arm Roast   ② Blade Roast
— Roast, Braise —

RIB

④ Boneless Rib Chop
④ Rib Chop
— Braise, Panfry —
④ Crown Roast
④ Rib Roast
— Roast —

LOIN

① Top Loin Chop
① Loin Chop
① Kidney Chop
— Braise, Panfry —
① Loin Roast
— Roast —

SIRLOIN

Cubed Steak**
① Sirloin Chop
— Braise, Panfry —
① Boneless Sirloin Roast
① Sirloin Roast
— Roast —

ROUND (LEG)

① ③ ④ Cutlets   ① ③ ④ Rolled Cutlets
Cutlets (Thin Slices)   ③ ④ Round Steak
— Braise, Panfry —
② Boneless Rump Roast
② Rump Roast   ③ ④ Round Roast
— Roast, Braise —

SHANK

⑤ Shank
⑤ Shank Cross Cuts
Braise, Cook in Liquid —

BREAST

⑥ Breast   ⑥ Stuffed Breast
— Roast, Braise —
⑥ Riblets   ⑥ Boneless Riblets   ⑥ Stuffed Chops
— Braise, Cook in Liquid —   — Braise, Panfry —

VEAL FOR GRINDING OR CUBING

Rolled Cube Steaks**   Ground Veal*   Patties*
— Braise —   — Roast (Bake) Braise, Panfry —
Mock Chicken Legs*   * City Chicken   Choplets*
— Braise, Panfry —

*Veal for stew or grinding may be made from any cut.   **Cube steaks may be made from any thick solid   piece of boneless veal.

Figure 14-3.

Veal Chart, showing where the retail cuts of veal come from and how to cook them. (National Live Stock and Meat Board)

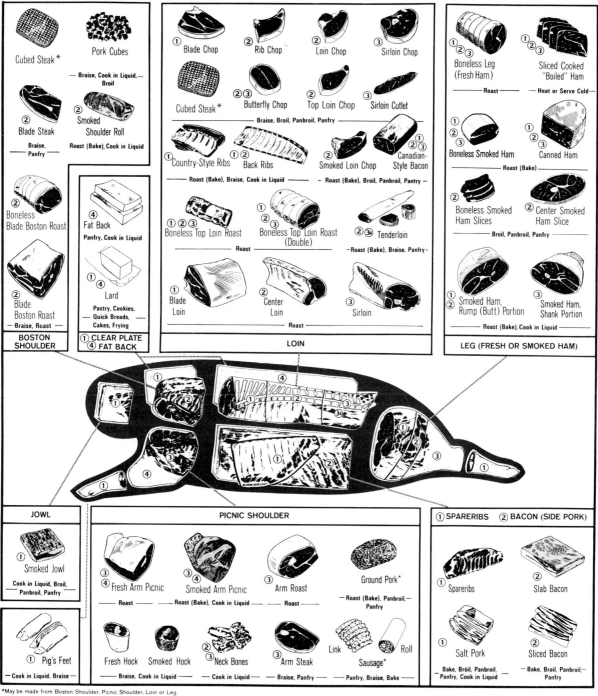

BOSTON SHOULDER

Cubed Steak*

Pork Cubes
— Braise, Cook in Liquid, — Broil

② Blade Steak
Braise, Panfry

② Smoked Shoulder Roll
Roast (Bake), Cook in Liquid

② Boneless Blade Boston Roast

② Blade Boston Roast
— Braise, Roast —

① CLEAR PLATE ④ FAT BACK

④ Fat Back
Panfry, Cook in Liquid

① ④ Lard
Pastry, Cookies, Quick Breads, Cakes, Frying

LOIN

① Blade Chop
② Rib Chop
② Loin Chop
③ Sirloin Chop

Cubed Steak*
② ③ Butterfly Chop
② Top Loin Chop
③ Sirloin Cutlet
— Braise, Broil, Panbroil, Panfry —

① Country-Style Ribs
① ② Back Ribs
② Smoked Loin Chop
① ② ③ Canadian-Style Bacon
— Roast (Bake), Braise, Cook in Liquid —   — Roast (Bake), Broil, Panbroil, Pantry —

① ② ③ Boneless Top Loin Roast
① ② ③ Boneless Top Loin Roast (Double)
② ③ ④ Tenderloin
— Roast —   — Roast (Bake), Braise, Panfry —

① Blade Loin
② Center Loin
③ Sirloin
— Roast —

LEG (FRESH OR SMOKED HAM)

① ② ③ Boneless Leg (Fresh Ham)
① ② ③ Sliced Cooked "Boiled" Ham
— Roast —   — Heat or Serve Cold —

① ② ③ Boneless Smoked Ham
① ② ③ Canned Ham
— Roast (Bake) —

② Boneless Smoked Ham Slices
② Center Smoked Ham Slice
— Broil, Panbroil, Panfry —

① ② Smoked Ham, Rump (Butt) Portion
③ Smoked Ham, Shank Portion
— Roast (Bake), Cook in Liquid —

JOWL

① Smoked Jowl
Cook in Liquid, Broil, Panbroil, Panfry

① Pig's Feet
— Cook in Liquid, Braise —

PICNIC SHOULDER

③ ④ Fresh Arm Picnic
③ ④ Smoked Arm Picnic
③ Arm Roast
Ground Pork*
— Roast —   — Roast (Bake), Cook in Liquid —   — Roast —   — Roast (Bake), Panbroil, — Panfry

Fresh Hock
Smoked Hock
③ Neck Bones
③ Arm Steak
Link   Roll Sausage*
— Braise, Cook in Liquid —   — Cook in Liquid —   — Braise, Panfry —   — Panfry, Braise, Bake —

① SPARERIBS   ② BACON (SIDE PORK)

① Spareribs
② Slab Bacon

① Salt Pork
② Sliced Bacon
— Bake, Broil, Panbroil, Panfry, Cook in Liquid —   — Bake, Broil, Panbroil, — Panfry

*May be made from Boston Shoulder, Picnic Shoulder, Loin or Leg.

Figure 14–4.

Pork Chart, showing where the retail cuts of pork come from and how to cook them. (National Live Stock and Meat Board)

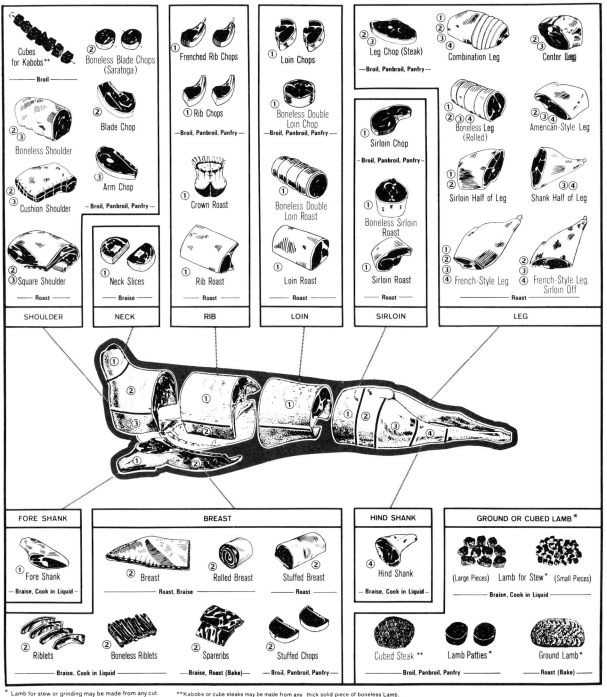

Figure 14-5.

Lamb Chart, showing where the retail cuts of lamb come from and how to cook them. (National Live Stock and Meat Board)

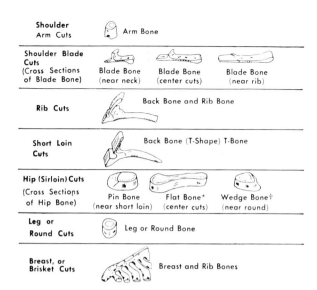

Shoulder Arm Cuts	Arm Bone		
Shoulder Blade Cuts (Cross Sections of Blade Bone)	Blade Bone (near neck)	Blade Bone (center cuts)	Blade Bone (near rib)
Rib Cuts	Back Bone and Rib Bone		
Short Loin Cuts	Back Bone (T-Shape) T-Bone		
Hip (Sirloin) Cuts (Cross Sections of Hip Bone)	Pin Bone (near short loin)	Flat Bone* (center cuts)	Wedge Bone† (near round)
Leg or Round Cuts	Leg or Round Bone		
Breast, or Brisket Cuts	Breast and Rib Bones		

*Formerly part of "double bone" but today the back bone is usually removed leaving only the "flat bone" (sometimes called "pin bone") in the sirloin steak.

†On one side of sirloin steak, this bone may be wedge shaped while on the other side the same bone may be round.

Figure 14-6.

Knowing the seven major bones of meat helps to identify various wholesale and retail cuts of meat. (National Live Stock and Meat Board)

loin muscle. Boneless tenderloin steak is sometimes called "filet mignon." Porterhouse steak contains a large portion of the tenderloin, the T-bone contains a lesser amount, and the club steak contains a very small portion. Sirloin steaks are cut from the sirloin section and are larger in size than other tender steaks. Rib steaks are cut from the rib section. Figure 14-7 shows some of the major tender cuts of steak.

Less tender steaks include the arm steak and the blade steak, cut from the chuck section; the flank steak, of which there are only two in a carcass, cut from the flank section; and cube and round steak cut from the round section. Round steak is sold as a full-cut round, or it is separated and sold as top round, which is the most tender, and bottom round, the least tender. However, the bottom round contains the eye-of-round, which is tender and is some-

times sold separately as thinly sliced steak. Figure 14-8 illustrates the full cut beef round steak, the top round and eye of round steaks.

The most tender roasts are the rib roast and the sirloin. Less tender roasts are the rump and heel-of-round from the round section, the arm or blade pot roasts from the shoulder section, as shown in Figure 14-9, and the brisket. A cross-rib roast is basically a pot roast, boned and tied together.

Other less tender cuts include the cross shank, beef plate, stew meat, and short ribs.

Veal

Veal cuts are similar in name to beef, except that a veal steak cut from the round is often called a cutlet, and other steaks are called chops. Veal cuts, except those from the loin section, are also not as tender as beef because they lack fat. One differing cut of veal is the breast, which is sold as a whole piece.

Pork

Tender pork steaks are called "chops" and come from the loin and rib sections, with the loin being preferred because of the tenderloin portion. The term *steak* is used when referring to the less tender arm or blade steaks. The Boston butt roast is similar to the beef blade pot roast. Fresh or smoked picnic shoulders will yield the most meat when they have a square shape, as this is an indication of plump muscles. The leg of pork is called ham and it is usually cured. The two roasts from ham are the shank and the butt portions. Center-cut ham slices also come from this section. Spareribs and bacon are the other two popular cuts of pork.

Lamb

Ground lamb is a flavorful form of meat. Lamb steaks are called chops; the rib and the loin

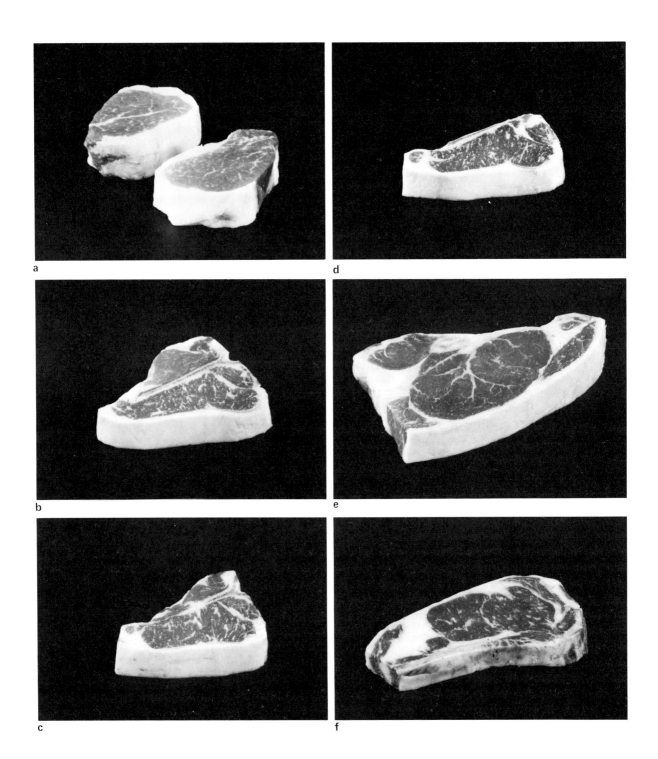

chop are the most tender and the most popular cuts.

The leg of lamb may be sold as one piece, or it may be cut and sold as the sirloin or shank portion. Other roasts are from the shoulder, rib, and loin sections.

Less expensive but flavorful cuts of lamb include the lamb breast, lamb shoulder chops, lamb riblets, and stew meat.

Variety Meats

All kinds of meat have a special segment called variety meats, which are the internal organs of the animal. Variety meats include the heart, liver, brains, kidneys, sweet breads, tongue, and tripe. Each form is highly nutritious and all are inexpensive forms of meat.

Purchasing

Meat consumes a major portion of the food budget for most people, but money can be saved by following some basic rules. Before shopping for meat, a decision must be made on the amount to buy, the tenderness desired, the time available for preparation, and the refrigerator and freezer storage available. It is also helpful, but not always possible, to become acquainted with the people from whom the meat is purchased.

Meat tenderness can be judged by the location of the cut, the shape of the bone, and the store brand or government grade appearing on the meat. Color is also an indicator of the quality and age of beef; beef from an older animal is a darker red. Veal, pork, and lamb are a pinkish color. Since less tender cuts of meat take a longer time to prepare, these cuts are

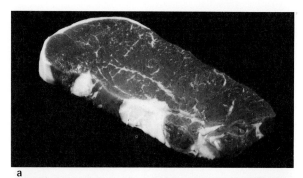

a

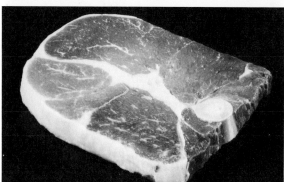

b

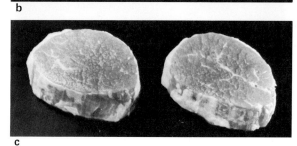

c

Figure 14-8.

A cut up round steak yields:
(a)   the top round
(b)   the round steak
(c)   the eye round
(Photos: National Live Stock and Meat Board)

Figure 14-7. [Opposite]

The tender cuts of beef steak are:

(a) Beef loin Tenderloin steak	*(d) Beef loin Toploin steak*
(b) Beef loin Porterhouse steak	*(e) Beef loin round bone sirloin*
(c) Beef loin T-bone steak	*(f) Beef rib steak small end*

(Photos: National Live Stock and Meat Board)

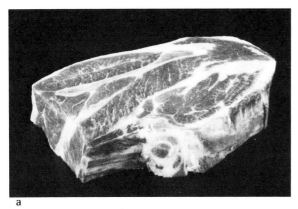

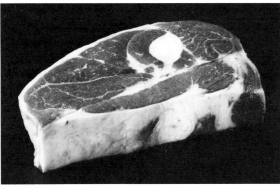

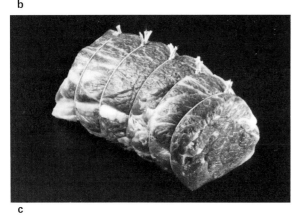

Figure 14-9.

Chuck is an economical cut of meat. The following cuts make excellent pot roast:

  (a) beef chuck blade roast
  (b) beef chuck arm roast
  (c) beef chuck cross-rib pot roast

(Photos: National Live Stock and Meat Board)

often not a wise purchase for the individual who is not home during the day, but a pressure cooker or a slow cooker can hasten the preparation of these cuts.

The usual meat serving is 3 ounces. However, some individuals will consume more meat and some will consume less. A young child would eat less, but a growing teenager would probably eat more. On the average, boneless meat, such as ground meat and flank steak, will yield four servings per pound; meat with small bone, such as round steak, will give three to four servings per pound; and meat with a large amount of bone and fat, such as steaks, spareribs, and short ribs, will yield only one to two servings per pound.

Cost Per Serving

Meat should always be purchased on a cost per serving basis, rather than cost per pound. The number of servings a particular cut of meat will yield per pound should always be figured. For example, a pound of spareribs may serve only one person, whereas a pound of lean ground beef could serve four people. In addition, a more tender, larger, and expensive cut of meat might be a better buy if storage is available because there are more servings per pound and less fat and bone waste. For example, a 3- to 4-pound blade cut pot roast at $1.89 per pound may not be as good a buy as a 4-pound boneless rump roast at $2.25 per pound.

Other Factors

Most stores have weekly meat "specials," which are usually $.10 to $.30 a pound less than the same meat at a regular price. It is smart to read the local food advertisements and plan menus accordingly.

In most recipes, two or three cuts of meat can be substituted for the cut or kind specified, and a decision of which cut to use can

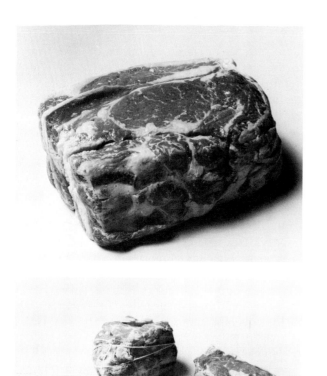

Figure 14-10.
(a) A arm bone roast is an economical beef purchase that can be cut into 3 separate portions to serve 1 or 2 people. (b) The roast can be cut to attain 2 tender steaks, beef chunks for a stew or stir-frying, and a small pot roast.

be made when the prices are checked. For example, bottom round steak, meat from an arm bone pot roast, or flank steak can be substituted for stew meat. Pork shoulder steaks can be substituted in recipes using pork chops and moist heat cookery, and beef cross shank could be substituted for short ribs cooked in a flavor-ful sauce. A lamb or pork shoulder roast can be interchanged with a beef pot roast. If adequate freezer storage is available, larger cuts may be purchased at a saving, cut into the necessary serving size portions, and then frozen. For example, Figure 14-10 shows the method in which a 7-blade pot roast of a 3-1/2″ to 4 inch thickness may be made into three meals for one or two people. Part of a pork loin may be cut into chops and the remaining portion can be used as a roast. A full leg of lamb can be cut in three sections with the large end cut into two or three steaks and the center portion used as a roast. The small end can be boned and the meat can be cut into cubes for kabobs or another lamb dish. Large hams can be cut into two or more roasts, or the center portion may be cut into ham steaks. The butcher will often do this for a small charge or as a courtesy to the customer.

Storage of Meats

Meat is a highly perishable food and all precautions must be taken to keep it safe for eating. The chapter on Food Safety should be reviewed to learn the dangers of unsafe food and bacterial growth.

Refrigerator

Meat should always be stored in the coldest part of the refrigerator or in a special meat compartment. Meat that is prepackaged in transparent wrap can be stored for 1 to 2 days. For storage up to 5 days, the meat should be unwrapped and lightly covered with waxed paper. Meats wrapped in heavy paper should be unwrapped and lightly covered with waxed paper before they are refrigerated.

All cured and ready-to-eat meats as well as canned meats that are marked *perishable* on the label, must be stored in the refrigerator. Most canned and ready-to-eat meats have a "use-by" date on the label, which should be followed to ensure safe eating.

Freezer

Meats are frozen at $0°$ F ($-18°$ C) or lower. Prepackaged meat, if it is to be stored longer than 2 weeks in the freezer, should be re-wrapped. Large quantities of meat should not be frozen at one time as this will raise the freezing temperature. Meats should not be stacked on top of one another until firmly frozen, as this results in slower and improper freezing.

Cured meats should not be frozen, because the seasonings used would cause the meat to become rancid. Meat that is thawed should not be refrozen, as the quality will be less than acceptable. However, frozen meat can be thawed, cooked, and then refrozen without abnormal signs of deterioration.

All fresh meats, except cured and ready-to-eat meats, freeze well and do not lose their quality if they are used within the recommended time period. A guide to freezer storage is provided in the chapter on Food Safety. Partial preparation of fresh meat before freezing can be a time-saver in thawing and food preparation. For example, ground meat can be shaped into patties, balls, or loaves, and other meats can be cut into serving portions or cubed before freezing. With all meats, freezer space can be saved if excess fat and bone are trimmed from the meat before freezing.

Most cooked meats and dishes that contain meat freeze well. These foods should be cooled in the refrigerator, properly packaged and wrapped in moisture- and vapor-proof materials, and frozen. Cooked meats should be used within 2 to 3 months so the date on which the meat was frozen should be clearly marked on the package. The freezing of meats and meat dishes is discussed in detail in the chapter on Food Preservation, which should be referred to.

Freezer Purchasing

When purchasing large amounts of meat for the freezer, several factors should be considered. First, is freezer space available for a large amount of meat? Second, is money available to purchase a large amount of meat without cutting the weekly food budget short for items needed other than meat? Third, how quickly can the meat be used?

Meat for the freezer is sold as a whole carcass, as a half, which includes a front and hind quarter, or as a quarter. Wholesale cuts such as a loin or chuck section may often be purchased. A carcass half or quarter is usually sold by its gross weight, which means that there is an average 25 per cent waste loss in cutting and trimming. It is important to know the cuts from each quarter because the forequarter will yield a large amount of ground beef and pot roasts, whereas the hindquarter will yield more steaks and roasts.

The cost of cutting, wrapping, and quick freezing may or may not be included in the price of the purchase. Meat for freezer storage should always be purchased from a reputable business to assure that what has been paid for is received.

Cookery

Meat is cooked to make it more flavorful and tender and to aid in eliminating bacterial contamination that may be present. However, not all bacterial toxins in meat are eliminated by cooking, so that only fresh meat should be cooked. Meat can be cooked by two methods; moist heat for less tender cuts and dry heat for tender cuts. With both methods the length of cooking time is affected by the grade or initial tenderness of the meat, its size and shape, and the kind of meat. For example, a choice grade of top round may be cooked by dry heat, or thin slices of veal may be cooked very quickly by moist heat. Meat cookery is not as precise as it is for certain baked products, because varying degrees of doneness yield an acceptable cooked meat, and the doneness of meat is mainly a matter of personal preference. However, overcooked meat has a dry texture and is not as flavorful and juicy.

Effect of Cooking

Certain changes take place in a meat's composition when it is exposed to heat.

Protein Structure. Protein is found in the muscle fibers and in the connective tissue of meat. When meat is heated, the protein in the muscle fibers toughens, but this is offset when the protein collagen, in the connective tissue, softens. The elastin in the connective tissue does not change. Consequently, tenderness of meat is, in part, affected by both the proper balance of protein and the length of cooking time.

Less tender cuts of meat have more connective tissue and thus more collagen and require a longer cooking time than tender cuts of meat that have less connective tissue. For example, an overcooked steak can be as tough as an undercooked pot roast.

Changes in Color. As meat is cooked, the interior changes from pink or red to a grayish color as a result of the heat acting on the pigments of the meat. The interiors of some beef and lamb roasts that are cooked to the rare or medium-rare stage still have a pink or reddish color, but the lean interior of veal and pork should show thorough cooking by a light-gray color. The exterior of all meat, whether it is seared or not, changes to a brownish or gray color because of the partial breakdown of fat, proteins, and pigments.

Juiciness and Tenderness. When meat is cooked at a low to moderately low temperature, the meat usually appears to be moist; extended cooking at low temperatures causes the meat to become dry. However, serving these meats in the cooking juices will make the meat more palatable. Meat cuts, such as steak, cooked at a high temperature for a short period of time are usually juicy and tender. Overcooking of these meats creates a dry and tough product. Other factors that affect the juiciness and tenderness of meat include the age of the animal, the length of time the carcass was aged and the amount of fat present. Young animals are more tender that the more mature animal; meat that is properly aged will be more juicy and tender; and the presence of fat around the meat seems to contribute to a meat's tenderness.

Effect of Pretenderization

It is often desirable to make less tender cuts of meat more tender by pretenderizing them. Pretenderizing the meat will also shorten the cooking time.

Pounding and Grinding. Less tender cuts of meat, such as round steak, can be made more tender by pounding the meat with the edge of a plate or with a specially designed malletlike instrument. This same process is done commercially by putting the meat through a machine that lightly grinds the surface. In these processes, both the connective tissue and the muscle fiber are broken down prior to cooking.

Meat Tenderizers. This product contains papain, an enzyme from the papaya fruit, which hydrolyzes the protein and thus makes the meat more tender. The tenderizer is sprinkled over the meat, which is then pierced with a fork to allow the tenderizer to enter the meat tissue. Meat tenderizers are not effective on thick cuts such as roasts. Care needs to be taken to use only the recommended amount of meat tenderizer, as too much tenderizer will make the meat soft and mushy. A commercial

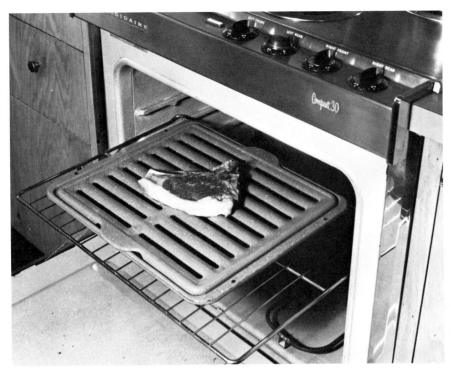

tenderizing method uses the same theory except that the substance is injected into the animal just before it is slaughtered.

Marinades. To induce tenderness and flavor, small chunks of meat or thin, less tender steaks, such as arm blade steak, may be placed in a liquid mixture and allowed to marinate for several hours. The marinating liquid, or marinade, may contain either an acidic food, such as tomato juice or vinegar, or an alcoholic ingredient, such as wine, together with other spices and herbs. Meats should always be marinated in the refrigerator and the marinating time may vary from 2 to 24 hours. An enzyme meat tenderizer may also be added to the marinade.

Dry Heat

Dry heat cooking, which means cooking without a cover and without additional liquid, is used for tender cuts of meat. Broiling, pan broiling, frying, and roasting are the four basic methods of dry heat cookery.

Broiling. To broil means to cook over or under direct heat. Meat that is to be cooked under direct heat is placed on a rack with a drip pan underneath to catch the drippings and melted fat. The meat is cooked 4 to 6 inches from the heat, as shown in Figure 14-11. The thickness or condition of the meat determines how close it should be placed to the heat source. Thick cuts and frozen meats should be placed farther from the heat source so that they cook evenly and do not form hard outer crusts. When the meat is browned on the top side, it is seasoned, if desired, turned over, and cooked to the desired degree of doneness. Doneness may be checked by making a small slash with a knife in the meat, or pressing the meat with a fork. Very rare meat will be soft, medium-done meat will be slightly firm, and well-done meat will be very firm. A meat thermometer may also be used to determine doneness. If the meat has a layer of fat encircling the outer edges, small slits made in the fat before broiling the meat will help to prevent the edges from curling. When broiling meat in an electric range, the door is left ajar for venting purposes; however, the door of a gas range should be left closed.

Cooking meat over direct heat from a wood fire, charcoal briquets, or a gas-ignited flame is a form of broiling, called *barbecuing*. An alternate form of barbecuing is called *rotisserie cooking*. A long rod is inserted into an evenly shaped large piece of meat, usually a roast, and the rod is attached to an electric motor that slowly turns the meat over the fire. Some ovens are equipped with rotisserie units.

When meat is barbecued, it is placed on a rack directly over the heat, and a drip pan is not used. The fat may drip onto the fire and cause the fire to flame up. Lightly spraying the flame with water will put out the flame and prevent the meat from becoming too seared before it is done. In rotisserie cooking it is sometimes possible to use a drip pan.

Meats that are most often broiled are tender beef and lamb steaks, ground meat patties, and bacon. Other cuts that can be broiled are liver, smoked ham, and roasts which are not more than 3- to 4-inches thick. Since veal has a minimum of fat, it is not broiled. Pork is usually not broiled unless it is precooked, since it is important that pork be thoroughly cooked. However, a thin pork chop, approximately 1/2-inch thick, can be satisfactorily broiled. The best results are achieved when other meats are at least 1-inch thick. Although broiling is usually used for tender cuts of meat, less tender cuts, such as blade pot roasts and blade steaks, are good when broiled if they have been first tenderized to help break down the less tender tissue.

Pan broiling. Pan broiling is done in a pan to which no fat or liquid has been added. The meat is placed in the pan and cooked over low heat, turning occasionally, so that both sides of the meat brown. As fat accumulates, it is poured off. When the meat has reached the desired stage of doneness, it is seasoned and served immediately. This method is particularly suited for small, thin pieces of tender meat and ground meat with a fair amount of fat.

Pan frying. Pan frying is a suitable method to cook meats that are low in fat, or meats which have been coated with flour, crumbs, or egg. To pan fry, a small amount of fat is heated in a heavy fry pan and the meat is cooked over moderate heat, turning occasionally, until it reaches the desired stage of doneness. Seasonings may be added during the cooking or after the cooking is completed.

Roasting. Roasting is done by placing the meat on a rack in a shallow roasting pan. The broiler drip pan makes a good roasting pan. If the meat has a fat covering, it should be placed on the rack with the fat side up so that the fat drips through the meat as it cooks.

The length of time to cook a roast is determined by the kind of meat, type of roast, and the weight. Many recipe books contain suggested timetables for roasting meat by minutes per pound. However, a more precise procedure than roasting by minutes per pound is to cook meat to a specified internal temperature by placing a meat thermometer in the thickest part of the roast, making sure that it does not touch any bone. Table 14–1 gives the internal temperature that meat should reach for a desired stage of doneness. The most satisfactory roast is obtained when it is cooked at 325° F (165° C). Figure 14–12 shows the proper placement of a roast on a rack and the insertion of a meat thermometer. When cooking a roast, the time schedule should allow the roast to finish cooking 15 to 20 minutes before serving time, since a roast is easier to carve when the juices have settled. A light covering

Table 14-1

Internal Temperatures of Meat Indicating Doneness

Meat	Internal Temperature
Beef, rare	140° F (60° C)
Beef, medium	160° F (71° C)
Beef, well done	170° F (77° C)
Veal, well done	170° F (77° C)
Lamb, medium	150° F (66° C)
Lamb, well done	180° F (82° C)
Pork, fresh	170° F–185° F (77°–85° C)
Ham, fully cooked when purchased	140° F (60° C)

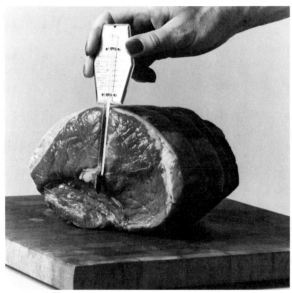

Figure 14-12.

A meat thermometer should be placed in the meaty portion of the meat at about the center, not touching any bone.

with foil helps keep the meat warm during this time period.

Beef cuts that are suitable for roasting include the sirloin tip, rib, and tenderloin. If the beef is of a prime or choice grade, the rump, top round, and eye of round may also be cooked by roasting. Veal cuts include those from the leg, loin, rib, and shoulder. Because lamb is so tender, most large cuts are roasted.

Cuts from pork include rib and loin roasts, spareribs, hams, and picnics.

Moist Heat

The term *moist heat* means to cook in some type of liquid, in trapped steam on top of the range, or in the oven. The meat needs to be cooked in a heavy pan with a tight-fitting lid, or it may be cooked in a slow cooker or in a pressure cooker.

Meats cooked by moist heat include those that have a large amount of connective tissue and little fat, as well as the less tender grades, standard and commercial. The length of cooking by moist heat depends on the cut of meat and varies from 1 to 4 hours. Pressure cookers take much less time; the slow cookers take longer but can be left unattended. The directions in the instruction books for the pressure cooker and slow cooker should be followed. Meats are tender when they are easily pierced with a fork.

The liquid used when cooking with moist heat may be water, stock or broth, vegetable juices, or a sauce such as a mushroom or tomato sauce. Some cuts of meat may not need additional liquid, but care should be taken to avoid excessive browning and the meat sticking to the pan. Meats can also be wrapped in heavy foil and cooked in the oven, or they may be cooked in special plastic bags designed for this purpose.

Because of the longer cooking time, meats develop a rich flavor when they are cooked by moist heat. Additional herbs such as thyme, rosemary, oregano, or basil may be added to achieve flavor variation. Other ingredients that may be added include garlic, onion, green pepper, celery, or carrot.

Braising

To braise is to brown the meat on all sides in a small amount of fat, cover, and cook over

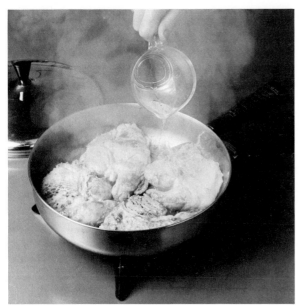

Figure 14-13.
A popular method for cooking pork chops is to brown them in a small amount of fat, add liquid, cover and cook by braising until tender.

low heat or in the oven at 300° F to 325° F (150° C to 165° C). If the meat is very fatty, additional fat may not be needed for browning. The meat may also be lightly coated with flour or crumbs before it is browned. It is better to add liquid, a small amount at a time, when meat is being braised. Figure 14-13 shows pork chops being prepared by the braising method.

Cuts of meat that are commonly cooked by braising include the less tender beef roasts, such as arm and blade pot roasts, and the rump roasts, round and flank steak, veal steaks and roasts, pork chops and roasts, lamb breast, shoulder cuts, and the shank.

Simmering

Less tender cuts of meats that are not browned first are covered with water or stock; the pan is then covered and the meat is cooked at a simmer until it is tender. Some cuts of meat cooked by simmering include corned beef brisket, pork hocks, and meaty soup bones.

Stewing

Stewing is cooking meat that has been cut into 1- to 2-inch cubes in enough liquid to cover the meat. During the last portion of cooking, vegetables such as carrots, onions, celery, and potatoes are added to the meat and cooked until tender. The meat may or may not be browned before the liquid is added.

Variety Meats

Variety meats are prepared either by moist or dry heat cookery, depending on the specific variety meat being used and whether it is beef, veal, pork, or lamb. They are simple to cook and provide a highly nutritious and flavorful variation to a meal. Table 14-2 gives the basic information necessary for the preparation of variety meats.

Cookery Variations

Some meat cuts can be stuffed or rolled with a flavorful dressing before they are braised or roasted. After the stuffing has been added, the meat is tied, skewered, or sewn together so that the stuffing does not fall out during cooking. Any kind of a thick steak or chop of a 1-1/2-inch thickness can be stuffed by cutting an opening or pocket in the muscle. Loin roasts can be stuffed in the same manner, and lamb or pork shoulder roasts can be boned, stuffed, and rolled. The flank steak and the full-cut round steak with the small bone removed can be spread with a stuffing, rolled, and tied. Individual portions of round steak are sometimes pounded flat, then stuffed and tied. Instructions for dressing preparation and ideas for dressing variations are given in the chapter on poultry. Figure 14-14 shows how a flank steak is stuffed and tied.

Table 14-2
Preparation of Variety Meats

Type	Preparation
Liver	Precook liver only if it is to be ground. Beef, veal, and lamb can be broiled or pan fried. Pork and beef liver are braised.
Kidneys	Wash, remove outer membrane, halve, and remove fat and white veins. Veal and lamb kidneys are simmered, braised, and broiled. Pork and beef kidneys are simmered and braised.
Heart	Trim out fibers at the top. Wash in cold water. Beef and veal may be stuffed and braised. Pork and lamb may be braised whole or cut in slices and braised.
Brains	Soak in salted cold water for 15 minutes. Precook in simmering water for 20 minutes. Add 1 teaspoon of salt and 1 tablespoon of lemon juice or vinegar to each quart of water used for precooking. After precooking, follow the recipe directions for serving.
Sweetbreads	Follow the same preparation as for brains, removing any loose outer membrane after cooking. Sweetbreads are braised, pan fried, broiled, or baked whole.
Tongue	Simmer in seasoned, salted water. After cooking, remove the outer skin.
Tripe	Precook in boiling, salted water until tender. Tripe is broiled, braised, or pan fried.

Meat entrées are varied by baking the meat in a pastry or biscuit crust. Cooked ground meat or other cooked meat may be used as the stuffing for a rolled-out rectangle of biscuit dough. The meat and dough are then rolled together, sliced, and baked, as shown in Figure 14-15.

Cooked ground meats and other cooked meats that have been chopped or ground are often used as the main ingredient for many casserole dishes, or a small portion of meat is used to make a complete protein for dishes using a substantial portion of a meat alternate.

Frozen Meats

Frozen meat can be completely or partially thawed, or it can be cooked in the frozen state. It is best to thaw meat in the refrigerator to eliminate the hazard of bacterial contamination. The microwave oven can also be used to defrost meat. For large cuts of frozen meat to cook completely, 1/3 to 1/2 more time must be allowed. Frozen meat that is to be broiled should be low from the heat of the broiler so that it will cook thoroughly without becoming too brown.

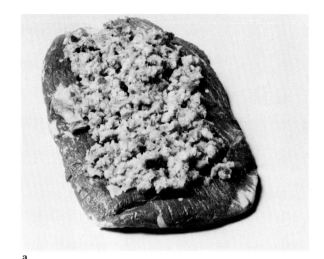

a

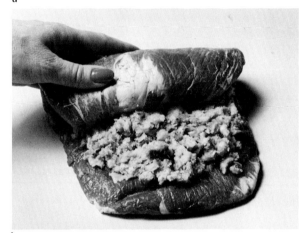

b

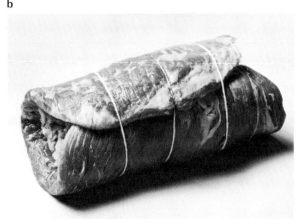

c

Microwave Cooking

The success of cooking meat in a microwave oven depends on the meat's size, shape, and tenderness. Cuts of meat, such as tender steaks and tender, evenly-shaped roasts, and slightly less tender cuts, such as round steak that has been pretenderized, can be successfully cooked in a microwave oven. Bacon, frankfurters, and ground meats are also good when cooked in a microwave oven. Other less tender cuts are not as palatable when they are cooked in a microwave oven because the meat is cooked too fast to allow the connective tissue to soften. However, some microwave ovens feature a slow-cook adjustment by which the cooking time is doubled; this is advantageous in cooking less tender meats. All frozen meats should be completely thawed before being cooked in a microwave oven. To permit even cooking of meat with bone in a microwave oven, the bone should be covered with foil during part of the cooking. If the bone is not covered, the heat absorbed by the bone is transferred to the meat and causes uneven cooking.

Meats that are cooked in a microwave oven in less than 10 minutes or are under 3 pounds do not brown as they do in conventional cooking. However, a mixture of dry onion soup mix and water brushed on the meat can aid in browning; some ovens feature a special "browning dish" that can be used to sear meats. Meats that are cooked longer than 10 minutes will brown, as a result of the changing composition of the meat.

When cooking ground meat in a microwave oven, it is important to keep the meat con-

Figure 14-14.

One example of a stuffed rolled roast is the flank steak which is (a) stuffed, (b) rolled, (c) tied, and cooked by braising until tender.

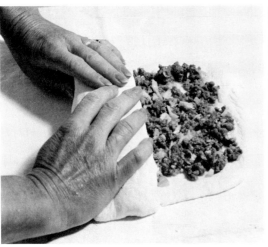
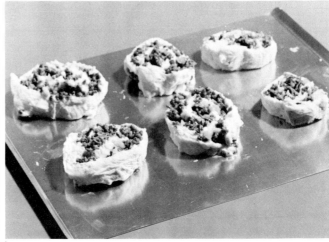

a   b

Figure 14–15.

Biscuit dough filled with cooked ground meat is an economical and nutritious dish to serve. (a) The dough is rolled into a rectangular shape, spread with stuffing, then (b) cut into slices and baked in the oven.

tinuously stirred to assure even cooking. Roasts need to be rotated one-quarter turn part way through the cooking time to assure even cooking and allowance for "carry-over" cooking is most important with all meat cooked in a microwave oven. When cooking roasts, a 10- to 15-minute carry-over time allows the temperature to equalize internally. A specially designed microwave oven meat thermometer may be inserted in the thickest portion of the roast prior to cooking, or a standard meat thermometer may be inserted at the beginning of the carry-over time. If the temperature does not rise sufficiently by the end of the carry-over time, the meat should be returned to the oven for more cooking. Standard meat thermometers must not be used in a microwave oven. Some ovens have a special temperature probe designed to show when the meat is done.

It is helpful to have a specially designed rack to keep a roast out of its own juices while it is cooking. If such a rack is not available, the juices should be poured off periodically while the meat is cooking.

RECIPES

———— **Panbroiling Ground Meat** ————

	Standard	*Metric*
Ground pork, beef, or lamb patties	4–1/2 inch thick	4
Seasoning to taste		

1. Heat a heavy fry pan over low heat, slightly.

Add the ground meat patties. Brown the meat on both sides, turning occasionally.

2. Pour off fat as it accumulates. Cook to desired degree of doneness. Season if desired. Serve immediately.

Yield: 4 servings

Pan Fried Veal Cutlets

	Standard	Metric
Veal cutlets	4, 1/2 inch thick	4
Salt and pepper	to taste	to taste
Fine bread crumbs	1 cup	250 mL
Eggs, slightly beaten	2	2
Fat	3 Tbsp.	45 mL

1. Season the cutlets with the salt and pepper and coat with the bread crumbs; dip into the egg; coat again with the bread crumbs.
2. Melt the fat in a heavy fry pan; add the cutlets and cook over a low heat until browned on both sides. Cooking time is approximately 30 minutes.

Yield: 4 servings

Beef Biscuit Roll

	Standard	Metric
Filling		
Ground beef	1 pound	454 gm
Chopped mushrooms	1 cup	250 mL
Chopped onion	1/2 cup	125 mL
Eggs, beaten	2	2
Salt	1–1/2 tsp.	7 mL
Parsley	1 Tbsp.	15 mL
Crust		
Master mix (refer to chapter on breads)	3 cups	750 mL
Water	1 cup	250 mL
or		
All-purpose flour, sifted	3 cups	750 mL
Baking powder	4–1/2 teaspoons	22 mL
Salt	1 tsp.	5 mL
Sugar	2 Tbsp.	30 mL
Shortening	1/2 cup	125 mL
Milk	1 cup	250 mL

1. Brown meat in a heavy fry pan; drain; add mushrooms, and onion. Cook over low heat until brown, stirring occasionally.
2. Remove from heat and add the egg, salt, and parsley. Cool.
3. If using a Master Mix, combine the dry ingredients and water and proceed with step number 5.
4. Sift the flour, baking powder, salt, and sugar together into a mixing bowl. Cut in the shortening and add the milk to make a soft dough.
5. Roll the dough out on a lightly floured pastry cloth or board to a 1/2 inch thickness.
6. Spread with the meat mixture and roll as for a jelly roll, sealing the ends.
7. Cut the roll into 1-inch thick slices, using a string, and place on an ungreased cookie sheet.
8. Bake at 425° F (220° C) for 20 to 25 minutes.

Yield: 8 servings

Broiled Liver

	Standard	Metric
Beef liver	4 slices, 3/4 to 1 inch thick	4
Salt	to taste	to taste
Pepper	to taste	to taste
Melted butter	3 Tbsp.	45 mL

1. Preheat the oven to broil.
2. Pretreat a broiler pan with a nonstick coating or melted shortening or oil.
3. Place the liver on the broiler pan and brush the top side with melted butter.
4. Cook the liver 2 to 3 inches from the heat source for 5 to 6 minutes. Turn. Brush the top side with melted butter and cook for another 5 minutes.
5. Season with salt and pepper.

Yield: 4 servings

Liver with Mushrooms

	Standard	Metric
Beef, calf, or pork liver	4 slices, 1/2 inch thick	4
Butter or margarine	4 Tbsp.	60 mL
Canned mushrooms	1 (4 oz.) can	1 (113 gm)
Lemon	1/2	1/2
Parsley	2 Tbsp.	30 mL
White wine	1/3 cup	75 mL

1. In a heavy saucepan or fry pan with a lid, melt the margarine. Add the liver and brown on both sides.
2. Add the mushrooms and the juice of the lemon over the liver; add the parsley and white wine. Cover and simmer 15 to 20 minutes or until fork tender.
3. Serve immediately.

Yield: 4 servings

Braised Pork Shoulder Steaks

	Standard	Metric
Pork shoulder steaks	4	4
Dehydrated onion	1 Tbsp.	15 mL
Mushroom Soup	1 (10 3/4 oz.) can	1 (305 gm) can

1. In a heavy fry pan with a lid or an electric skillet, brown the steaks on both sides over a low heat.
2. Add the mushroom soup and onion; cover; cook over a low heat until tender; approximately 1 hour.

Yield: 4 servings

Veal Scallopini

	Standard	Metric
Veal, thin slices	8	8
Flour	1/4 cup	60 mL
Butter or margarine	1/4 cup	60 mL
Onions, sliced thin	2	2

Garlic clove, minced	1	1
Beef bouillon cubes	2	2
Water, boiling	1 cup	250 mL
Dry mustard	1 tsp.	5 mL
Paprika	1 Tbsp.	15 mL
Chopped parsley	2 Tbsp.	30 mL
Butter or margarine	1/4 cup	60 mL
Sour cream	1-1/2 cups	375 mL

1. Lightly coat the veal with flour. Melt the butter or margarine in a heavy fry pan and sauté the onion and garlic until the onion is tender.
2. Dissolve the bouillon cubes in hot water; add the dry mustard and papriks. Set aside.
3. Melt the additional butter in a saucepan; brown the floured veal on both sides over low heat.
4. Pour the bouillon mixture over the veal; add the onion and garlic; cover and cook over low heat for 30 minutes.
5. Stir in the sour cream; heat; serve immediately.

Yield: 4 servings

Individual Stuffed Steaks

	Standard	Metric
Top round steak	4 (4 inch × 4 inch) pieces	4
Dry bread crumbs	1-1/2 cups	375 mL
Grated onion	3 Tbsp.	45 mL
Thyme	1 tsp.	5 mL
Milk	1/3 cup	75 mL
Worcestershire	1 tsp.	5 mL
Catsup	2 Tbsp.	30 mL
Egg, beaten	1	1
Fat	2 Tbsp.	30 mL
Water	1/2 cup	125 mL

1. With a wooden mallet, pound the steak to a 1/4-inch thickness.
2. Mix together the bread crumbs, onion, thyme, milk, Worcestershire sauce, catsup, and egg.
3. Spread the stuffing on each piece of meat. Roll as for a jelly roll and tie with string.

4. Melt fat in a heavy fry pan with a lid. Add the meat rolls and brown over low heat. Add the water and cover.
5. Bake at 350° F (175° C) for 30 minutes or until tender.

Yield: 4 servings

--------------------- Beef Stroganoff ---------------------

	Standard	Metric
Butter or margarine	3 Tbsp.	45 mL
Mushrooms, drained	2 (4 oz.) cans	2 (227 gm)
Chopped onion	1	1
Flank steak	1-1/2 pounds	680 gm
Flour	1/3 cup	75 mL
Butter or margarine	2 Tbsp.	30 mL
Horseradish sauce	1 Tbsp.	15 mL
Water	1/2 cup	125 mL
Worcestershire sauce	1 tsp.	5 mL
Salt	1-1/4 tsp.	6 mL
Pepper	1/4 tsp.	1 mL
Sour cream	1 cup	250 mL

1. Melt the butter or margarine in a heavy fry pan with a tight-fitting lid. Add the mushrooms and onion and sauté until the onion is tender. Remove the onion and mushrooms to a dish.
2. Cut the meat on the diagonal, across the grain, into 1-inch pieces. Coat lightly with the flour.
3. Add the 2 Tbsp. of butter or margarine to a fry pan; melt. Over moderate heat, brown the meat on all sides.
4. Place the onion-mushroom mixture on top of the meat. Add the water, Worcestershire sauce, salt, and pepper. Cover and cook over low heat 1-1/2 hours or until the meat is tender.
5. Just before serving, stir in sour cream.

Variation
1. Bottom round steak or meat pieces cut from an arm bone or blade pot roast may be used. These meats are not cut on the diagonal.

Yield: 4 servings

--------------------- Fruited Lamb Shoulder Chops ---------------------

	Standard	Metric
Fat	2 Tbsp.	30 mL
Lamb shoulder chops	4	4
Orange, thinly sliced	1	1
Lemon, thinly sliced	1/2	1/2
Brown sugar	2 Tbsp.	30 mL
Orange juice	1/2 cup	125 mL

1. Melt the fat in a heavy fry pan with a lid; add the lamb chops and brown on both sides over moderate heat.
2. Layer slices of the orange and lemon over the chops; sprinkle the brown sugar over the top; pour the orange juice over all.
3. Cover and cook over a low heat on top of the range or in the oven at 325° F (165° C) for 1-1/2 hours or until tender. Add more orange juice if needed.

Yield: 4 servings

--------------------- Foil-Wrapped Pot Roast ---------------------

	Standard	Metric
Blade cut pot roast	2 pounds	907 gm
Onion soup mix	1 envelope	1
Butter or margarine	2 Tbsp.	30 mL

1. Preheat the oven to 325° F (165° C).
2. Roll out a piece of aluminum foil long enough to wrap the meat securely.
3. Put 1 Tbsp. of butter or margarine in the center of the foil. Sprinkle one half of the onion soup mix on the foil.
4. Place the meat on top of the butter and soup mix.
5. Place 1 Tbsp. butter on top of meat. Sprinkle the remaining soup mix over the top of the meat.
6. Seal the edges of the foil tightly together. Bake for 2 hours.

Yield: 4 to 6 servings

Meat Loaf

	Standard	Metric
Ground beef	1-1/2 pounds	680 gm
Oats, uncooked	3/4 cup	175 mL
Dehydrated onion	1 Tbsp.	15 mL
Salt	1 tsp.	5 mL
Pepper	1/4 tsp.	1 mL
Tomato juice	1 cup	250 mL
Worcestershire sauce	2 tsp.	10 mL
Egg, beaten	1	1

1. Preheat the oven to 350° F (175° C).

2. Place the ground beef, onion, salt, and pepper in a mixing bowl.

3. Combine the tomato juice, Worcestershire sauce, and egg and pour over the meat ingredients. Mix the ingredients together until thoroughly blended.

4. Pack the meat mixture into an ungreased loaf pan, 8-1/2 × 4-1/4 × 2-1/2 inches and bake for 1 hour. To cook in the microwave oven the meat mixture is shaped into a circle in a glass baking dish and a glass is placed in the center of the ring. The loaf is cooked 6 minutes; the drippings spooned out.

Yield: 4 to 6 servings

Baked Stuffed Pork Chops

	Standard	Metric
Diced apple	1 cup	250 mL
Cooked and finely chopped prunes	1/3 cup	75 mL
Soft bread crumbs	3/4 cup	175 mL
Salt	1/2 tsp.	2 mL
Sugar	1 Tbsp.	15 mL
Butter or margarine	2 Tbsp.	30 mL
Onion, minced	1 Tbsp.	15 mL
Hot water	3 Tbsp.	45 mL
Pork rib chops	4, 1-1/2 inch thick with pocket	4
Water	1/2 cup	125 mL

1. Combine the apple, prunes, bread crumbs, salt, and sugar together in a bowl.

2. Melt the butter or margarine in a heavy fry pan; add the onion and cook until tender.

3. Add the cooked onion and hot water to the apple mixture and blend.

4. Fill the pocket of each pork chop with the stuffing mixture and skewer or close with toothpicks.

5. Add the water to the fry pan; add the pork chops; cover with the lid and bake at 375° F (190° C) for 1 hour. Remove the cover the last 45 minutes. In the microwave, cook uncovered 10 minutes per pound. Rotate cooking dish halfway through cooking time.

Yield: 4 servings

Barbecued Spareribs

	Standard	Metric
Spareribs	3 pounds	1360 gms
Onion, chopped	1	1
Catsup	1 cup	250 mL
Worcestershire sauce	2 Tbsp.	30 mL
Chili powder	1 tsp.	5 mL
Salt	1 tsp.	5 mL
Vinegar	2 Tbsp.	30 mL
Water	1-1/2 cup	375 mL

1. Preheat the oven to 350° F (175° C).

2. Cut the spareribs into serving-size pieces and place in a shallow roasting pan.

3. In a mixing bowl blend together the onion, catsup, Worcestershire sauce, chili powder, salt, vinegar, and water.

4. Pour the sauce over the spareribs and bake for 1 hour or until tender. Baste the ribs with the sauce every 15 minutes. To cook in the microwave oven, arrange ribs in a shallow baking dish with the meaty side toward the outer edge of dish. Add 1/4 c. water and cook 2-1/2 minutes, covering ribs with paper towel and lid. Rotate dish 1/4 turn and cook 2-1/2 minutes; pour off water. Repeat procedure 2 more times. Cover with barbecue sauce and cook 5 minutes.

Yield: 4 servings

Lamb Stew

	Standard	Metric
Fat	3 Tbsp.	45 mL
Lamb, cubed	2 pounds	907 gm
Flour	2 Tbsp.	30 mL
Thyme	1 tsp.	5 mL
Salt	1/2 tsp.	2 mL
Pepper	1/2 tsp.	2 mL
Water	1-1/2 cups	375 mL
Sliced carrots	1 cup	250 mL
Potatoes, quartered	2	2
Onion, sliced	1	1

1. Melt the butter in a heavy fry pan with a lid. Coat the lamb with the flour and brown on all sides in the fat over moderate heat.
2. Sprinkle with the thyme, salt, and pepper. Add the water and cook over low heat for 1-1/2 hours.
3. Add the carrots, potatoes, and onion and cook 30 minutes or until tender.

Yield: 4 servings

Corned Beef

	Standard	Metric
Corned beef	4 pounds	1814 gm
Onion, peeled	1	1
Cloves	4	4
Peppercorns	6	6
Carrot, peeled	1	1
Celery stalk	1	1
Parsley	2 Tbsp.	30 mL

1. Place the corned beef in a large deep kettle and cover with cold water. Bring to a boil and skim off the foam that may accumulate.

2. Stick the whole cloves into the onion and add to the corned beef along with the peppercorns, carrot, celery, and parsley.
3. Cover and cook 3-1/2 to 4 hours or until tender. Remove from the liquid, slice, and serve. To cook in the microwave oven, the corned beef and other ingredients are placed in a casserole dish and covered. The corned beef is cooked for 1 hour, 45 minutes; dish is rotated 1/4 turn each 15 minutes.

Yield: 6 to 8 servings

Spiced Fresh Tongue

	Standard	Metric
Tongue	3 to 4 pounds	1360 to 1814 gm
Vinegar	1/3 cup	75 mL
Salt	2 tsp.	10 mL
Sugar	3 Tbsp.	45 mL
Bay leaves	3	3
Onion	1	1
Whole cloves	12	12
Grated lemon rind	1 Tbsp.	15 mL

1. Place the tongue in a deep pan; add water to cover. Add the vinegar, salt, sugar, and bay leaves.
2. Stud the onion with the cloves and add to the pan together with the lemon rind.
3. Cover the pan and bring to a boil. Simmer over a low heat until the tongue is tender, about 3 hours.
4. Remove the skin. Serve warm or cold.

Yield: 6 to 8 servings

LEARNING ACTIVITIES

1. Plan two 3-day menus in which the average male and female obtain the RDA requirement for protein from meat and two glasses of milk.

2. Plan a menu in which the entrée casserole contains two-thirds plant protein and one-third animal protein; then calculate the total grams of protein pro-

vided in a 3-ounce and a 6-ounce serving of the casserole.

3. Plan a menu that includes liver as the entrée and calculate the milligrams of iron provided in a 3-ounce serving.

4. Calculate your total calorie intake for 1 day and determine what percentage is derived from meat or dairy products. Decide if this percentage is below, above, or within the recommended daily total protein calorie contribution of 13 to 15 per cent.

5. If your total calorie intake is above the recommended percentage, decide how your diet could be changed.

6. Plan four menus using either beef, veal, pork, or lamb as the entrée for each menu. Write an analysis of how the meat, its cut, and its preparation contribute to the shape, flavor, and texture of the menu.

7. Research the reasons why meat prices continue to rise in relation to land availability and food and labor costs, and report to the class.

8. Organize a panel discussion for the class on the pros and cons of why Americans should eat less meat. Present the discussion to the class or to an organized group.

9. Plan a menu and a time schedule by which an individual could complete the cooking of a less tender cut of meat the day before it is to be served for dinner.

10. Investigate local markets in your area to determine if they have instigated the standardized meat-labeling system for retail cuts. Whether the markets have or do not have this system, interview the owner or manager to get his feelings on the effectiveness of the system.

11. Investigate the information provided on labels of cured meats at a local market and report to the class on what you find. Suggest label information that could be more helpful to the consumer.

12. Go to the meat market and determine if you can recognize from the cuts of meat offered the tenderness of the meat and a method for its preparation. Consult your text to see if you were correct.

13. Learn the main bones as illustrated in this text, and see if you can locate these bones on retail cuts of meat.

14. At a local market check the price of a T-bone, sirloin, and flank steak, and decide which would be the best buy for one, three, or four persons, on a cost per serving basis.

15. If a local market carries a roast labeled cross-rib, compare the cost of this roast with a pot roast and determine which would be the best buy on a cost per serving basis.

16. Compare the cost of a beef blade pot roast, arm pot roast, and a boneless rump roast on a cost per serving basis; determine which would be the best buy.

17. Plan a menu using a less tender cut of meat as the entrée. Make a list of different cuts of meat that could be used in place of the one called for in the recipe. Check at the market to determine which meat would be the best purchase on a cost per serving basis.

18. Plan three menus around a store's weekly meat "specials." Calculate the savings between using the meat at a special price and at its regular price.

19. Divide a piece of top round steak into three sections. Cook one piece to the rare stage, one to the medium-rare stage, and one to the well-done stage. Com-

pare the difference in texture, flavor, juiciness, and palatability. Decide which piece is most desirable according to your personal preference.

20. Cut a piece of bottom round steak into three pieces. Marinate one piece for 24 hours in a marinade. The second day tenderize one piece of the steak by pounding and a second piece with a meat tenderizer. Broil all three pieces and determine which is the most flavorful, juicy, and tender.

21. Cut an arm bone pot roast into four sections. Cook one section by the roasting method; do the second section by the braising method, on top of the range adding water as needed; cook the third section by the braising method, using vegetable juice as needed for the liquid; and cook the fourth section in a pressure cooker, following the cooker instructions. Evaluate each piece for tenderness, textural characteristics, flavor and palatability, and length of time to cook. Determine which piece is the most acceptable for your preference.

22. Prepare as a class the different forms of variety meats; taste each form to learn that they are acceptable and flavorful types of meat.

23. Make a list of the ways a cooked meat could be used in a variety of preparations.

24. If a microwave oven is available, prepare a cut of meat in the microwave oven and by a comparable, conventional cooking method. Compare the difference in texture, taste, and palatability.

25. Pan broil a frozen meat patty and a fresh meat patty of the same weight. Compare the length of time that it takes to cook each one.

REVIEW QUESTIONS

1. What makes meat a high-quality protein?
2. What is the average difference between animal and plant protein digestibility?
3. What three factors determine the fat content of meat?
4. What meat is the best source of thiamine?
5. Which cuts of meat are richest in iron?
6. Why should meats not be considered a major source of energy?
7. What are four ways that shape variety can be achieved by using meat in a menu?
8. What are the flavor and texture characteristics of overcooked meats?
9. Why does meat continue to be expensive?
10. What does the stamp "U.S. Inspected and Passed" tell the consumer?
11. Who pays for the federal grading of meat?
12. What is the difference between quality and yield grading?
13. What are the five major grades of beef?
14. Since choice and commercial grades of beef contain the same proportion of fat, why is a commercial grade less tender?
15. What are the four components of meat?
16. What are the two substances of which connective tissue are made?
17. How are these substances changed in cooking?
18. How can the age of an animal be judged by the bone's appearance?

19. What is the difference in the compositions of an animal that is entirely grass-fed and one that is partially fed in a feed lot?
20. What is meant by baby beef?
21. What is the difference between veal and beef?
22. How is meat cured?
23. Why do less tender cuts of meat come from the shoulder and leg sections of an animal?
24. What does the standardized meat label tell the consumer?
25. What is the maximum percentage of fat that ground beef can contain under the standardized labeling system?
26. Why is the porterhouse steak so tender?
27. What are two tender beef roasts and three less tender beef roasts?
28. From what cut of veal does the cutlet come?
29. What is the difference between a pork loin chop and a pork shoulder steak?
30. How can the tenderness of meat be judged when it is purchased?
31. How many servings will meat with a large amount of fat and bone average?
32. How long can fresh meat be safely stored in the refrigerator?
33. Why should meat be purchased on a cost per serving basis?
34. Why are weekly meat "specials" considered a good buy?
35. What three cuts of meat can be substituted for stew meat in a recipe?

36. What three factors should be considered when planning the purchase of a large amount of meat for the freezer?
37. What should be known before purchasing a hind- or a forequarter of beef for the freezer?
38. How should prepackaged meat be wrapped for refrigerator storage after 2 days?
39. How does a long cooking time affect the tenderness of tender and less tender cuts of meat?
40. What are two methods of making less tender cuts of meat more tender before cooking?
41. What are the four basic methods of dry heat cookery?
42. What cuts of meat are particularly suited to pan broiling?
43. What is the difference between pan broiling and pan frying?
44. How is a roast cooked by dry heat? What is the best method to tell when it is done?
45. How does moist heat cookery differ from dry heat cookery?
46. What does braising mean?
47. How does braising differ from simmering?
48. Approximately how much longer than usual should a frozen roast be cooked?
49. Why are less tender cuts of meat not recommended for microwave cooking?

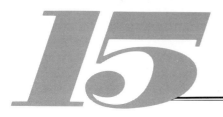

15

Poultry

Poultry is the general term for domestic birds including chickens, turkeys, ducks, geese, and Rock Cornish game hens. In past years, poultry, mainly chickens, were sold as by-products of the egg industry and other kinds of poultry were available only for the Thanksgiving and Christmas holidays. Modern food technology has greatly increased the availability of all kinds of poultry through scientific breeding and mass production.

Poultry can be served in a variety of ways and it is a popular food to serve for entertaining. It is the main ingredient of many casseroles, hearty salads, and flavorful soups, and is delicious when cooked by such methods as frying, barbecuing, and roasting. It has been said that there are more recipes for cooking chicken than for any other kind of food.

Nutritional Factors and Menu-Planning Points

Poultry is a complete protein food, containing all nine essential amino acids. It contains a small amount of carbohydrate and has a lower fat content than other meats. Poultry is an excellent source of the B vitamins, thiamine, riboflavin, and niacin. Because of poultry's low fat content, its calorie content is less than that of the red meats. Turkey, goose, duck, and dark meat have a higher fat content than the flesh of chickens and white meat.

Inherent Factors

Balance. Because of poultry's complete protein value, it can provide the nutritional balance for any meal. For example, two fried chicken legs will provide an average of 24 grams protein and 176 calories. The lower calorie content of poultry is helpful to the weight-watcher who is planning balanced meals.

Flavor. The delicate flavor of young chickens and turkeys makes them excellent foods to combine with more flavorful and pungent herbs, spices, and other strongly flavored foods. Vegetables such as Brussels sprouts or broccoli, which have a rather strong flavor, make good accompaniments to serve with chicken and turkey. The older, more mature chickens and turkeys have a stronger flavor. The broth from cooking older birds makes an excellent base for soups and sauces.

Duck and goose have a stronger flavor and are complemented when they are served with a special addition such as an orange- or plum-flavored coating.

Texture. The texture of poultry, when it is cooked properly is tender and moist. Duck and goose have a slightly drier texture than chicken and turkey, and the older, more mature birds have a tougher and more fibrous meat texture.

External Factors

Chicken is always a good choice to serve as an entrée since most people enjoy this fowl. Chicken has a high degree of digestibility and its texture and flavor have appeal to all ages and all cultures.

Economically, chicken is a wise purchase to help the food budget, and its many available forms provide a variety of choices in menu planning.

Because fresh and frozen poultry needs adequate storage, larger birds should not be purchased if storage space is not available. However, poultry pieces, roasts, and smaller birds such as the Rock Cornish game hens do not take up large amounts of space in the freezer.

If poultry is frozen, the time schedule for meal preparation must allot ample time for thawing. The average time of preparation for ready-to-cook poultry is about 1 hour, but the larger birds that are cooked by roasting may take up to 4 hours to cook.

Poultry Grading

The U.S. Department of Agriculture has set quality-grading standards for poultry, but before poultry can be federally graded it must be inspected for wholesomeness by a federal or federally trained state inspector. Poultry is graded on the basis of its overall appearance, the amount of meat and fat present, and its freedom from skin defects and bruises. Federal grading of poultry is paid for by the processor. For more information on poultry grading see Chapter 3, "Food Safety."

Most birds sold to the consumer are Grade A in quality. Grade B and Grade C poultry are most often sold without the grade mark and are either sold in supermarkets or are used in commercially prepared poultry dishes. The lower grades of poultry are less attractive birds that have less meat and fat.

Specially processed raw forms of poultry such as poultry roasts may also carry the USDA grade.

Kinds of Poultry

Each kind of poultry has several groupings that are based on breed, weight, and age, with the younger poultry having the most tender meat. Chicken and turkey have both dark and light meat and are the most popular, but ducks and geese, which are composed of dark meat, are equally good and nutritious.

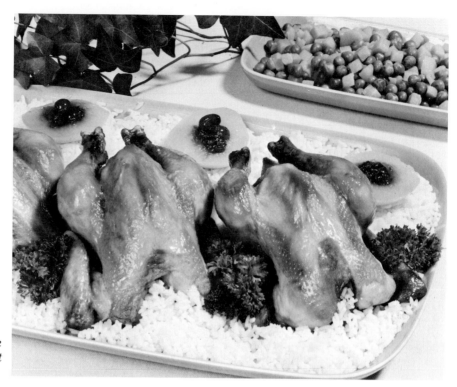

Figure 15-1.
One method to cook Rock Cornish game hens is to roast them (Swift & Co.)

Chicken

There are five different groups of chicken, based on age, weight and sex.

1. The broiler-fryer is the most common and most available. It is a young chicken, 9 to 12 weeks of age and weighs from 1-1/2 to 3-1/2 pounds.
2. The capon is a large desexed rooster, 12 to 18 weeks of age, and weighing 4 to 7 pounds. It has a large amount of white tender meat.
3. The roaster chicken, 12 to 18 weeks of age, usually weighs 3-1/2 to 5 pounds. It has tender meat.
4. The Rock Cornish game hen, 5 to 7 weeks of age and weighing 2 pounds or less, is shown in Figure 15-1.
5. The stewing chicken is a mature bird weighing 2-1/2 to 5 pounds. It has more fat than the others and is less tender.

Turkey

There are two general groupings of turkeys. The young hen and the young tom turkeys are under 15 months of age and average in size from 8 to 15 pounds. Mature or yearling turkeys are older, more mature turkeys, which weigh 15 pounds or more.

Duck

The most common grouping of duck is broiler, fryer, or roasting ducklings. Each is under 6 months of age and averages in weight between 4 and 6 pounds.

Goose

Most geese sold commercially are under 16 weeks of age and weigh from 6 to 12 pounds.

Purchasing

Poultry is sold whole, in pieces, or as roasts or rolls. The kind and amount of poultry to buy depends on the price per pound, the storage facilities available, the desired number of servings, the intended use, the time available for preparation, and personal preference. In purchasing larger birds, such as whole turkeys, the amount of desired planned-overs must also be considered.

Whole

Whole poultry is most often the best buy in price and servings per pound.

If there is personal preference for white or dark meat, or if storage space is not available, purchasing a whole bird would not be economical because of food waste and the small pieces may not be eaten, causing food waste.

The following table gives the approximate amount to plan for each serving when purchasing whole poultry.

Fryers or broilers	1/4 lb. to 1/2 bird
Roasters	1/2 lb. to 3/4 lb.
Stewing fowl	1/2 lb. to 3/4 lb.
Rock Cornish game hen	1/2 to 1 hen

Cuts

Chicken and turkey are most often available in cut form. Chicken and turkey cuts include halves, breasts, legs, thighs, wings, and necks. Chicken and turkey are either sold as whole cut-up birds, or in special groupings such as legs and thighs or wings and necks. Ground turkey meat is also available. The giblets, which are also sold separately, are the liver and giz-

zard of poultry. Figure 15-2 shows the various cut pieces of chicken.

Roasts and Rolls

The most common poultry roast, the quartered turkey roast, includes a leg and a portion of the body. Turkey rolls are available as dark meat, white meat, or a combination. They are relatively expensive, but are quicker to prepare than a whole bird and no waste is involved.

Selection

Fresh poultry should have a creamy-white skin, which does not look coarse or purplish in color and the flesh should feel plump and firm. The skin of frozen poultry should not exhibit any dry areas, and no package of fresh or frozen poultry should be purchased that has been torn or is leaking, since a torn or leaky package creates the danger of microorganisms.

Female poultry has more usable meat per pound and has a better flavor than that of the male in more mature birds, although this has no significance in younger birds. Specially bred "broad-breasted" birds also yield more meat per pound.

Chickens are available fresh, frozen, canned, and dehydrated. There is no difference between the fresh and frozen birds, but if the chicken has been frozen, it should not be refrozen until it is cooked. Canned chickens should be purchased under a familiar label. Because of its cost, dehydrated chicken is a good purchase only when there is a special need or when storage is at a premium, as for a camping or hiking trip.

Most whole turkeys are sold frozen, which increases their availability throughout the entire year. Fresh turkeys are most readily available during the Thanksgiving and Christmas holiday seasons. Some whole turkeys are specially processed with a self-basting solution of butter, broth, or an oil and water solution.

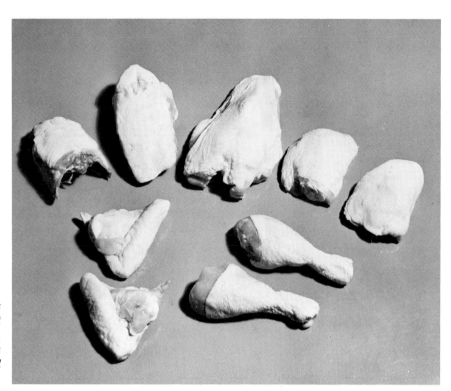

Figure 15-2.
Common cuts of chicken as shown from left to right include the chicken wings, back in two sections, the chicken breast, thighs, and legs.

Increasingly more turkeys are being sold with a built-in heat gauge that "pops-up" to tell when the bird is done. Stuffed frozen turkeys, which are also sold, must not be thawed before they are cooked, and the instructions on the package must be followed carefully. As with most foods, these convenience features add to the cost of purchase.

Because ducks and geese are grown domestically in only certain parts of the country, they are most often sold in whole, frozen form.

Method of Cutting and Deboning Poultry

It is much more economical to cut a whole bird into pieces than to purchase the pieces separately if time is not a hindering factor and if all the pieces will be eaten. Some specialty recipes call for pieces of chicken to be deboned. This too is more economical if done at home, although sharp knives and/or a pair of poultry shears must be on hand to perform these tasks.

Cutting

Before cutting poultry, the giblets and neck are removed from the body cavity. The directions for cutting up and deboning a whole chicken are given and illustrated in Figures 15-3 and 15-4.

After the meat is deboned, it may be flattened to make a cutlet or spread with a stuffing,

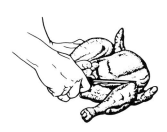

1. Begin by cutting off legs. Cut skin between thighs and body of chicken.

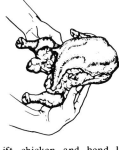

2. Lift chicken and bend legs, grasping one leg with each hand. Bend legs until hip joints are loose.

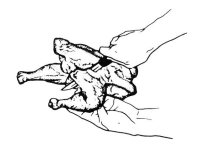

3. Remove leg from body by cutting from back to front as close as possible to the back bone.

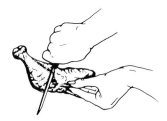

4. Separate thigh and drumstick. Locate joint by squeezing between thigh and drumstick. Cut through joint.

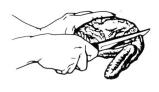

5. To remove wing from body, start cutting on inside of wing just over the joint. Cut down and around the joint. To make the wing lie flat, make a small cut on the inside of the large wing joint. Cut just deep enough to expose the bones. Repeat with wing on other side.

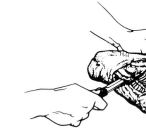

6. To cut the body into breast and back sections, place the chicken on neck end and cut from the tail along each side of back bone through rib joints to neck. Cut through the skin that attaches the neck-and-back strip to the breast. Place neck-and-back strip skin side up on cutting board. Cut into two pieces just above the spoon-shaped bones in the back. Another method is to separate the back from the breast by cutting between the breast and back ribs from the shoulder to the tail end. Bend the back away from breast to separate the shoulder joints.

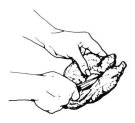

7. Place breast skin side down on cutting board. Cut through white cartilage at the V of the neck.

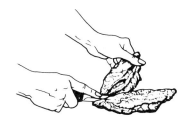

8. Hold breast firmly with both hands and bend back both sides. Push up with fingers to snap out the breastbone. Cut breast in half lengthwise.

Figure 15-3.

How to cut up a chicken. (From: Jeanne H. Freeland-Graves, Principles of Food Preparation: A Laboratory Manual. *New York: Macmillan, 1979, p. 196.)*

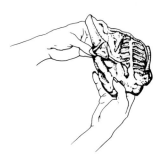

Bend and break keel bone.

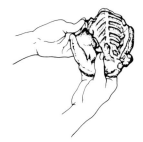

Run thumb between meat and keel bone.

Figure 15-4.
How to bone chicken breasts. (From Jeanne H. Freeland-Graves, Principles of Food Preparation: A Laboratory Manual. *New York: Macmillan, 1979, p. 197.)*

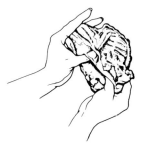

Separate breast from rib cage.

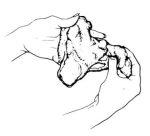

Remove skin and trim.

rolled and fastened together, and deep-fried or baked. Deboned meats are also used in many ways, as for stir-fry cooking and food kabobs.

Storage

Fresh, frozen, and cooked poultry all need to be carefully stored to prevent contamination by microorganisms and to preserve the flavor and texture.

Fresh

Fresh poultry should be refrigerated immediately after being purchased and used within 1 to 2 days thereafter. If the poultry is wrapped in heavy paper, it should be unwrapped and placed on a platter with the giblets stored in a separate container. The poultry and giblets should both be covered with waxed paper or plastic wrap. Specially packaged poultry in a transparent wrap does not need to be unwrapped for short storage.

Frozen

Frozen poultry is stored at a temperature of 0° F (–18° C) or less until it is ready to use. Frozen poultry that is to be later thawed, should always be left in its moisture-proof wrapping.

The safest and most recommended method for thawing poultry is to place the frozen poultry on a platter or tray and then thaw the poultry in the refrigerator. Small birds will take 1 or 2 days and larger birds will require 2 or 3 days to thaw in the refrigerator.

Cooked

Cooked poultry is always stored in the coolest part of the refrigerator. It is important that cooked poultry be quickly cooled to prevent microorganism growth. The meat should be cut from the bone of a large bird and stored in small quantities. All cooked poultry should be loosely covered, and gravy and broth must be covered and promptly refrigerated. The proper way to care for stuffing is discussed in this chapter under the section, roasting.

Cooked poultry can also be frozen. When it is properly wrapped in an airtight package, cooked poultry can be stored for 2 to 4 months. The flavor of frozen cooked poultry may not be quite as good as the unfrozen variety but it is still nutritious. Stuffings should not be frozen as they lose their flavor and texture.

Canned and Dried

Canned and dried poultry should be stored at room temperature. Properly processed dried poultry can be stored for up to 2 years, and canned poultry can be successfully stored for up to 12 months.

Basic Methods of Cookery

Poultry can be cooked in a variety of ways and most kinds of poultry can be used interchangeably in most recipes that call for poultry. The method chosen for cooking poultry may depend either on the age of the bird or the special flavor and texture that are desired from the cooked product. For example, a mature, less tender bird is most often cooked by a moist-heat method. Different tastes can be achieved by using such cooking methods as broiling, drying, or roasting.

Whatever cooking method is chosen, poultry should be completely cooked. Poultry must not be partially cooked on 1 day and the cooking completed on the next day, since microorganisms grow readily in partially cooked foods. The flesh of some cooked poultry, even though it is completely cooked, may have a pinkish color. This is a chemical reaction and does not make the food unsafe to eat.

Dry Heat

All kinds of young tender poultry can be cooked without additional moisture being added or by the use of dry heat.

Broiling. Although all cuts of poultry can be broiled, the flesh pieces including the breasts, drumsticks, and thighs are best suited for broiling. Poultry may also be halved or quartered and broiled. The poultry is placed 7 to 9 inches from the broiler element on a broiler rack. More flavor and skin moisture is attained by basting the poultry with a marinade sauce or fat during the cooking process. The meat should be turned every 10 to 20 minutes and basted as necessary. To baste means to lightly brush the surface with a liquid.

Broiling poultry takes approximately 45 to 70 minutes, depending on the size of pieces being cooked. If poultry pieces of varying size are cooked together, smaller pieces will be finished first and should be removed from the heat.

Barbecuing. The same procedure that is used for broiling is also followed in barbecuing except that the meat is cooked over the coals rather than under the heat, as illustrated in Figure 15-5. The time for cooking is about the same as for broiling but may vary depending upon the warmth of the fire and climatic conditions. Also, the poultry pieces need to be rotated to assure even cooking over concentrated heat.

Frying. Poultry pieces may be pan fried, oven fried, or deep fried. Pan-fried and oven-fried chicken may be coated to give the chicken a

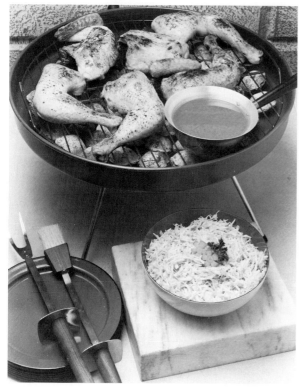

Figure 15-5.

Barbecued chicken is more flavorful when basted with a seasoned sauce during cooking. (Karo Corn Syrup)

crisp exterior surface and a moist interior, or it may be thoroughly dried and fried in a small amount of fat. Flour mixed with salt, pepper, and other seasonings is the most common coating used for pan and oven frying. The easiest way to coat the chicken is to place the coating mixture in a paper or plastic bag, add one or two pieces of poultry, close the top, and shake until the pieces are coated.

Deep-fried chicken is dipped in a batter or coated before it is cooked. The basic directions for deep frying are discussed in Chapter 5, "Fats."

To oven fry chicken the oven is preheated to 350° F (175° C), and enough fat is melted in a baking pan to reach a depth of 1/8 inch. The chicken pieces are placed in the pan and turned to coat all sides in the fat. The poultry is baked for 20 to 25 minutes, turned, and baked for an additional 25 to 30 minutes or until it is tender.

To pan fry poultry a heavy frying pan is used and enough fat is melted in the pan to reach a depth of about 1/8 inch. The poultry is added to the fat and cooked over moderate heat for approximately 50 minutes or until tender. The chicken needs to be turned frequently to assure adequate cooking and browning.

Poultry is deep fried at 350° F (175° C) for 10 minutes or until tender. Only a few pieces of chicken should be cooked at any one time, and after they are cooked the pieces of chicken need to be drained on absorbent toweling.

Roasting. All kinds of poultry may be roasted in whole form, in halves, or in quarter sections. Whole poultry may be cooked with or without stuffing. Unstuffed poultry cooks in less time than stuffed poultry.

If poultry is to be stuffed, the following important rules must be followed to prevent unsafe bacterial growth.

1. Stuff bird just before cooking. Poultry should never be stuffed and then frozen except in commercially prepared form.

2. Stuffing ingredients may be prepared the day before, but perishable foods must be refrigerated, and meat and broth should not be added to a stuffing until just before it is ready to use. Table 15-1 gives some suggested ideas for stuffings.

3. Remove the stuffing immediately after cooking and store it separately. Leftover stuffing needs to be thoroughly reheated before it is served and should be used within 2 to 3 days.

4. The stuffing should not be packed tightly into the bird as the dressing expands

Table 15-1

Suggested Ingredients for Rice and Bread Stuffings (5 Cups)

Ingredients	
Apple-Raisin	2 cups chopped apples; 1/2 cup raisins
Corn, whole-kernel, drained	1 cup
Giblets	Cooked gizzard and liver, chopped
Green pepper	1/2 cup chopped green pepper, sautéed
Ham	1 cup cooked ham, finely minced
Orange	2 teaspoons grated orange rind
Mushrooms	1/2 cup fresh mushrooms, sliced and sautéed or 1 (3 oz.) can sliced mushrooms, drained
Nuts	1/2 cup almonds, walnuts, or filberts
Olives	1/2 cup green olives, sliced
Oysters	1 cup oysters, drained and chopped
Sausage	1 cup sausage, cooked
Water chestnuts	1 cup canned water chestnuts, drained and sliced

during the cooking as moisture from the bird is absorbed. Approximately 1/2 cup of stuffing is allowed for each pound of bird.

The stuffing may also be cooked separately in a baking dish. The neck and giblets found in the bird cavity are flavorful additions. After being cooked at a low temperature for 1-1/2 hours, the broth and chopped giblets can be used in making stuffing or gravy.

The following is the proper way to prepare a bird for roasting, as illustrated in Figure 15-6.

1. The bird is rinsed with water, patted dry, and the interior cavity is rubbed lightly with salt.

2. The neck cavity is stuffed lightly and fastened with a metal skewer that is a long, pin-shaped prong. The body cavity is stuffed lightly and the legs are either tied together with string or, as in most marketed poultry, a piece of skin is left below the cavity for the legs to be tucked under.

The wings are held close to the body by tieing with a piece of string.

3. The bird is placed on a roasting rack in a shallow baking pan. The broiler pan makes a suitable baking dish for large birds. If a rack is not available, peeled potatoes may be used to hold the bird in place.

4. Poultry is roasted at 325° F (165° C). A timetable chart for poultry is the best reference to determine the length of cooking time for the poundage and kind of poultry.

5. Poultry should reach an internal temperature of 180° F (82° C) to 185° F (85° C) to be completely cooked; the stuffing should reach 165° F (74° C). A meat thermometer is the best guide for meat doneness. The thermometer is inserted where it does not touch a bone, preferably in the meaty portion of the inner thigh or in the breast. Another way to determine doneness is to move the drumstick back and forth. If it moves easily and the meat

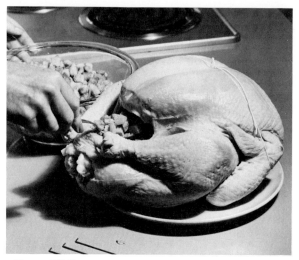

Figure 15-6.
Poultry dressing is lightly packed into the bird. After the front cavity has been skewered or sewn shut, the wings and legs can be tied to the body with string.

feels soft the poultry is probably done. If the dressing has not reached a temperature of 165° F (74° C) when the bird is done, the dressing should be removed from the bird cavity, placed in a baking dish, returned to the oven, and allowed to complete cooking.

6. To assure even cooking, the skin or string holding the legs of the poultry together should be cut two thirds of the way through the cooking time. If the bird seems to be browning too rapidly, those portions may be covered with a moist, thin cloth or with aluminum foil.

Figure 15-7 shows a roasted turkey ready to serve.

Moist Heat Cookery

Cooking poultry in liquid, thereby using moist heat, is an excellent way to tenderize older birds and a good way to cook less meaty pieces of poultry. Young poultry may also be cooked by moist heat. Poultry that is cooked by moist heat may be left on the bone or the meat may be removed from the bone and used in casseroles, soups, and salads. It is quicker to cook poultry pieces by moist heat than to cook the whole bird unless it is very small.

Simmering. Poultry is simmered by adding 1 or more cups of liquid to the pan and cooking over low heat on top of the range or in the oven at 350° F (175° C) for 45 minutes to 3 hours or until the poultry is tender. Poultry may be browned in hot fat before it is simmered; this process is called braising. Cooking

Figure 15-7.
Roasted to a golden brown and attractively garnished, the turkey is ready to be carved and served. (Armour & Company)

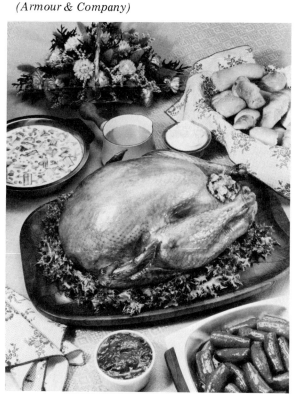

time is dependent on the quality of the meat, the size and kind of the poultry pieces, and the method of cooking.

Stewing. Stewing is a version of simmering in which other vegetables and seasonings are added to the broth and meat. Vegetables commonly used in stewing include onions, carrots, and celery. Other seasonings may be added including salt, pepper, thyme, and bay leaves.

Microwave Cooking

All kinds of poultry, with the exception of mature poultry, can be successfully cooked in a microwave oven. To achieve even cooking in a microwave oven, whole or poultry pieces, or the dish holding them, should be rotated during the cooking. It is best to prick the skin of poultry with a fork prior to cooking, and to cover the meat with waxed paper during the first half of cooking time. Poultry browns to a certain extent just by being cooked, but if deeper browning is desired, paprika, soy sauce, or seasoned coating mixes may be used.

Whole poultry cooked in a microwave oven should first be cooked breast down, then turned over and cooked breast-side up. Either stuffed or unstuffed poultry may be roasted in a microwave oven. A casserole lid with a lip serves as a good rack to hold the bird, but the drippings should be drained off periodically because the accumulation of liquid can retard the cooking.

Mature poultry, such as stewing chickens, is not successfully cooked in a microwave oven because of the prolonged cooking time needed to tenderize the tissue. However, the cooked meat can be used in casserole dishes that are to be cooked in a microwave oven.

Thawing of poultry is successfully done in a microwave oven. It is important to allow for "carry-over" or extended cooking time with poultry as with other foods.

Convenience Products

Many convenience foods contain poultry as a main food or ingredient. Frozen products include ready-to-heat-and-eat fried chicken, frozen dinners with poultry as the entrée, and frozen food dishes with poultry as a main ingredient, such as chicken and noodles. Canned and cooked whole chickens and canned products with chicken as a main ingredient are also available. Dehydrated chicken is used in dried soup mixes, and special poultry accompaniments, such as ready-to-mix stuffings and gravies, are also marketed.

RECIPES

————— Stewed Chicken —————

	Standard	Metric
Celery tops	3	3
Bay leaf	1	1
Carrot, diced	1	1
Sprig parsley	1	1
Stewing chicken, cut into pieces	1 (4 lb.)	1,814 gms
Boiling water	4 cups	1,000 mL
Salt	2 tsp.	10 mL
Onion, sliced	1	1

1. Cut a 6 inch × 6 inch square of cheesecloth and place the celery tops, bay leaf, carrot, and parsley in the center. Tie up the cheesecloth with a piece

of string to form a sack. (This is called an herb bouquet.)

2. Place the chicken in a large pan; add the water, salt, onion, and herb bouquet of vegetables.

3. Cover; bring to a boil; reduce heat to a simmer. Cook 2-1/2 hours or until tender. Remove the herb bouquet.

4. The stewed chicken may be used to prepare the stewed chicken and dumpling recipe that follows, or the meat may be removed from the bones and used for chicken casseroles; the chicken and broth may be used for chicken soups.

Yield: 4 to 5 servings

Stewed Chicken and Dumplings

	Standard	Metric
All-purpose flour, sifted	1-1/2 cups	375 mL
Baking powder	2 tsp.	10 mL
Salt	3/4 tsp.	4 mL
Milk	3/4 cup	175 mL
Recipe, stewed chicken	1	1

1. Sift the flour, baking powder, and salt together.

2. Add the milk and stir only until well blended.

3. Bring the stewed chicken and broth to the boiling point.

4. Dip a metal tablespoon into the boiling liquid and then into the dumpling mixture. Using this procedure drop spoonfuls of the mixture into the liquid.

5. Cover the pan and cook for 12 minutes, keeping the mixture at a moderate boil. The lid should not be removed while the dumplings are cooking.

6. Remove the chicken and dumplings to a platter; serve with the liquid remaining in the pan.

Yield: 4 to 5 servings

Chicken Fricasse

	Standard	Metric
Recipe, stewed chicken	1	1
Butter or margarine	3 Tbsp.	45 mL
Flour	3 Tbsp.	45 mL
Half-and-half	3/4 cup	175 mL
Chicken broth	1-1/2 cups	375 mL
Sprigs parsley	4	4

1. When the chicken is tender, remove it to a serving platter and cover to keep warm.

2. Strain the broth through a sieve lined with cheesecloth to remove the fat or carefully take a spoon and skim the fat off the top of the liquid.

3. Melt the butter in a heavy skillet and blend in the flour.

4. Combine the chicken broth and the half-and-half and stir it gradually into the flour-butter mixture. Stir constantly until the mixture thickens and is smooth.

5. Pour the sauce over the chicken and garnish with parsley.

Yield: 4 servings

Chicken and Macaroni

	Standard	Metric
Elbow macaroni	1/2 cup	125 mL
Diced celery	1/4 cup	60 mL
Chicken broth	1/2 cup	125 mL
Condensed cream of celery soup	1 (10 3/4 oz.) can	1 (305 gm) can
Cooked chicken, diced	1 cup	250 mL
Minced parsley	2 Tbsp.	30 mL
Worcestershire sauce	1/2 tsp.	2 ml
Salt	1/4 tsp.	1 mL
Soft bread cubes	1/2 cup	125 mL
Butter or margarine	1 Tbsp.	15 mL

1. Cook the macaroni according to the package directions. Drain.

2. Preheat the oven to 350° F (175° C).

3. Cook the celery in the chicken broth for 5 minutes.

4. Combine the macaroni, celery, broth, soup, chicken, parsley, Worcestershire sauce, and salt in a greased 1-1/2-quart casserole. Sprinkle with the bread cubes and dot with butter.

5. Bake for 30 to 40 minutes.

Yield: 4 servings

Chicken or Turkey à La King

	Standard	Metric
Recipe, stewed chicken or 2 cups cooked chicken or turkey	1	1 or 500 mL
Butter or margarine	4 Tbsp.	60 mL
Chopped green pepper	1/4 cup	60 mL
Mushrooms, sliced	1 (4 oz.) can	1 (113 gm)
Milk	1 cup	250 mL
Chicken broth	1 cup	250 mL
Egg yolk, slightly beaten	1	1
Chopped pimiento	2 Tbsp.	30 mL
Flour	1/4 cup	60 mL
Salt	1 tsp.	5 mL

1. Remove the meat from the bones of the cooked chicken and cut into small pieces to yield 2 cups.

2. Melt the butter or margarine in a heavy skillet and sauté the green pepper and mushrooms for 5 minutes.

3. Blend in the flour. Combine the milk and broth and stir gradually into the flour mixture until it is thickened and smooth.

4. Blend a small amount of the sauce into the egg yolk and then blend the egg yolk mixture into the sauce, stirring constantly. Cook 2 minutes.

5. Add the chicken, pimiento, and salt to the sauce. Cook until the mixture is hot.

6. Serve over biscuits, rice, or cornbread.

Yield: 4 to 5 servings

Chicken Vegetable Soup

	Standard	Metric
Stewing chicken, cut in pieces	1 (3 to 4 lb.)	1 (1360 to 1814 gm)
Onion	1	1
Water	8 cups	2,000 mL
Rice	1/4 cup	60 mL
Parsley, chopped	1 Tbsp.	15 mL
Salt	1 tsp.	5 mL
Diced carrots	1/2 cup	125 mL
Diced celery	1/2 cup	125 mL
Tomato, diced	1	1
Butter or margarine	1 Tbsp.	15 mL
Flour	1 Tbsp.	15 mL
Milk, heated	1 cup	250 mL

1. Place the chicken pieces, onion, and water in a large pan. Bring to boiling; reduce the heat to simmer; cover. Cook 2 hours or until the chicken is tender.

2. Remove the chicken; cool; and remove meat from the bones.

3. Strain the broth in a cheesecloth-lined sieve to remove the fat.

4. Measure 5 cups of the broth and return to the saucepan. Add the rice, parsley, salt, carrots, celery, and tomato. Bring the mixture to a boil; reduce the heat to low and cook for 15 minutes.

5. In a heavy skillet melt the butter or margarine and blend in the flour. Gradually stir in the milk and cook, stirring constantly, until thickened. Gradually stir the thickened sauce into the broth mixture and cook for 5 minutes.

Yield: 4 to 6 servings

Turkey Tetrazzini

	Standard	Metric
Spaghetti	4 oz.	113 gm
Butter or margarine	3 Tbsp.	45 mL
Sliced fresh mushrooms	1/2 cup	125 mL
Flour	3 Tbsp.	45 mL
Chicken bouillon	1 cup	250 mL
Milk	3/4 cup	175 mL

	Standard	Metric
Diced cooked turkey	2 cups	2 mL
Thyme	1/2 tsp.	2 mL
Dehydrated onion	1 tsp.	500 mL
Grated parmesan cheese	1/2 cup	125 mL

1. Preheat the oven to 400° F (205° C).
2. Cook the spaghetti as directed on the package. Drain.
3. Melt the butter or margarine in a heavy fry pan. Add the mushrooms and sauté for 5 minutes. Blend in the flour.
4. Combine the bouillon and milk and add gradually to the flour mixture; cook until thickened, stirring constantly.
5. Combine the spaghetti, turkey, thyme, onion, and sauce. Turn into a greased casserole dish. Sprinkle with cheese and bake 25 minutes or until bubbly. In microwave oven cook for 15 minutes, rotating dish 1/2 turn 8 minutes through cooking time.

Yield: 4 to 6 servings

Turkey Divan

	Standard	Metric
Cooked turkey	8 slices	8
Frozen broccoli spears, cooked and drained	1-10 oz. pkg.	1 (284 gm)
Condensed cream of chicken soup	3/4 can	3/4 can
Grated sharp cheddar cheese	1/2 cup	125 mL

1. Preheat the oven to 375° F (190° C).
2. Arrange the turkey slices on the bottom of a greased casserole dish.
3. Cover with a layer of broccoli.
4. Pour the cream of chicken soup over the broccoli and turkey.
5. Sprinkle cheese over the top.
6. Cook for 20 minutes or until lightly browned. In microwave oven cook for 10 minutes, rotating dish 1/4 turn after 5 minutes of cooking.

Yield: 4 servings

Chicken Cacciatore

	Standard	Metric
Fryer-broiler chicken, cut in pieces or enough pieces to equal weight	1 (2-1/2 lb.)	1 (1,270 gm)
Flour	1/2 cup	125 mL
Salt	1 tsp.	5 mL
Pepper	1/4 tsp.	1 mL
Fat	1/4 cup	60 mL
Chopped onion	1/2 cup	125 mL
Minced garlic clove	1	1
Tomato paste	1 (6-1/4 oz.) can	1 (176 gm)
Canned tomatoes	2-1/2 cups	625 mL
Bay leaf	1	1
Oregano	1/2 tsp.	2 mL
Basil	1/2 tsp.	2 mL
Lemon juice	1-1/2 Tbsp.	22 mL
Worcestershire sauce	1/2 tsp.	2 mL

1. Combine the flour, salt, and pepper in a paper bag and add a few chicken pieces; close the bag and shake to coat.
2. Melt the fat in a heavy skillet and brown chicken. Remove the chicken pieces to a platter. Add the onion and garlic and sauté for 5 minutes.
3. Add the tomato paste, tomatoes, bay leaf, oregano, and basil to the skillet and bring to a boil. Add the chicken, lemon juice, and Worcestershire sauce. Cover the pan and simmer for 45 to 60 minutes or until the chicken is tender. Remove the bay leaf.
4. Serve over a cooked pasta.

Yield: 4 servings

Chicken Kiev

	Standard	Metric
Whole chicken breasts, skinned and deboned	4 large	4
Chopped green onions	1 Tbsp.	15 mL
Parsley, minced	1 Tbsp.	15 mL
Salt	1 tsp.	5 mL
Butter, chilled	1/2 cup	125 mL
Egg, beaten	1	1
Water	1 Tbsp.	15 mL
Flour	1/2 cup	125 mL
Dry bread crumbs	1/2 cup	125 mL

1. Cut the chicken breasts in half lengthwise. Place between two pieces of waxed paper or plastic wrap and pound with a wooden meat mallet to 1/4 inch in thickness.
2. Sprinkle each chicken piece with the onion, parsley, and salt.
3. Place 1 tablespoon of butter or margarine on top of the filling.
4. Roll up, tucking in the sides; fasten with toothpicks.
5. Combine the egg and water; dredge the chicken rolls in flour; dip in the egg mixture; and roll in the bread crumbs. Chill for 1 hour.
6. Fry in deep fat at 375° F (190° C) until the chicken rolls are light brown, about 5 minutes.

Yield: 4 to 8 servings

Roast Duckling

	Standard	Metric
Duckling	1 (4 lb.)	1 (1814 gm)
Garlic clove, peeled and cut in half	1	1
Salt	1 tsp.	5 mL
Pared, cored, and quartered apples	2 cups	500 mL
Raisins	1 cup	250 mL
Orange juice	1 cup	250 mL
Honey	1/2 cup	125 mL

1. Preheat the oven to 325° F (165° C).
2. Wash the duck; pat dry with toweling.
3. Season the cavity of the duck by rubbing with the garlic clove and sprinkling with salt.
4. Combine the apples and raisins and fill the cavity.
5. Place on a rack in a shallow roasting pan and roast, uncovered.
6. Combine the orange juice and honey and baste every 15 minutes.
7. Cook for 1-1/2 hours.

Yield: 4 servings

Note: Duck does not carve well and is easier to serve if cut into quarters.

Broiled Rock Cornish Game Hens

	Standard	Metric
Currant jelly	1/2 cup	125 mL
Orange juice	1/4 cup	60 mL
Rock Cornish game hens, cut in half	2	2

1. Preheat the oven to broil.
2. Melt the currant jelly over a low heat. Combine with the orange juice.
3. Place the Rock Cornish game hen halves on the broiler rack of a broiling pan.
4. Cook 7 inches from the broiler, basting and turning every 15 minutes. Broil until tender, approximately 45 to 60 minutes.

Yield: 2 to 4 servings

Bread Stuffing

	Standard	Metric
Butter or margarine	1/2 cup	125 mL
Onion, chopped	1	1
Chopped celery	3/4 cup	175 mL
Parsley, chopped	1/4 cup	60 mL
Thyme	1 tsp.	5 mL
Salt	1 tsp.	5 mL
Pepper	1/2 tsp.	2 mL
Dried bread cubes	5 cups	1250 mL

1. Melt the butter or margarine in a heavy skillet. Add the onion and celery and cook over low heat until tender.
2. Combine the cooked celery-onion mixture with the parsley, thyme, salt, pepper, and bread cubes. Toss lightly to mix.
3. If desired, add a small additional amount of poultry broth or melted fat. The dressing should be moist but not soggy.

Yield: 5 to 6 cups

LEARNING ACTIVITIES

1. Compare the cost of fresh cut-up fryers, fresh whole fryers, and frozen ready-to-cook fryers. Determine which form would be the best buy for a single person living alone and a family in which both adults are working.
2. Compare the cost of whole canned chicken and a fresh ready-to-cook chicken.
3. Make a list of times when canned chicken might be a good item to have on hand.
4. Plan a luncheon and dinner menu using stewed chicken.
5. Plan a dinner menu with roast turkey as the entrée.
6. Plan three menus using planned-over turkey as the entrée.
7. Select a frozen turkey or chicken dinner at the grocery store. Prepare a meal from basic ingredients that is the same as the frozen dinner. Keep a chart of the time involved in preparation and the total expense. Cook the frozen dinner and do a flavor comparison between the fresh and frozen dinners.
8. Do a cost and time analysis of the two dinners prepared in number 7 and decide which is the best preparation method for a specific situation of your own choice.
9. Demonstrate to the class how to cut up a whole chicken.
10. Demonstrate to the class how to debone a chicken breast or chicken thigh.
11. Make a list of recipes for which it would be advisable to use deboned meat or for which deboned meat is necessary.
12. Make a list of sauces that can be used in broiling or barbecuing chicken. Prepare a kind of poultry by broiling or barbecuing with one of the sauces.
13. Do a research paper on the modern production methods used for raising poultry and present your report to the class.
14. Prepare a bread stuffing and divide it into three portions. Add different ingredients to each portion. Bake in the oven at 350° F (175° C) for 30 minutes; taste; and decide which is the most acceptable.
15. Plan an oven meal with oven-fried chicken as the entrée. Prepare the chicken and make a chart of preparation time and a cost analysis.
16. Prepare a rolled turkey roast. Compare the number of servings available from the roast as compared to the number of servings from a 10 lb. turkey.
17. Investigate the different kinds of poultry that are available at the local market and make a chart on the price per pound. If possible, prepare a goose or duck by a cooking method of your choice.
18. Many restaurants and fast-food outlets will prepare fried chicken for a crowd. Compare the cost of obtaining ready-to-eat chicken for 25 people from one of

these outlets versus the cost of home preparation of fried chicken for 25 people. What are the food safety precautions that must be taken with either choice?

19. Demonstrate to the class how to wrap poultry for freezer storage. Use either uncooked or cooked meat. Refer to Chapter 3.

20. Plan a foreign recipe that uses chicken as the main ingredient. Prepare the foreign dish and tell the class the types of other foods that would be served with it as a part of a cultural menu.

REVIEW QUESTIONS

1. What has caused the increased availability of poultry on the market?
2. What accounts for poultry's low calorie content in comparison to the red meats?
3. What kinds of other foods can be combined with poultry?
4. What three characteristics of poultry are looked for when poultry is federally graded?
5. What is the difference between a broiler-fryer chicken and a Rock Cornish game hen in age?
6. Which chicken has the largest amount of white meat?
7. What are five factors that determine the amount and kind of poultry to purchase?
8. What determines whether poultry is purchased in whole or cut-up form?
9. What is the advantage of the turkey roll?
10. What appearance factors should be looked for when purchasing fresh poultry?
11. How long can fresh poultry be stored before it is cooked?
12. What is the recommended method for thawing frozen poultry?
13. What is the proper way to care for cooked meat from a large bird?
14. How long can cooked poultry be satisfactorily frozen?
15. Which pieces of poultry are most suitable for broiling?
16. Why is poultry most often coated before it is fried?
17. What are four important rules to remember about stuffings?
18. What is the internal temperature that a roasted bird must reach to be completely cooked?
19. What is the temperature that stuffing must reach to be cooked?
20. Where is the best place to insert a meat thermometer in a bird?
21. What group of poultry must be simmered or stewed to be palatable?
22. What vegetables and seasonings are added when poultry is cooked by the stewing method?
23. What ingredients can help achieve a deeper browning when poultry is cooked in a microwave oven?
24. What types of convenience products using poultry as a main ingredient are available?

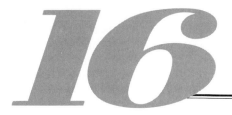

Fish and Shellfish

Since the beginning of recorded time, fish and shellfish have been common foods for people living near coastal or inland waters. The development of modern methods of fish harvesting, processing, and packaging has made fish and shellfish available throughout the country on a year round basis. Because of the favorable nutrient composition of this food and its many available forms, fish adds a wide diversity to planning appetizers, accompaniment foods, and entrée dishes.

Although man still hunts fish and shellfish, many fish farms are now in operation to make certain kinds of fish and shellfish more available and to assure a continuous restocking of the supply of fish in both inland and coastal waters. As land for growing other high-quality protein foods becomes scarce, fish will become

of increasing importance to a daily meal pattern.

Nutritional Factors to Consider

Carbohydrate, Fat, and Protein

Fish contain no carbohydrate but shellfish contain a small amount. The fat content of fish varies with the species. Most fish contain less than 5 per cent fat, but some fish, such as halibut, mackerel, or salmon, have a fat content ranging up to 25 per cent. However, the fat is mainly unsaturated, which makes fish a desirable food choice for low-calorie and low-cholesterol diets. Shellfish contain varying amounts of cholesterol and are therefore not usually recommended for low-cholesterol diets. The protein in fish and shellfish is a high-quality, complete protein that is comparable to other meats, poultry, eggs, and milk.

Vitamins and Minerals

Fish and shellfish are good sources of the B vitamins. Oysters and the fatter fish have a relatively high amount of vitamin A, and fish-liver oils such as cod-liver oil are a rich source of vitamin D.

Saltwater fish and shellfish have a high content of the mineral, iodine, and all fish contain the minerals phosphorus and potassium. With the exception of oysters, all fish and shellfish are low in iron; unless fish are cured in salt, their sodium content is low.

Calories

Fish foods are not high in calories except when they are cooked in additional fat or served in rich sauces. A 3-1/2-ounce serving of most fish will average about 150 to 200 calories.

Menu-Planning Points

Inherent Factors

Balance. Because of the nutritional qualities of fish and its many marketed forms, fish can balance any menu. Fish and shellfish are served as the entrée portion of a meal and can be prepared in many ways as appetizers and ingredients for soups and salads.

Color. Fish and shellfish range in color from white to varying shades of pinkish-red; this must be considered when planning a menu. The flesh of such fish as cod, sole, halibut, and mackerel and of all shellfish is white. The surface color of cooked shrimp has a pinkish tinge; salmon is of varying shades of pink,

depending on the species. The white-fleshed species of fish and shellfish need the addition of other more colorful foods to make the meal attractive. For example, a menu featuring oyster stew is more tempting when it is served with a relish tray of crisp bright vegetables.

Shape. Fish come in a variety of sizes and shapes and are marketed in a variety of forms. Smaller fish, such as trout as an individual serving, or a larger fish, such as salmon served on a platter, add interesting shape to any meal. Fish fillets can be stuffed and rolled for shape variation as shown in Figure 16–1, and fish steaks and fish sticks are other form variations. Many interesting shapes are added to a meal when oysters, clams, crabs, or lobsters are served in or out of the shell. Cooked, shelled shrimp served in a salad, or scallops broiled on skewers are other shapes that make a meal interesting.

Flavor and Texture

Most fish has a delicate flavor, unless it has been specially cured, and is complemented when garnished with a slice of lemon or lime and served with other foods that are more highly seasoned. Fish is also complemented when served with sweeter foods, such as fruits, or cold food dishes, such as fruit ices and sherbets. Because the texture of fish is soft, some crisply textured foods need to be included in the menu.

External Factors

Age. Because of the nutrient quality, delicate flavor, and soft texture of fish, it is a highly acceptable food for people of any age. If fish is cooked with the bones still in the fish, care must be taken to remove them before the fish is served to children or others who cannot separate the bone from the flesh before eating.

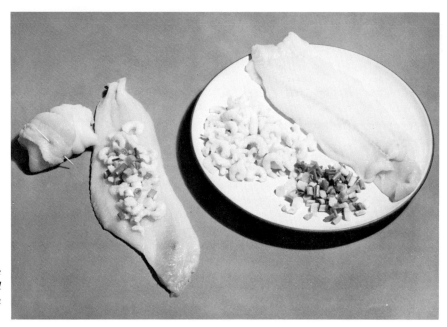

Figure 16-1.
The stuffing is placed on the center of the fillet, rolled and held together with a wooden pick while it cooks.

Culture. More than 240 fish are marketed around the world, and many peoples have certain customs of eating fish that are a part of their heritage. For example, many Asiatics eat fish raw and Scandinavians eat raw fish like herring after the fish has been marinated.

Economics. The cost of fish is variable, depending on geographical location. Saltwater fish and shellfish are less expensive along the coastal areas where they are harvested; the price of freshwater fish is also variable for the same reason.

Food Availability. Most fish is readily available throughout the year either fresh, frozen, or canned. Because fish is a highly perishable food, it will not be available fresh in many regions.

Space and Equipment. No special equipment is needed for fish cookery. However, many gourmet types of cookware and serving dishes are available that are made especially for fish.

Time Scheduling. All fish and shellfish cook very quickly, with the exception of large, whole fish that when baked take approximately 1 hour to cook. Some specialty fish dishes may require a longer preparation. Certain forms of shellfish, such as crab and shrimp, can be purchased precooked and ready-to-eat. Time scheduling should allow for fish to be cooked just before serving time, as fish that is overcooked or held before serving will become dry and unflavorful.

Kinds of Fish and Shellfish

Fish are classified as fin fish if they have skeletal bone and shellfish if they live in a shell and have no bone. Fin fish are further divided by whether they are from fresh water or salt water. Examples of freshwater fish are catfish, bass, perch, and trout. There are more varieties of saltwater fish, including cod, halibut, haddock, herring, mackerel, red snapper, salmon, smelt, swordfish, turbot, and tuna.

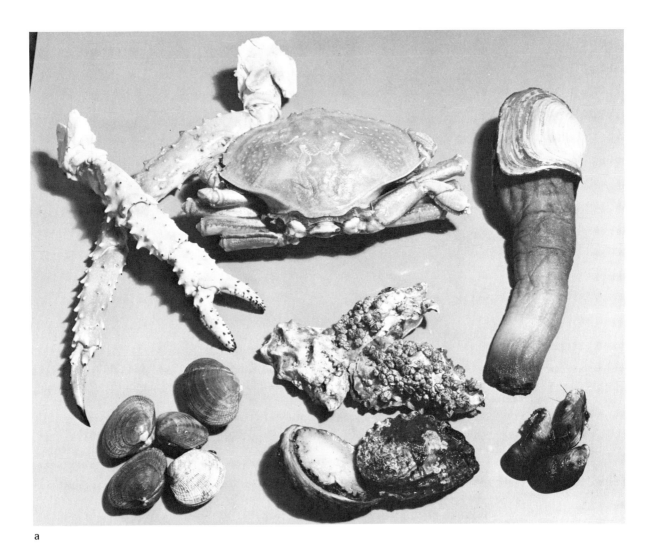

a

All shellfish live in salt water and are further categorized as mollusks and crustaceans. Mollusks, those shellfish that live in a hard shell and have an unsegmented body, include clams, mussels, oysters, and scallops. Crustaceans, such as crabs, lobster, and shrimp, live in a hard shell and have a segmented body. Several species of the crustaceans and mollusks are found either along the Pacific or Atlantic seaboards. A variety of shellfish from the Pacific and Atlantic coasts are pictured in Figure 16–2(a) and (b).

Pacific Coast

Clams common to the Pacific coastal region are the butter, razor, pismo, and geoduck varieties. Butter clams are usually steamed and eaten, whereas other varieties of clams are mostly used for chowders. The oyster is called the "Pacific" oyster and is marketed in small, medium, and large sizes. These are eaten raw, fried, or used in soups and in a variety of other food dishes. A rarer, small and delicate oyster is called the "Olympia" oyster.

Figure 16–2.

(a) [Opposite] Shellfish common to the Pacific coast include (starting from top left and proceeding clockwise): Alaskan King crab, Dungeness crab, geoduck, mussels, oysters, clams, and in the middle is abalone in its shell. (b) Shellfish common to the Atlantic coast include (starting top right and proceeding clockwise): Blue crab, shrimp, cherrystone clams, steamer clams, sea scallops, bay scallops, oysters, and mussels. A Maine lobster is in the middle (Courtesy Elizabeth Belfer and Pisacane Midtown, New York City)

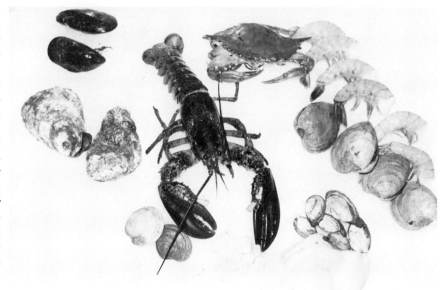

b

Abalone are found in California and Alaska. Mussels are similar to the flavor of the butter clam but are much smaller in size and often an overlooked delicacy.

The two kinds of crab from the Pacific coast are the dungeness and the king. The meat of the king crab, principally from the leg, is stringy in texture, whereas that from the body and leg of the dungeness is more flaky and of a sweeter flavor. Lobsters found off the California coast are called the "rock or spiny" lobster, in which the edible meat is found only in the tail. There are several sizes and varieties of Alaskan and California shrimp.

Atlantic Coast

Small, hard-shelled clams are called "littlenecks" and "cherrystones" and are usually eaten raw; the larger sizes are used for soups and chowders. A soft-shelled variety is steamed or fried. The oyster species is called "Eastern." Scallops are found only along the Atlantic seaboard and are taken either from the deep waters or bay areas. The only portion of the scallop that is eaten is the muscle which opens the shell.

The blue crab of the Atlantic coast is a smaller-sized crab than those from the Pacific. A true lobster, characterized by its two large, hard-shelled forward claws, is found in the northern waters of the Atlantic. Because the meat is spread throughout the body, the true lobster is sold whole, rather than just the tail, as with the rock lobster of the Pacific. Small shrimp are also harvested in northern waters, and larger sizes of shrimp come from the warm waters of the Gulf of Mexico.

Forms of Fish

Fresh and frozen fin fish are available in several different forms, dependent upon the size of the fish, its bone structure, and its shape. Small flat fish, such as the sole and red snapper, are either sold whole or cut into thin fillets. Larger and rounder fish are cut into thick fillets,

Forms of Fish **269**

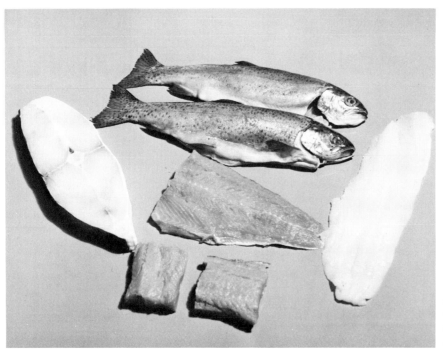

Figure 16-3.

Forms of fish commonly available for purchase are steaks, whole fish, fillets, and chunks of fish.

steaks, or chunks, or they may be sold whole. Examples of larger fish are salmon and halibut. The forms of fish are illustrated in Figure 16–3.

Whole

A whole fish includes the head, tail, fins, scales, and entrails. Fish are not available in this form unless they have just been caught. Whole fish with the entrails, scales, and usually the head, tail, and fins removed are called "dressed" fish.

Fillets

A fish fillet is a lengthwise piece of flesh cut away from the backbone. A butterfly fillet has both sides of the fish held together by the uncut flesh and skin of the belly. A fillet contains few, if any, bones. Filleting a whole fish is illustrated in Figure 16–4.

Steaks

A fish steak is a crosswise cut that contains a section of the backbone. Fish steaks are 5/8 to 1-inch thick and are usually cut from those fish weighing 3 or more pounds.

Chunks

Chunks of fish are crosswise cuts that are thicker than steaks and can be called fish roasts. The center cuts and those near the head have more flesh than those near the tail.

Fish Portions and Sticks

Fish portions are cut from frozen fish blocks and are coated with a batter and then breaded. Some fish are partially cooked before they are packaged and frozen; others are not.

Fish sticks are prepared in the same manner as the partially cooked fish portions. Each of

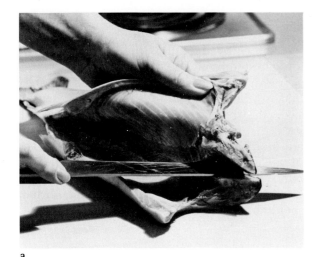

a

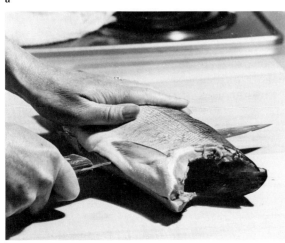

b

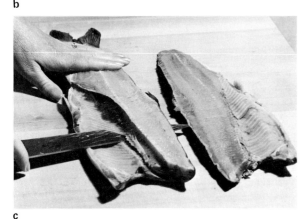

c

these fish cuts is regulated by the U.S. Department of the Interior in weight, size, and the percentage of fish contained.

Other Forms

Many varieties of fish are canned and some are cured by smoking, salting, or marinating.

Purchasing

The price of fish varies with the form in which it is purchased, the harvest season, the marketability of the fish, and consumer demand. Marketability is influenced by the fact that many people buy only fish whose name they recognize, even though other available fish may have similar characteristics and be cheaper in price. Some fish and shellfish, such as salmon, crab, or lobster, are always high in price because they are considered by many to be choice foods.

Just as with some cuts of meat, fish may sometimes be a better buy when the unedible portion is not included in the price. For example, crabmeat may be a better buy than a whole, unshelled crab; cooked and shelled shrimp may be a better buy than raw shrimp in the shell; and a chunk of fish may be a better buy than a whole fish. These factors are also dependent upon how the fish is to be cooked and served.

A serving portion of fish should equal 3 to 3-1/2 ounces, but the amount to purchase will vary with the amount of edible meat, based

Figure 16-4.
(a) The first step is to cut down to the backbone just in back of where the head was. A sharp knife is essential to filleting. (b) With the knife on the top side of the backbone, lay the fish flat and cut one half of the flesh away. (c) Slip the knife under the backbone on the second part and remove the backbone. Remaining rib bone must be removed in a separate step.

upon its purchased form. One serving equals 1/2 pound from dressed fish; 1/3 pound from fillets, steaks, or fish portions; 1/4 pound from fish sticks; and 1/6 pound from canned fish.

Other factors should be considered when purchasing fish and shellfish.

Fresh

When purchasing fillets, steaks, chunk portions, or a whole fresh fin fish, certain characteristics should be looked for. The fish should have a firm flesh, and if the form contains bone, the flesh should cling to it. If the head remains, the eyes should be bright and bulging and the gills should be red. The fish skin should be shiny, with markings of its characteristic color. All fish should have a mild, not "fishy," odor. The smell of fish is a strong indication of its freshness.

Fillets cut from larger fish, like salmon or halibut, are usually more expensive forms to purchase than steaks or chunks; however, fillets from smaller fish, such as red snapper or sole, are a better buy, because there is less waste than in the whole fish.

Fresh shellfish may be purchased live or freshly cooked at the time of purchase. Fresh lobsters and crabs must show signs of life, such as moving their legs. If the lobsters or crabs do not move, they are probably dead and should not be purchased. The shells of oysters and clams should be tightly closed, and fresh shrimp and scallops should have a mild, nonammonia-like odor. Uncooked shrimp should be firm-fleshed and be a grayish-green color. Scallops should be cream-colored.

Oysters and clams in the shell are usually sold by the dozen, whereas unshelled and uncooked crab, lobster, and shrimp are usually sold by the pound.

Oysters and clams taken from the shell should be plump and the liquid surrounding oysters should be clear. Shucked, meaning taken from the shell, oysters and clams are sold either by the pint, quart, or pound. Scallops are sold by the quart or pound.

Freshly cooked crab and lobster have a shell that is bright red, and the meat taken from the shell is white with a reddish tinge on the surface. Crab legs may be sold separately and are more expensive than the chunks or flakes of meat. Cooked shrimp may or may not be removed from the shell, but the surface color should have a pinkish tinge and the shrimp should have a mild odor.

Frozen

All forms of fin fish can be purchased frozen, but care should be taken to purchase only frozen fish that is wrapped in moisture and vapor-proof material that shows no signs of leakage or damage.

Lobster and shrimp are the only shellfish that are available frozen in the shell. The meat of other shellfish that can be purchased frozen includes crab, clams, oysters, scallops, and shrimp. Some meat may be breaded and frozen or chopped.

Canned

The most popular forms of canned fish are tuna and salmon. Tuna is sold as solid, chunk, flaked, or grated, and may be packed in oil or water. Chunk and solid are the more expensive forms of tuna and salmon and should be purchased if appearance is important, as in a salad, but all kinds are acceptable for eating. The label will designate this information.

Salmon is packed according to the species and this information is on the label. The more expensive and deeper red-colored flesh of sockeye or chinook breaks into large flakes, whereas the silver or pink salmon breaks into smaller flakes. Use often determines the kind of salmon that is purchased. For example, silver or pink salmon is better for making a salmon loaf or salmon patties.

Other canned fish, such as sardines, mackerel, and herring, are often packed in different flavored sauces and in chunks, pieces, fillets, or whole forms.

Crab, oysters, clams, lobsters, and shrimp are also available canned; this is often a better purchase than fresh or frozen varieties. Crab-meat is sold as chunks, flakes, or legs; oysters are sold whole; shrimp are sold whole and in varying sizes; clams may be whole or chopped; and lobster meat is available in chunks. These shellfish may also be canned in a special sauce or have been through a curing process.

Cured

All kinds of fish and some shellfish are cured by drying, salting, smoking, and marinating. Lox salmon is an example of a fish that is salted and smoked. Kippered salmon has been salted and dried, and is sometimes smoked. Pickled herring is an example of a marinated fish. Cured fish products are most often expensive and should be purchased in small amounts.

Storage

Fresh and frozen fish and shellfish are highly perishable foods that must be properly stored to prevent spoilage. For refrigerator storage, fresh fish and shellfish must be tightly wrapped in a moisture- and vapor-proof material, such as plastic wrap or foil. If the fish is purchased in heavy butcher paper, the fish must be unwrapped and recovered. It is important to cover the fish tightly to prevent microorganisms from entering and to prevent a fishy odor from penetrating other foods.

Fresh, uncooked fish and shellfish must be used within 1 to 2 days, but the flavor and quality of the fish will be best if prepared the day of purchase. Live crabs or lobsters must be immediately cooked and the meat removed from the shell and refrigerated. Cooked fish and shellfish may be stored in a covered container for 3 to 4 days.

Frozen fish and shellfish should be thawed in the refrigerator; once thawing has been completed, the fish must be used immediately. It takes approximately 24 hours for a 1-pound package of frozen fish to thaw.

Fish and shellfish that are purchased frozen, freshly frozen, or cooked and frozen, must be stored at $0°$ F ($-18°$ C). Fish should not be frozen for longer than 4 to 6 months, and cooked fish and shellfish should be frozen for not longer than 2 to 3 months, since the quality and flavor of fish and shellfish rapidly deteriorate with longer storage.

All forms of fresh fish may be frozen. To save freezer space, when the flesh is dressed, all inedible sections, such as the fins, should be removed. Small whole fish freeze best in an ice block; this is done by placing the fish in a watertight container, cover the fish with water, and then freezing. Large fish may be tightly wrapped and frozen, or the fish may be frozen in an ice glaze. An ice glaze is formed by dipping a frozen fish in cold water, freezing until an ice coating forms on the fish, and repeating the process until the ice glaze is 1/8 inch thick.

With the exception of shrimp or lobster, all shellfish are frozen without the shell. Shrimp may be frozen cooked or uncooked, and frozen lobster may be partially or fully cooked. Crab is cooked and the meat removed from the shell for freezing. Oysters, clams, and scallops are removed from the shell and frozen without prior cooking.

Canned fish and shellfish are stored in a cool, dry area and should be used within 1 year. Specially cured products are stored in the refrigerator and will keep for several weeks.

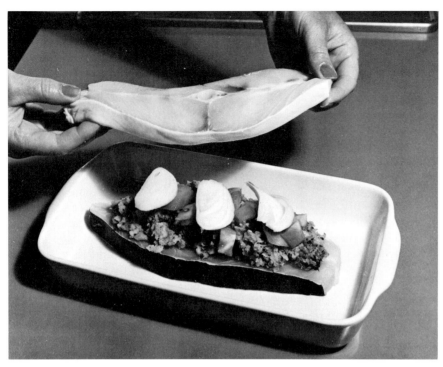

Basic Methods of Fish Cookery

Fish is cooked to make it more palatable, to develop the flavor, and to break down the small amount of connective tissue that is present. The same methods used in cooking meat and poultry are used for cooking fish, but because there are no less tender cuts of fish, the cooking time for all methods of fish cookery is short. Most types of fish can be interchanged in recipes calling for fish as an ingredient.

As fish cooks, it loses its translucency, the juices become milky, and the flesh develops an opaque, whitish appearance. Fish is done when it is easily flaked with a fork.

Dry Heat

Because fish is naturally tender and cooks quickly, baking, broiling, and frying are all popular methods for preparing fish.

Baking. Whole fish, steaks, fillets, and chunks can be baked. A whole fish may be stuffed and baked or a stuffing may be placed between fillets or steaks, as illustrated in Figure 16-5. The temperature range for baking fish is between 350° F (175° C) and 400° F (205° C). The higher temperature is sometimes more preferable for larger, whole fish, and smaller pieces should be baked at the lower temperature. Because fish has a low fat content, it is brushed with melted butter or margarine, topped with strips of bacon, or baked in a sauce spooned over the top to keep the surface moist. The cooking surface needs to be lightly greased to prevent the fish from sticking.

Broiling. Forms of fish suitable for broiling are fillets and steaks. Fish with a higher fat content, such as salmon, swordfish, or trout, are better for broiling than leaner fish. It is preferable to have the fish cuts at least 1-inch thick, but not always possible with fillets.

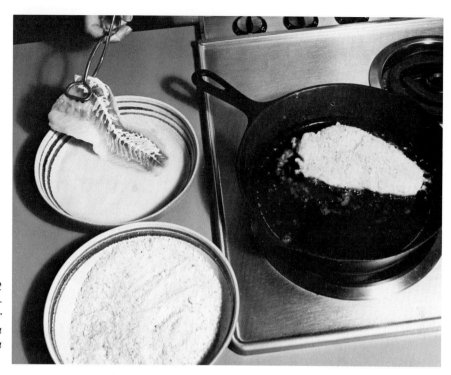

Figure 16-6.
Fish may be fried by first dipping in egg and then rolling in bread, cereal or cracker crumbs. It is cooked in a small amount of fat in a heavy pan.

The fish is laid on a lightly greased broiler rack and placed in the oven so that it is 3 to 4 inches from the heat. Prior to being cooked, the fish should be coated with melted butter, margarine, or a sauce to prevent it from drying out. Halfway through the cooking time, thick cuts of fish are turned and the surface is again coated with fat. Thin fillets do not need to be turned. The time for broiling fish is determined by the thickness of the cut and ranges from 8 to 15 minutes.

The fatter, more full-flavored fish, such as salmon or trout, may also be barbecued. Thinner cuts of fish are more easily barbecued when they are placed in a holding rack or on top of a finely meshed wire.

Frying. Fish may be pan fried, oven fried, or deep-fat fried. Suitable fish forms are fillets, steaks, and small fish.

Fish that is to be pan or deep fried may first be dipped in a mixture of 1/4 cup milk and slightly beaten egg, and then rolled in dry bread or cereal crumbs. Pan-fried fish may also be cooked in a small amount of fat without the additional coating. Fish to be deep fried may also be dipped in a batter.

To pan fry fish, a small amount of fat is melted in a heavy fry pan and the fish is cooked over moderate heat. When one side of the fish is browned, the fish is turned over and the other side is cooked. Pan frying of breaded fish is shown in Figure 16-6. Because of the lower smoking point of animal fats, it is advisable to use fat or oils of vegetable origin. A good combination to use is 1/2 butter or margarine and 1/2 vegetable oil.

When using a method called oven frying, the fish are first dipped in salted milk, and then rolled in dry bread crumbs. The proportion of milk to salt is 1/2 cup milk to 1 teaspoon salt. The fish is then placed in a well-greased shallow baking pan, coated with melted butter or margarine, and baked at 500° F (260° C) for

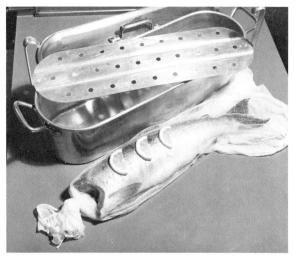

Figure 16-7.

A fish will hold its shape better when first wrapped in cheese cloth before poaching. Pictured here is a fish poacher or poissonière.

10 to 15 minutes. The fish is done when it is brown and flakes easily with a fork.

Moist Heat

Simmering and steaming are the two methods of moist heat cookery that can be used to cook fish.

Simmering. This method is sometimes called "poaching" and is used for cooking small whole fish, fillets, steaks, and chunks. Lean fish, like cod, bass, or red snapper, are easier to poach because the flesh of lean fish is firm and does not fall apart readily. Fish may be tied in cheesecloth before cooking to help retain its shape, as shown in Figure 16-7.

The fish is cooked at a simmer in barely enough liquid to cover the fish until it flakes easily with a fork. This usually takes 5 to 10 minutes for small cuts of fish, but a whole fish will take about 20 minutes, depending on its size. Various liquids may be used, including water, milk, or a mixture of white wine and water. Additional seasonings are often added to the liquid, like onion, garlic, carrot, lemon juice, bay leaf, and various spices and herbs. After the cooked fish has been carefully removed from the liquid, the liquid may be thickened and served as a sauce for the fish, or the fish may be used as a main ingredient for casseroles, salads, or soups.

Steaming. Fish is cooked by steaming when it is placed on a greased rack over boiling water and the pan is tightly covered. This fish is done when it flakes easily with a fork. Fillets steam in 3 to 4 minutes; steaks in 6 to 8 minutes; and a 3-pound whole, dressed fish in about 20 minutes. The fish is then served as when it is prepared by simmering.

Basic Methods of Shellfish Cookery

Shellfish may be cooked in the shell or out of the shell, depending on the type of shellfish, but all shellfish are cooked by the principles of moist and dry heat cookery. Clams and oysters are sometimes eaten without being cooked, but most people prefer them cooked. In most shellfish recipes, the various species can be interchanged, but particularly crab meat can be substituted for lobster meat and scallops for oysters.

Cooking with the Shell

Shellfish cooked in the shell include hard shelled crabs, lobsters, clams, oysters, and shrimp.

Dry Heat. Shellfish may be cooked by dry heat without prior cooking. Oysters are cooked on a rack over an open fire until the shells open. Actually, the oysters steam in their own liquid when this method is used. Clams with cleaned shells may be baked in a casserole in the oven. Any shells that do not open should be discarded. Crab, lobster, and shrimp may be broiled or baked after the shell is opened and unedible parts removed.

Moist Heat. Crabs, lobsters, clams, mussels, and shrimp in the shell are usually cooked by moist heat. Before they are cooked, the shells must be scrubbed with a brush in clean, fresh water; clams that have been dug in the sand are soaked in fresh water to which salt has been added. Cornmeal added to the soaking water helps to eliminate sand inside the shell. Lobster, crabs, and clams need to be alive when they are cooked. The geoduck is most often ground and cooked in chowders.

The basic moist heat cookery method for these shellfish is to plunge them into boiling water and cook just until they are done. Clams are cooked when the shell opens, and lobster, crabs, and shrimp are completely cooked when the shell turns pink for shrimp and deep red for crabs and lobsters.

Cooking Without the Shell

Shellfish cooked out of the shell include clams, soft-shelled crabs, oysters, shrimp, and scallops. Oysters and clams both must be shucked, and the shell of shrimp must be peeled off. Scallops are marketed without the shell.

Dry Heat. There are many recipes for cooking clams, oysters, shrimp, and scallops by frying, broiling, and baking, but in all recipes these shellfish need to be coated with a fat to prevent their surfaces from drying out.

Moist Heat. Oysters, shrimp, and scallops may be simmered for a short period of time. Specific recipes indicate the length of cooking time, but it is usually not longer than 1 to 4 minutes.

RECIPES

————————— **Whole Baked Fish** —————————

	Standard	Metric
Fish, whole, dressed	3 to 5 pounds	1,361–2,268 gm
Butter, cut in 3 slices	1/4 pound	113 gm

1. Preheat the oven to 375° F (190° C).
2. Place the fish on a greased shallow baking pan. Cut three 1/4-inch gashes on top of the fish and insert slices of butter or margarine.
3. Bake at 375° F (190° C) for 50 minutes or until it is easily flaked with a fork.

Yield: 6 to 8 servings

Variations

1. The fish may be stuffed with a bread or vegetable stuffing.
2. The fish may be basted with a butter and lemon juice or white wine mixture during the cooking time.
3. Fish may be wrapped in foil and cooked in this manner.

Baked Fish Steaks

	Standard	Metric
Thinly sliced onion	1/2 cup	125 mL
Fish steaks, 1-inch thick	2 pounds	907 gm
Chopped mushrooms	2 cups	500 mL
Chopped tomato	1/2 cup	125 mL
Chopped green pepper	3 Tbsp.	45 mL
Chopped parsley	2 Tbsp.	30 mL
Lemon juice	1/3 cup	75 mL
Salt	1/2 tsp.	2 mL
Dill weed	1/4 tsp.	1 mL
Butter or margarine	1/4 cup	60 mL

1. Preheat the oven to 350° F (175° C).
2. Arrange the onion slices on the bottom of a greased 9 X 12-inch casserole dish and place the fish steaks on top of the onion.
3. Mix together the mushrooms, tomato, green pepper, parsley, lemon juice, salt, and dillweed and place on top of the steaks.
4. Pour the melted butter or margarine on top of the vegetable steak mixture and bake for 30 minutes or until it is easily flaked with a fork. To cook in microwave oven cover fish with waxed paper and cook for 12 minutes, rotating dish 1/4 turn after 6 minutes cooking time.

Yield: 6 servings

Fish with Broiled Topping

	Standard	Metric
Butter or margarine	3 Tbsp.	45 mL
Fillets or shellfish	2 pounds	907 gm
Sour cream	2 cups	500 mL
Lemon juice	1-1/2 Tbsp.	22 mL
Grated Parmesan cheese	2/3 cup	150 mL
Minced chives	1-1/2 tsp.	7 mL
Minced parsley	1 Tbsp.	15 mL

1. Turn on the broiler unit of the oven.
2. Melt the butter or margarine in a heavy fry pan and brown the fish on both sides. Set aside.

3. Combine the sour cream, lemon juice, parmesan cheese, chives, and parsley.
4. Place the fish on a greased broiler rack and spread with the sour cream mixture. Heat just until bubbly and serve immediately.

Yield: 6 servings

Spicy Broiled Fish Fillets

	Standard	Metric
Fillets	2 pounds	907 gm
Salt	1 tsp.	5 mL
Sharp, grated cheddar cheese	1 cup	250 mL
Prepared mustard	1 Tbsp.	15 mL
Horseradish	1 tsp.	5 mL
Chili sauce	2 Tbsp.	30 mL
Melted butter or margarine	1/4 cup	60 mL

1. Preheat the broiler unit of the oven.
2. Combine the cheese, prepared mustard, horseradish, and chili sauce.
3. Place the fish on a greased broiler rack and sprinkle with salt.
4. Brush the fish with butter or margarine and broil for 5 minutes; turn and brush again with butter or margarine; broil for 5 minutes.
5. Place the cheese mixture on top of the fish and broil for 1 to 2 minutes or until bubbly. Serve immediately.

Yield: 6 servings

Broiled Scallops

	Standard	Metric
Olive oil	1/4 cup	60 mL
White wine	1/4 cup	60 mL
Lemon juice	2 Tbsp.	30 mL
Parsley	1 Tbsp.	15 mL
Scallops	1 pound	453 gm

1. Turn the oven unit to broil.

2. Combine the olive oil, white wine, lemon juice, and parsley together in a bowl.
3. Dip the scallops into the olive oil mixture and arrange on a broiler pan or place on individual metal skewers and place on a broiler pan. Broil 8 to 10 minutes or until the scallops are cooked through, turning half way through cooking time. Serve immediately.

Yield: 4 servings

Variation:

1. Use chunks of halibut in place of the scallops.

Poached Fish

	Standard	Metric
Fresh salmon, bass, or red snapper	3 pounds	1361 gm
Water	3 cups	750 mL
Peppercorns	4	4
Lemon slices	2	2
Salt	1 tsp.	5 mL
Celery	1 stalk	1
Carrot, scraped	1	1
Onion	1 medium	1
White wine	1 cup	250 mL
Butter or margarine	1/4 cup	60 mL
Flour	1/4 cup	60 mL

1. Place the fish on a rack that will fit in the pan or tie fish in cheesecloth.
2. Combine the water, peppercorns, lemon slices, salt, celery, carrot, and onion in a large saucepan with a lid and bring to a boil.
3. Add the fish to the boiling liquid and pour the wine over the fish. Cover and simmer for 20 minutes or until the fish flakes easily with a fork. Remove the fish from the liquid.
4. Strain the liquid and set aside.
5. Melt the butter or margarine in a saucepan. Add the flour and cook until smooth, stirring constantly. Add the strained liquid and cook over low heat until thickened, stirring constantly. Serve the sauce over the fish.

Yield: 4 to 6 servings

Fried Fish in Herbed Sauce

	Standard	Metric
Flour	1/4 cup	60 mL
Salt	1/2 tsp.	2 mL
Pepper	1/8 tsp.	0.5 mL
Vegetable oil	1/4 cup	60 mL
Fish fillets or steaks	2 pounds	907 gm
Tomatoes, peeled and chopped	4	4
Garlic clove, minced	1 small	1
Butter or margarine	1 Tbsp.	15 mL
Tarragon	1/2 tsp.	2 mL
Salt	1/4 tsp.	1 mL
Pepper	1/8 tsp.	0.5 mL
Blanched, slivered, and toasted almonds	1 cup	250 mL

1. Mix together the flour, salt, and pepper. Dip the fish in the mixture to coat all sides.
2. Heat the vegetable oil in a heavy fry pan and cook the fish for 2 or 3 minutes over moderate heat to brown both sides. Set aside.
3. Combine the tomatoes, garlic, butter or margarine, tarragon, salt, and pepper in another heavy saucepan and cook over moderate heat until the mixture is bubbly.
4. Pour the tomato mixture over the fish and heat until it is just warmed. Serve immediately.

Yield: 6 servings

Oyster Pan Roast

	Standard	Metric
Butter or margarine	3 Tbsp.	45 mL
Chopped green onion	1 Tbsp.	15 mL
Finely chopped green pepper	1/4 cup	60 mL
Sliced mushrooms	1/2 cup	125 mL
Chicken broth	1/3 cup	75 mL
Butter or margarine	3 Tbsp.	60 mL
Oysters, medium-sized	18	18

1. Melt the butter or margarine in a heavy fry pan.

Add the chopped green onion, chopped green pepper, and sliced mushrooms. Cook until tender. Add the chicken broth. Put the mixture into a bowl and set aside.

2. Melt the second amount of 3 Tbsp. of butter or margarine in the fry pan. Add the oysters to the pan and cook over medium heat for 2 minutes.

3. Add the green onion mixture to the oysters and cook an additional 2 minutes. Serve immediately.

Yield: 3 to 4 servings

———————— Clam Patties ————————

	Standard	Metric
Minced clams	1 (8-1/2 oz.) can	1 (241 gm)
Egg, slightly beaten	1	1
Flour	1 cup	250 mL
Vegetable oil	2 Tbsp.	30 mL
Butter or margarine	2 Tbsp.	30 mL

1. Drain the clams and combine with the egg and flour.

2. Heat the vegetable oil and butter or margarine until bubbly, in a heavy fry pan.

3. Drop the clam mixture by the spoonful into hot fat. Cook until crispy on one side, turn, and cook the other side, about 3 minutes on each side.

Yield: 4 servings

———————— Deep Fried Fish ————————

	Standard	Metric
White fish fillets, flounder, cod, sole	2 pounds	907 gm
Egg	1	1
Lemon juice	1 Tbsp.	15 mL
Dry bread or cereal crumbs	3/4 cup	175 mL
Salt	1 tsp.	5 mL
Pepper	1/4 tsp.	1 mL

1. Cut the fish into serving pieces.

2. Beat the egg and lemon juice together.

3. Mix together the bread or cereal crumbs, salt, and pepper.

4. Dip the fish into crumbs, then into egg mixture, and again into crumbs. Set on a piece of waxed paper.

5. Heat the fat in a deep fryer to 375° F (190° C). Fry the fish in deep fat until brown and crisp, about 5 minutes.

6. Drain the fish on paper toweling. Serve immediately.

Yield: 6 servings

———————— Crust Pan Fried Fish ————————

	Standard	Metric
Fish fillets, cod, red snapper, or halibut	2 pounds	907 gm
Yellow cornmeal	1/2 cup	125 mL
Flour	1/2 cup	125 mL
Pepper	1/4 tsp.	1 mL
Salt	1/2 tsp.	2 mL
Buttermilk	1/2 cup	125 mL
Butter	1/4 cup	60 mL
Hydrogenated shortening	1/4 cup	60 mL

1. Cut the fish into serving pieces.

2. Combine the yellow cornmeal, flour, salt, and pepper in a bowl; pour the buttermilk into a separate bowl.

3. Dip the fish into the buttermilk and coat with the flour mixture. Set on a piece of waxed paper.

4. Melt the butter and shortening in a heavy fry pan. Brown the fish on both sides and cook until the fish flakes easily with a fork, about 5 minutes.

Yield: 6 servings

———————— Shrimp Stuffed Fillets ————————

	Standard	Metric
Chopped green onion	1/4 cup	60 mL
Small shrimp	3/4 cup	175 mL
Dill weed	1/2 tsp.	2 mL
Fish fillets	6	6

	Standard	Metric
Butter or margarine	3 Tbsp.	45 mL
Flour	3 Tbsp.	45 mL
Salt	1 tsp.	5 mL
Milk	1 cup	250 mL

1. Preheat the oven to 350° F (175° C).
2. Combine the chopped green onion, small shrimp, and dill weed.
3. Spread the mixture evenly between the six fillets and roll the fillets, securing with a wooden pick. Place in a shallow, greased baking dish.
4. Melt the butter in a heavy saucepan; stir in the flour and cook until the mixture is smooth. Add the milk and salt and stir until the mixture thickens. Pour over the fillets and bake for 20 minutes. In the microwave oven, bake for 10 minutes, rotating dish 1/4 turn after 5 minutes cooking time.

Yield: 6 servings

Salmon Casserole

	Standard	Metric
Peas, cooked	1-1/2 cups	375 mL
Salmon	1 (16 oz.) can	1 (454 gm)
Ripe olives, sliced	1/2 cup	125 mL
Onion, dehydrated	1/4 cup	60 mL
Butter or margarine	1/4 cup	60 mL
Flour	1/4 cup	60 mL
Milk	1-1/2 cups	375 mL
Salt	1/2 tsp.	2 mL
Pepper	1/8 tsp.	0.05 mL
Bay leaf	1	1
Beef bouillon cubes	2	2
Dry bread crumbs	1/4 cup	60 mL
Cheddar cheese, sharp, grated	1/2 cup	125 mL

1. Preheat the oven to 350° F (175° C).
2. Drain the peas and drain and flake the salmon. Add the onions and olives to the pea mixture. Set aside.
3. Melt the butter in a heavy saucepan; add the flour and stir until the mixture is smooth; add the milk, and stir constantly over low heat until the mixture is thickened. Add the salt, pepper, bay leaf, and beef bouillon cubes; stir to mix.
4. In a 9 × 9-inch greased casserole dish put the pea, salmon, onion, olive mixture. Remove the bay leaf from the sauce and pour the sauce over the mixture in the casserole dish. Sprinkle with the bread crumbs and the cheese. In the microwave oven bake for 10-12 minutes, rotating dish 1/4 turn after 6 minutes cooking time.
5. Bake for 30 minutes.

Yield: 6 servings

Deviled Crab

	Standard	Metric
Crab meat	2 cups	500 mL
Lemon juice	2 Tbsp.	30 mL
Cream of mushroom soup	1 (10-1/2 oz.) can	1 (306 gm)
Worcestershire sauce	1-1/2 tsp.	7 mL
Prepared mustard	1 tsp.	5 mL
Cayenne pepper	1/8 tsp.	0.5 mL
Butter or margarine	2 Tbsp.	30 mL
Sliced mushrooms	1 cup	250 mL
Butter or margarine	2 Tbsp.	30 mL
Fresh bread crumbs	1/2 cup	125 mL
Parmesan cheese	1/2 cup	125 mL

1. Preheat the oven to 400° F (205° C).
2. In a mixing bowl, combine the crab meat, lemon juice, cream of mushroom soup, Worcestershire sauce, prepared mustard, cayenne pepper, and sautéed mushrooms. Turn into a greased, 2-quart baking dish.
3. Melt the butter or margarine in a heavy fry pan and sauté the mushrooms until they are lightly browned.
4. Melt the remaining 2 Tbsp. of butter or margarine in a pan. Add the bread crumbs and cheese and toss lightly with a fork until blended.
5. Sprinkle the crumb mixture over the crab and bake for 20 minutes or until heated through.

Yield: 4 servings

Variations:

1. The mixture may be baked in a dungeness crab shell or in individual shell ramekins.

————————— Pickled Shrimp —————————

	Standard	Metric
Celery leaves	1/2 cup	125 mL
Mixed pickling spices	1/4 cup	60 mL
Salt	1 tsp.	5 mL
Shrimp, raw	2 pounds	907 gm
Sliced onions	2 cups	500 mL
Bay leaves	8	8
Salad oil	1-1/2 cups	375 mL
White vinegar	3/4 cup	175 mL
Celery seeds	2-1/2 tsp.	12 mL
Salt	1-1/2 tsp.	7 mL
Tabasco sauce	2 drops	2 drops

1. Bring 3 quarts water to a boil in a large saucepan. Add celery leaves, mixed pickling spices, salt, and shrimp. Cook 8 minutes or until the shells turn pink.

2. Drain the water from the shrimp. Remove the shells from the shrimp and the black line down the back.

3. Layer the shrimp, sliced onion, and bay leaves in a large shallow pan.

4. Combine the salad oil, vinegar, celery seeds, salt, and Tabasco sauce. Pour the marinade mixture over the shrimp and refrigerate for 24 hours. Baste the shrimp occasionally with the marinade.

5. Serve as an appetizer or salad ingredient.

Yield: 4 cups

LEARNING ACTIVITIES

1. Investigate at a local market the kinds and forms of fish and shellfish that are available.
2. If both fresh and frozen fish and shellfish are available, compare the prices of various forms to determine the best buy.
3. Make a list of the kinds of fish that you have tasted. Plan a menu around one of these kinds of fish.
4. Make a list of the kinds of shellfish that you have tasted. Plan a menu around one of these.
5. If possible, cook a fish that you have never sampled. Then develop a menu using the fish as an entrée.
6. Investigate the different kinds and the prices of canned fish and shellfish that are available at a local market. Plan a menu around the least expensive canned fish and a variety of shellfish.
7. Plan breakfast, lunch, and dinner menus for 3 days that include fish as the main source of protein for at least one menu each day. Decide what other foods would have to be included to assure an adequate supply of iron.
8. Prepare a research paper to present to the class on the various kinds of fish farming that take place in the United States.
9. Prepare a chart that shows the amount of fish consumed in the United States as compared to that consumed in three other countries of the world.
10. Prepare a fish fillet by broiling, pan frying, and deep frying. Decide which method yields the most flavorful fish and which is the most time-consuming.
11. Make a list of sauces that would be a flavorful addition to serve with fish.
12. If possible, demonstrate to the class the proper method to fillet a fish or shuck an oyster as learned by experience or by reading another book on this subject.

REVIEW QUESTIONS

1. Why is fish a choice food for some diets?
2. How does the protein quality of fish and shellfish compare with that of meat or eggs?
3. In what two minerals is fish low?
4. How might the answer to number three affect menu planning?
5. What are four menu-planning factors that must be considered when planning other foods to accompany a fish entrée?
6. What must be planned in time scheduling for a menu that has fresh fish as an entrée?
7. Why is fish considered an acceptable food for people of any age?
8. What are the two categories of fish and shellfish?
9. What is the difference between a mollusk and a crustacean?
10. What is a dressed fish?
11. How do a fish fillet and a steak differ?
12. What are four factors that influence the price of fish?
13. What are four factors that indicate a healthy, fresh fish?
14. What should be the appearance of fresh crabs and lobster at the time of purchase?
15. What is the most expensive form of tuna fish?
16. How is canned salmon sold and which is the most expensive kind of salmon?
17. How should fresh fish be stored in the refrigerator and for how many days?
18. How long can cooked fish be stored in the refrigerator?
19. How should frozen fish be thawed?
20. What is the recommended time for freezing fresh fish and cooked fish?
21. What are three methods for preparing fish for freezing?
22. What are three signs of fish being completely cooked?
23. Which types of fish are most preferred for broiling?
24. What are the three methods for frying fish?
25. Why is it suggested not to use all animal fat as the fat for frying?
26. What is the method for simmering or poaching fish?
27. How is a poached fish served?
28. How does steaming fish differ from simmering fish?
29. What is the sign that clams or oysters have completed cooking in the shell?
30. What is the sign that live crabs or lobsters have completed cooking?
31. What is a scallop?

17

Bread

The age-old saying that bread is the staff of life has not changed. In some homes bread is the single source of food, and in other homes, bread is a principal food served at every meal, including snacktime. The life and health of many people is dependent upon the world's yearly production of wheat, the principal grain used in making bread.

Although most forms of bread are readily available for purchase in the United States, there is nothing like the aroma of freshly baked bread in a home. The individual who prepares bread also receives a great deal of satisfaction from creating the product.

Two categories of bread, quick breads and yeast breads, are discussed in this chapter, along with the basic functions of other major

ingredients used in bread making and other flour mixtures.

Nutritional Factors to Consider

Carbohydrate and Fat

Bread is a major source of energy-providing carbohydrate in the diet. Although fat is an important ingredient in most breads, it is not present in a large enough amount to be a major contributor to energy needs.

Protein

Bread is a major contributor of protein to the diet. Although the cereal grains from which bread is made are incomplete sources of protein, most breads contain other complete proteins, such as milk and eggs, which help to balance the protein content. Breads are also eaten at a meal with other complete protein foods such as meat, milk, eggs, cheese, or fish.

Vitamins and Minerals

Breads made from whole grain and enriched white flour are a major source of the B vitamins, thiamine, riboflavin, and niacin, and the mineral iron. Breads using milk as the major source of liquid and commercially made breads containing milk solids are a good source of calcium.

Calories

Considering the major nutrients that bread provides for the human diet, it is not high in calories. The average slice of enriched white bread contains only 76 calories, whereas an 8-ounce glass of whole milk contains 159 calories and a medium-sized apple contains 80 calories. A meat sandwich made with two slices of bread contains approximately 300 calories, and a regular-sized candy bar contains approximately 150 calories.

Menu-Planning Points

Inherent Factors

Balance. Breads supply balance in a meal by providing the additional nutrients needed to meet one's daily requirement.

Color. Color can be achieved or balanced in a meal by using a variety of breads. Enriched white bread provides balance for a meal of brightly colored foods, whereas a bread made from the whole grains, such as whole wheat or rye, provides a warm, brown color to contrast more blandly colored foods.

Shape. Both yeast breads and rolls and quick breads can be made into a variety of shapes to provide added interest to a meal. For example, yeast breads may be baked in small, individual loaves or baked in a cylindrical shape by using a can as the baking container. Many different shapes of yeast rolls can be made, including fan tans, bow knots, and snails. The classic muffin and biscuit add their own shape variety to a meal.

Flavor. Many flavor variations are possible in breads. The use of different flours provides a wide array of flavors, from the pungent sourness of rye to the nutty flavor of whole wheat. Additional flavor variations are possible by using a variety of herbs and spices in breads. For example, adding dill weed or caraway seed to a bread made from enriched white flour provides a distinctive flavor. Adding cheese to biscuits or nuts and chopped cranberries to muffins provides different flavor variations.

Texture. The texture of a meal can be complemented by the kind of bread that is served. A meal that has an entrée of soup is complemented in texture by serving a crunchy French bread or bread sticks. The soft-textured dinner yeast roll complements a meal featuring roast beef as the entrée.

External Factors

Age and Culture. There is neither an age nor a culture that does not enjoy bread in some form. However, young children should not be given crunchy breads that they may choke on, and senior citizens may have difficulty chewing the coarser-textured breads. Many cultures have their own specific breads. For example, many of the people in South America prefer a thin, crisp bread made from corn flour, whereas many European cultures prefer the heavy texture and flavor of breads made from rye flour.

Economics. Making bread at home is slightly less expensive than purchasing bread at the market. However, time is often a factor in making a decision on whether or not to bake bread at home. Many bakeries and supermarkets offer day-old bread, which is an economical purchase. Specialty breads are more expensive than the standard loaf but offer variety to meals.

Space and Equipment. Bread begins to stale immediately after it is baked and should be purchased only in amounts that can be used in one week if freezing is not possible. Certain equipment is essential for successful bread making, and attempting a project without adequate equipment can be an economic loss to the food budget.

Time Scheduling. All bread preparation takes a certain amount of time. If time is short, the commercial convenience mixes or the home-prepared mixes save many steps in bread preparation. Refrigerator dough or battery yeast doughs can save time and still allow the preparation of bread in the home.

Storage of Bread

Bread is a perishable food and is susceptible to staling, bread mold, and ropiness. The exact length of time that bread can be stored without its eating quality being affected depends upon several factors, including the chemical preservatives added to commercially baked bread to retard spoilage, the conditions under which it is stored at home, and the humidity and warmth of the weather.

Signs of staling bread are a loss of flavor and aroma and the development of a firm, crumbly, and harsh texture. This is best prevented by storing bread in its original wrapper, or if home-baked, by wrapping the bread in moisture-resistant paper, plastic bag, or foil. Bread must be stored in a clean, dry and well-ventilated container or drawer. The container should be kept away from heat-producing units, such as ranges, refrigerators, and radiators.

Bread may be stored in the refrigerator, but the cool temperature will increase staling. Refrigeration storage helps to decrease mold growth in hot, humid weather. All kinds of baked bread can be frozen satisfactorily at 0° F (–18° C) and then thawed at room temperature. Freezing stale bread does not restore its freshness.

Ropiness in bread is caused by a bacterial growth in the dough and is noted by an off-color, a sticky interior, and an odor similar to overripe soft fruit. Ropiness is most likely to occur in bread in hot, humid weather.

Bread that is stored for an excessive period of time will dry out. Although stale bread is not palatable for eating, it can be further dried and ground or rolled into crumbs to be used as a topping for casseroles, a breading for such foods as pork chops or fish fillets, or a meat extender in such food dishes as a ground meat loaf. Stale bread that is cut into cubes makes a good bread pudding. Dry bread crumbs can be stored indefinitely in a tightly closed container in a clean, dry storage area.

Ingredients and Their Functions

All breads contain a flour and a liquid. Other ingredients such as eggs, fat, a leavening agent, sugar, and salt are added to make different kinds of bread. Additional ingredients such as herbs, spices, nuts, fruits, and cheese may be used to further vary the flavor, color, and texture of breads.

Flour

Flour is the product resulting from the grinding or milling of a cereal grain. Standards of identity have been established by the FDA for both varying types of flour and the enrichment of flours made from other than whole-grain flours. Since 1941, the enrichment of white flour with the B-vitamins, thiamine, niacin, and riboflavin and with iron has been a practice of the food industry. Today more than half of the states require enrichment of flour and bread products.

The most common kind of flour used in making breads and other baked products is made from wheat. Wheat flour is highly desirable in bread making because it contains the two proteins, gliadin and glutenin. When wheat flour is mixed with water, these two proteins combine to make gluten, which is the strong, sticky, and elastic part of a flour-liquid mixture. The protein quality of flour that is made from hard wheat is greater than that made from soft wheat.

Flour made from wheat may be bleached to improve the color and the baking quality. If flour has been bleached by a government-approved bleaching agent, the word "bleached" must be clearly shown on the label. Flours made from other grains are used in breads in which texture and volume are not desirable characteristics of the product, or are used in combination with wheat flour to yield a product differing in flavor, texture, and volume from that containing only wheat flour. The one exception is rye flour, which contains the two proteins necessary for making gluten but in a differing proportion. A bread made from rye flour has a much firmer texture and a lesser volume than a bread made from wheat flour.

Several different kinds of wheat flour are used in breads and other baked products.

All-purpose Flour. This flour, suitable for all food products requiring flour as an ingredient, is the most common kind of flour used in bread making. All-purpose flour is made from a blend of hard or soft wheats. Hard-wheat flours have a higher proportion of protein and are better for yeast-leavened breads. Soft-wheat flours bake into a more tender product and are more desirable for quick breads such as muffins.

Instant-Blending Flour. This an an all-purpose flour that has been further processed into a more granulated and pourable form, which does not pack down when stored. Instant-blending flour does not need to be sifted before it is used, and it combines more readily with a liquid as in the making of sauces.

Self-rising Flour. This flour contains leavening ingredients and salt which, if mixed with a liquid, produce the leavening agent carbon dioxide. Specially developed recipes should be used when using this flour.

Cake Flour. This flour is made only from soft wheat and is a very finely ground, silky-textured flour. Because cake flour has a low protein quality, the gluten-forming properties of cake flour are poor; thus cake flour is not suitable for making bread, but it can be substituted for other baking purposes by using 2 extra tablespoons per cup.

Whole-wheat Flour. This flour is made from the entire wheat berry. A loaf made from whole-wheat flour is smaller in size and more compact than bread made from all-purpose flour, because the bran in whole-wheat flour inhibits the rising power of the dough.

Eggs

Eggs provide added nutrients, color when the egg yolk is used, and a richer flavor to bread. In addition, eggs help to make a fine crumb and a tender crust and eggs help to distribute the fat in a mixture because of their emulsifying properties. Eggs serve as a leavening agent in breads that are beaten by incorporating air into the mixture. Then as the mixture is heated, the egg protein coagulates and traps the increased volume.

Fat

All kinds of fat may be used in bread making including hydrogenated fats, cooking oils, butter, margarine, and lard. The kind of fat used in bread making will vary with specific recipes. The addition of fat to a bread mixture makes a more tender product because the fat coats the flour particles and keeps them separated. Fat also contributes to making a moister and softer product.

Leavening Agents

A leavening agent is air, steam, and/or the gas carbon dioxide, which is produced from baking soda, baking powder, or yeast. When a leavening agent is incorporated into bread and other baked products, the resulting baked food is light and porous. Baked products that do not contain a leavening agent or which contain an insufficient amount are compact and have a tough texture. Likewise, too much of a leavening agent produces a baked product with a poor flavor and a coarse texture.

Baking Soda. Baking soda, when combined with an acid, produces carbon dioxide. Common acidic foods, which are normally combined with baking soda in making breads and other baked products, include sour milk, buttermilk, fruit juices, and molasses. Baking soda will produce carbon dioxide when it is heated alone, but a highly undesirable flavor results.

Baking soda can be substituted for baking powder in a recipe if an acidic food is also added. The equivalent measurement is 1/4 teaspoon soda to 1 teaspoon baking powder. To this proportion, 1/2 cup sour milk or buttermilk is substituted for 1/2 cup sweet milk.

Sweet milk may be made sour by adding 1-1/2 teaspoon vinegar or lemon juice to 1/2 cup sweet milk.

Baking Powder. Baking powder is a mixture of baking soda, an acid powder, and a starch. The soda and acid powder are mixed in proportions to release carbon dioxide from the baking soda. The starch is used to absorb any moisture that may be present during storage and thus prevent the soda and acid from combining before use. It is important to keep baking powder tightly covered during shelf storage, to store it in a cool, dry place, and to purchase it in small amounts to avoid deterioration.

Baking powders are classified as single-acting or double-acting powders. Single-acting powders produce carbon dioxide at room temperature when they are mixed with a liquid. Breads and other baked products that use a single-acting powder need to be quickly mixed and baked to prevent an excessive loss of carbon dioxide before the baking process is completed. Double-acting powders contain two acid powders; one reacts with the soda at room temperature to produce carbon dioxide when mixed with a liquid and the other produces carbon dioxide when exposed to heat. Double-acting powders are usually more desirable for home baking because of interruptions that may occur to slow the mixing-baking process.

Yeast. Yeast is a living plant that can only be viewed under a powerful microscope. As a leavening agent, yeast produces carbon dioxide along with alcohol by using sugar as its source of food. This process is called *fermentation.* For reproduction and growth of the yeast cell, moisture and warmth in addition to the food, sugar, need to be present. Yeast cells grow best at a temperature of 85° to 90° F (30°-32° C). An excessive amount of salt or sugar can cause the yeast cells to lose water and make them less active.

Fermentation and the production of carbon dioxide continues during the "raising" period of bread, which follows the mixing and/or kneading of a bread dough and is the time when the yeast cells continue to give off carbon dioxide and cause the dough to expand until it is nearly double in volume. This action gives bread its porous appearance. As the bread is baked, its structure is set and the carbon dioxide and alcohol are driven off. Yeast also helps to make the gluten of flour more soft, elastic, and digestible, and contributes to the characteristic flavor of bread.

Yeast is sold in two forms. Compressed yeast is sold in a small cake form and is composed of moist, living cells with a small amount of starch added to bind the cells together. Compressed or cake yeast is perishable and needs to be refrigerated, or it may be frozen for up to 3 months.

Active dry yeast is a dried, granular form that is not as perishable as compressed yeast. It can be stored at room temperature, or it may be frozen for several years. Active dry yeast is sold in foil packets with each packet containing 1 tablespoon, or it is available in some markets in bulk form that needs to be refrigerated after being opened. Active dry yeast labels contain a "use-by" date after which time the yeast should not be used.

Air and Steam. Air and steam are additional leavening agents that always help to make a more light and porous baked product. Air is always used in combination with another leavening agent. Incorporation of air into a mixture occurs in the general preparation and mixing of ingredients. For example, beating any form of egg or beating a mixture incorporates air, creaming of fat and sugar entraps air, and the heating or baking of a mixture entraps the air in the cells and causes the mixture to expand.

Steam, is a common leavening agent in all breads and other baked products because they contain water which evaporates as the mixture is heated. When steam is the main leavening agent, as it is in popovers, the temperature of the oven must be very high to cause the liquid to rapidly evaporate and produce steam.

Liquids

A liquid is an essential ingredient of all breads and other baked products containing flour. The principal functions of a liquid are to hydrate or combine with the starch and gluten in flour, to help dissolve the sugar and salt, to activate and dissolve the leavening agents other than air and steam, and to serve as a leavening agent by producing steam.

Several liquids are used in preparing breads and other baked products. Most breads use milk in some form because a softer texture is achieved. However, French bread with its characteristic coarser texture uses water as its liquid. Nonfat dry milk, a very economical and nutritious milk to use in bread making, can be reconstituted or mixed in with the dry ingredients and water in the proper proportion used as the liquid. Evaporated milk may also be used when diluted with water in the proper proportions.

Breads and other baked products that are noted for their special flavor may use such liquids as the water in which pared potatoes are cooked, fruit juices, or coffee.

Sugar

Breads and other flour mixtures may or may not contain sugar. When sugar is included, it has several important functions. Sugar provides flavor and contributes to the tenderness of a product and aids in the browning of the crust. When yeast is used as the leavening agent, the sugar provides food for the yeast. Granulated sugar is most often the sugar used but some recipes may call for other sweeteners, such as molasses, honey, or brown sugar.

Salt

Salt enhances the flavor of bread, and when yeast is the leavening agent, it helps to control the action of the yeast in gas formation.

Quick Breads

Quick breads are those breads that are leavened by an agent other than yeast. Food products included under the heading of quick breads include muffins, biscuits, pancakes, popovers, crepes, waffles, and breads, such as corn bread, tea breads, and some coffee cakes. With the exception of some tea breads, quick breads have their best eating quality when they are served immediately after they have finished baking. Tea breads most often have their best eating quality after they have been completely chilled and their additional ingredients have had time to mellow.

Methods of Preparation

The method for preparing a quick bread is dependent upon the amount of liquid used in proportion to the flour. Pancakes, crepes, waffles, and popovers have a high proportion of liquid to flour and are classified as pour batters. Muffins, drop biscuits, coffee cakes, and tea breads have a lesser amount of liquid and are classified as drop batters. Rolled biscuits have even less liquid and are classified as a dough.

Muffin Method

Ingredients for quick breads mixed by the muffin method are combined by (1) sifting the dry ingredients together into a mixing bowl;

(2) melting the fat and letting it cool slightly, or oil may be used; (3) beating the eggs slightly and combining with the fat and liquid; (4) adding the liquid ingredients all at once to the dry ingredients and stirring only until the dry ingredients are moistened. Overmixing and beating these types of quick breads develops the gluten of the flour and makes a product that has a coarse texture and an interior which has holes or tunnels rather than a fine grain texture. Figure 17-1 shows the interior texture of an overmixed muffin and a muffin that was mixed properly. Table 17-1 lists the quality characteristics of some quick breads. The one exception for extended mixing is a very rich quick bread that needs more mixing.

Waffle batters may be prepared using the whole egg or by separating the eggs and beating the egg yolks and whites separately. In this method, the stiffly beaten egg whites are folded into the batter just before cooking the mixture in a waffle iron. Waffles may also be mixed by the conventional method as discussed in chapter 18 "Cakes".

The batter for popovers is beaten in order to form a smooth batter that is free of lumps. Adding the liquid gradually at first, helps to prevent lumps from forming. Popover batter cannot be overmixed because the ratio of flour to liquid is such that the gluten strands do not develop. There are many variations on mixing crepe batters but one standard method is to mix the eggs into the dry ingredients. The liquid is added and then the fat. Crepe batters are allowed to rest 1 hour or more before they are cooked to allow the gluten strands to soften.

Biscuit or Pastry Method

The following method of preparation is called the biscuit or pastry method; this procedure may be followed for the making of most pour and drop batter recipes.

The dough for rolled biscuits is prepared by

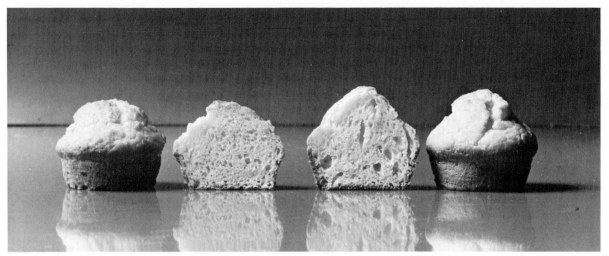

Figure 17-1.
The interior of muffin. Right muffin illustrates the characteristics of a quick bread that is improperly mixed, Left muffin illustrates the characteristics of a properly mixed quick bread.

sifting the dry ingredients together into a bowl. The fat is then cut into the flour mixture by using a pastry blender or two table knives. Cutting in the fat helps to separate the gluten strands of the flour and to produce a flaky, layered biscuit.

The liquid is added all at once to the flour-fat mixture and the dough is mixed with a fork until all the dry ingredients are well moistened. The dough is then turned out onto a lightly floured pastry cloth and lightly kneaded for approximately 30 seconds to develop some of the gluten. The proper method for kneading dough is discussed in the section Methods of Preparation for yeast breads in this chapter, but biscuit kneading should be much lighter. The dough is then rolled to a thickness of 1/2 to 3/4 inch, depending on the desired height of the biscuit, and is then cut with a floured biscuit cutter.

Table 17-1
Quality Characteristics of Some Quick Breads

Product	Characteristics
Muffins	Even grain with air cells of same size
	Well-rounded tops with pebbled surfaces
	Tender crumb
Pancakes	Light brown in color
	Moist on the interior
Popovers	Thick, crusty walls
	Hollow interiors
Rolled Biscuits	Light, golden brown surface color
	Straight sides
	Moist and tender crumb
	Small grain and air cells
	Peels off in layers

Convenience Quick Bread Mixes

Quick breads can also be prepared by using commercially purchased or home-prepared mixes. These mixes, which contain the dry ingredients and sometimes the fat, require only the addition of egg, liquid, and sometimes fat. The recipe section of this chapter contains a recipe for a home-prepared mix from which many quick breads can be made. Refrigerated roll biscuits require only baking.

Baking Quick Breads

All quick breads with the exception of biscuits need to be baked as soon as they are mixed so that they do not lose the air that was incorporated into the product as a leavening agent during the mixing. Biscuits may be held at room temperature for 1/2 hour or in the refrigerator for 2 to 3 hours before baking. If biscuits are refrigerated, they should be brought to room temperature before being cooked.

Quick breads with the exception of rolled biscuits are baked in greased or nonstick coated pans or in pans that have been sprayed with one of the nonstick coatings. Rolled biscuits are baked on ungreased baking sheets. If glass baking containers are used, the oven temperature should be reduced by 25° F (10° C) For example, a recipe calling for an oven temperature of 350° F (175° C) should be reduced to 325° F (165° C) if a glass baking dish is used. Paper baking cups set into muffin tins are also suitable containers for baking quick breads from batters. If all sections of a muffin tin are not filled with batter, they should be partially filled with water to assure even cooking of the muffins. Because quick breads need moderately high to hot ovens for successful baking, it is important to preheat the oven.

Other special factors should be considered when cooking various quick breads.

Popovers. Popovers are baked either in 5-ounce greased glass custard cups, in muffin tins, or in specially designed iron popover pans that have fairly straight sides and are 2 to 3 inches deep. The initial baking of popovers must be done in a very hot oven to allow the liquid to evaporate and the crust to set.

Pancakes. Pancakes are cooked on top of the stove in a heavy fry pan, a special griddle, or an electric fry pan or griddle. The batter is poured onto a medium-hot cooking surface that has been greased with a small amount of fat. Pancakes are cooked on one side until small bubbles form and remain and are then turned to the other side until they are lightly browned. The length of cooking time depends on the thickness of the batter and the heat of the griddle.

Waffles. Waffles are baked on a special iron that has been sprayed with a nonstick spray coating or which has been lightly greased. Some nonstick coated irons do not need a fat coating. Waffles are cooked when the lid of the iron raises easily and the desired stage of crispness has been reached.

Crepes. Crepes are cooked on top of the stove in a heavy skillet, approximately 6 inches in diameter, or in a special crepe pan. If the pan is of the nonstick variety, it should be lightly greased and the excess fat removed with a paper towel before cooking the crepes. Figure 17-2 shows the cooking of a crepe.

Tea Breads and Coffee Cakes. Tea breads are usually baked in loaf pans and need to be cooled for approximately 10 minutes on a cooling rack before they are removed from the pan. Most coffee cakes are left in the baking pan until it is time to serve them.

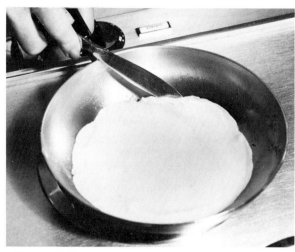

Figure 17-2.
Crepes are cooked in a very lightly greased heavy sauce pan and flipped when the edges set.

Rolled Biscuits. Rolled biscuits are baked on ungreased baking sheets.

Muffins and Drop Biscuits. Muffins and drop biscuits are baked in greased muffin tins or in paper baking cups set in muffin tins.

Yeast Breads

Yeast breads are made from the same basic ingredients as quick breads except that they are mainly leavened by yeast. The dough is mixed thoroughly by stirring, beating, and sometimes kneading it to completely develop the gluten in the flour. Yeast breads can be categorized into stiff doughs and batters. Breads and sweet and dinner rolls are made from both stiff doughs and batters. The dough from which rolls are made usually requires less kneading and is of a softer consistency than bread dough. A sweet dough contains an increased amount of sugar, fat, and eggs. The gluten development in yeast breads allows for expanded volume, and the elasticity in yeast doughs allows the creation of many shapes. With the exception of batter yeast breads, these breads do not need to be served immediately.

Methods of Preparation

Yeast doughs may be prepared by any one of five methods. The choice of which method to use is mainly dependent on an individual's time schedule and the kind of bread desired. Since each of the methods uses slightly different ingredient proportions, it is advisable not to change methods within a recipe.

The two major causes for failure in making a successful yeast bread are dissolving the yeast in too hot water and failing to cool the ingredients sufficiently before adding them to the yeast mixture. Compressed yeast is dissolved in lukewarm water at a temperature of 95° F (35° C) and active dry yeast is dissolved in warm, not hot, water at a temperature of 105 to 115° F (40 to 46° C). It is easier to dissolve dry active yeast when it is sprinkled on top of the water. Active dry yeast and compressed yeast may also be blended with the flour in specific recipes, and the warmed liquid may be combined with the sugar, salt, and fat and added to the dry ingredients.

If fresh milk is the liquid used in the recipe, it needs to be scalded to help prevent some of the protein that is present in milk from softening the gluten of the flour. However, pasteurized, reconstituted dry milk and evaporated milk need only to be warmed. Milk warmed to the scalding point, 190° F (88° C) facilitates the melting of fat.

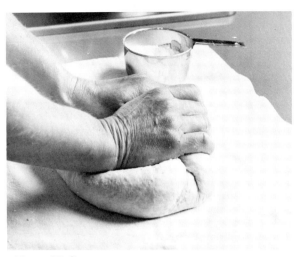

Figure 17-3.

Yeast dough is best kneaded with the heel of the hand as demonstrated here.

Straight Dough Method

In the straight dough method the milk is warmed and then poured over the sugar, salt, and shortening in a large mixing bowl and stirred until the fat is melted and the sugar and salt are dissolved. To this mixture 1 cup of flour is beaten in to further cool the mixture. If eggs are used, they are beaten into the mixture, which is then tested to determine if it has reached a lukewarm temperature. When the mixture has reached the right temperature, the yeast is stirred in. It is easier to add the remaining flour in 1 cup equivalents, beating the mixture until it is smooth after each addition of flour. The amount of flour used to make a dough that comes away from the sides of the bowl will vary slightly, depending on the working conditions, so that a little more or less flour may be needed than called for in the recipe.

The dough is then turned out onto a lightly floured surface or a pastry cloth and is then kneaded until it is smooth. Dough is kneaded by folding the dough over, pressing it away with the heel of the hand, making a 1/4 turn

of the dough, and then repeating the process. Figure 17-3 shows dough being kneaded. Kneading causes the gluten to become flexible so that as the dough rises and the yeast makes more gas, the dough can expand and trap the gas.

In the initial kneading of bread dough, additional flour may be added to the surface on which the dough is being kneaded to prevent the dough from sticking to the surface. The dough has been kneaded sufficiently when it has become a smooth satiny ball with small bubbles on the surface and is springy and elastic. The dough should not stick to the hands or to the kneading surface. This takes approximately 8 to 10 minutes.

The kneaded ball of dough is placed in a greased bowl and is then turned over so that the entire surface is glossy. The grease helps to keep the exterior of the dough soft as it rises. The bowl is then covered with a clean cloth, towel, or waxed paper.

It is important to have a warm temperature of about 85° to 90° F (29° to 32° C) to achieve the proper fermentation of the yeast. Dough needs to rise until it has doubled in bulk, which usually takes from 1-1/2 to 2 hours. The dough should be free from drafts while it is rising and should not be over a direct source of heat or in direct sunlight.

Three methods work satisfactorily to create the proper atmosphere for rising dough. One is to place the bowl of dough in a cold oven with a large pan of warm water underneath the dough, or the bowl may be placed in a deep pan of water that feels just warm to the touch. The third method is to set the bowl near a range, heat vent, or radiator, but never on top of a direct source of heat.

The dough has risen sufficiently when it has doubled in bulk and when the indentation of a finger pressed into the dough remains as illustrated in Figure 17-4. The dough is now punched down by making a fist and pushing into the center of the dough as illustrated in

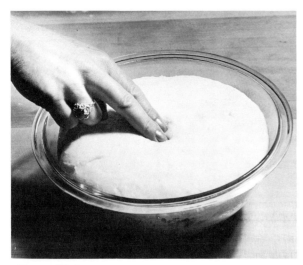

Figure 17-4.
The dough has risen adequately when a finger indentation remains in the dough.

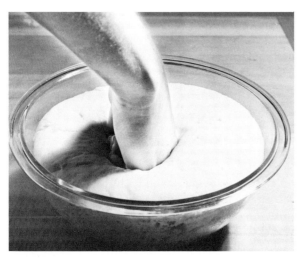

Figure 17-5.
Punching down risen dough is an important step in preparing yeast doughs.

Figure 17-5. Punching the dough down releases some of the gas and speeds up the yeast activity and makes a finer textured product by breaking the larger air pockets into smaller ones. Some doughs are punched down and allowed to rise again before shaping.

The dough is then shaped into rolls or loaves, allowed to rise a second time, and then baked. After the dough is punched down and before it is shaped, it should be allowed to rest on the working surface for about 10 minutes. Resting makes the dough easier to handle and helps the product better hold its shape.

Sponge Method

The sponge method for making yeast doughs includes three rising periods and two steps in mixing. In the first stage of mixing the yeast is dissolved and combined with part of the flour, some sugar, and the liquid. This mixture is then allowed to rise until it is spongy and bubbly. The second stage of mixing involves combining the sponge with the remaining ingredients and the flour, then mixing as with the straight dough method to make a dough that can be kneaded. Following the kneading stage, the dough rises a second time. It is then shaped and rises for a third time.

Batter Method

The batter method for making yeast breads eliminates two steps; there is no kneading and no shaping of the dough. Batter yeast breads contain a higher proportion of liquid to flour and are mixed more quickly than stiff yeast doughs. The basic steps in mixing the ingredients are similar to the straight dough method; however, following the mixing of ingredients, the batter either rises in its original mixing bowl or in its baking pan and is then baked.

Batter breads because of the softer texture have a better eating quality when served soon after being baked.

Refrigerator Method

Refrigerator doughs are basically mixed in the same manner as a straight dough. Refrigerator dough recipes may or may not require kneading. Only recipes designed for refrigeration should be used because the proportions of sugar and salt are such that the action of the yeast is extended over several days. The advantage of a refrigerated dough is that portions may be used over a period of 4 to 5 days, with the rest being kept refrigerated.

Cool-Rise Method

In the cool-rise method, the yeast is mixed in with the flour, salt, sugar, and fat, and the warm liquid is added to the mixture, which is then beaten vigorously by hand or with an electric mixer. Additional flour is added and the process is repeated. The last amount of flour is added and mixed in by hand. The dough is kneaded and then covered on the working surface with plastic wrap and a towel and allowed to rise for approximately 20 minutes. The dough is then punched down, shaped into form, and placed in the baking pan. The dough is allowed to rise in the refrigerator for 2 to 48 hours before baking.

Convenience Yeast Breads

All kinds of yeast breads and rolls are available in bakeries and in the bread sections of grocery stores. Packaged yeast bread and roll mixes are also available together with frozen yeast breads that need only to be baked. Partially baked rolls called "brown and serve rolls" are also available.

Shaping of Doughs

Stiff yeast dough is shaped either into bread loaves or rolls. It is helpful to have the following equipment laid out before beginning to shape loaves or rolls: a washable ruler which helps to determine form size, a rolling pin, a pastry brush, a small amount of melted butter

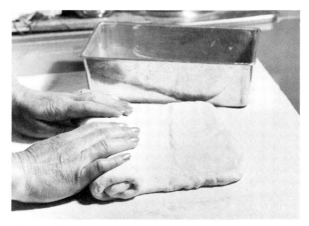

Figure 17-6.
A bread loaf is shaped for the pan by tightly rolling dough the width and length of the pan, and pinching and turning the edges under.

or margarine, and the proper size pans. Using the right pan size is important for bread to attain the proper volume and shape in rising. Pans used in loaf and roll baking include a baking sheet, a muffin tin, a loaf pan, and round or square cake pans. All pans should be greased lightly when they are used in baking bread.

To cut dough into usable amounts for shaping, the dough is turned out onto a cutting board and evenly cut through with a sharp knife into equal amounts. While one portion of dough is being shaped, the other portion is returned to the bowl and covered. Unused portions of refrigerator dough should be returned to the refrigerator.

To shape a loaf of bread, the dough is first rolled out to a width that is equal to the length of the bread pan. The dough is rolled up tightly and the edge is pinched to the roll to form a tight seal. Figure 17-6 illustrates the shaping of a loaf. The ends of the dough are pressed down firmly and folded under. The rolled loaf is placed in the center of the greased pan with the seam-side down.

To shape rolls yeast dough is rolled in three basic forms: a rectangle usually 9 × 12 inches,

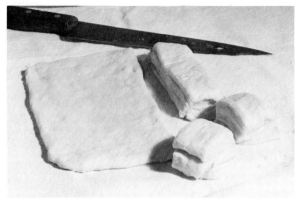

Figure 17-7.
Fan tans are shaped by cutting a rectangular piece of dough into strips 1-1/2 inches wide, stacking 4 to 6 layers atop one another and cutting the stacks into 1-1/2 inch sections.

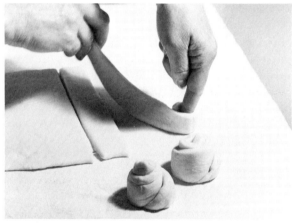

Figure 17-8.
Pinwheels are made by coiling narrow strips of dough around a finger and turning the end underneath.

a circle 9 inches in diameter, or a 9-inch roll. If more shapes are desired, the sizes of the forms must be altered.

Fan Tans

To make fan tan rolls the dough is rolled into an 11 × 9 inch rectangle and brushed lightly with melted butter or margarine. The dough is cut into seven equal strips approximately 1-1/2 inches wide, and the strips are piled atop one another. The dough is then cut into six equal pieces about 1-1/2 inches long and placed in a greased muffin tin with the cut-side up. Fan tan rolls are illustrated in Figure 17-7.

Pinwheels

To make pinwheels the dough is rolled into a rectangle, 9 × 12 inches, and brushed with melted butter or margarine. The dough is cut with a sharp knife into 12 equal strips approximately 1-inch wide. The pinwheel is made by holding one end of the strip firmly down on a greased baking sheet and coiling the strip around and around. The end is tucked firmly underneath the shaped roll. Pinwheels are illustrated in Figure 17-8.

Cinnamon or Filled Rolls

To make cinnamon or filled rolls the dough is rolled into a rectangle, 9 × 12 inches, and brushed with melted butter or margarine. One half cup of sugar is mixed with 1-1/2 teaspoon cinnamon and sprinkled over the dough. If desired, 1/3 cup of raisins may be added. The dough is then rolled as for a bread loaf and the edge is pinched to the roll. The roll is cut into slices by sliding an 8-inch piece of string under the roll, bringing the ends up over, and crossing the string ends to cut through the roll as illustrated in Figure 17-9.

Crescents

Crescents are made by rolling the dough into a circle that is 9 inches in diameter and approximately 1/4-inch thick, as shown in Figure 17-10. The dough is brushed lightly with butter or margarine and cut into eight pie-shaped pieces. Each piece is rolled tightly from the wide end and the point is sealed firmly

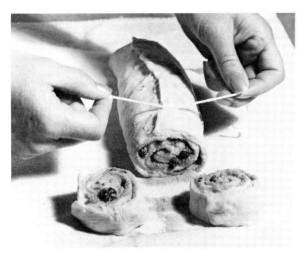

Figure 17-9.
Cinnamon rolls are easily sliced by using a piece of string.

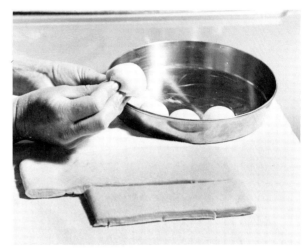

Figure 17-11.
Pan rolls are shaped by forming smooth chunks of dough into balls.

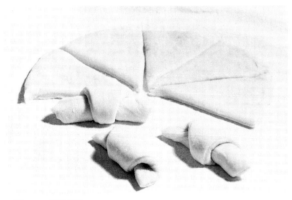

Figure 17-10.
Crescent rolls are made by cutting pie-shaped wedges of dough from a circle of dough, rolling the wedge from the wide end, sealing the point underneath.

underneath. The rolls are placed on a greased baking sheet with the point-side underneath and slightly curved to form a crescent.

Parker House

Parker House rolls are made by rolling the dough into a circle 9 inches in diameter and cutting the dough into rounds with a biscuit cutter. With the dull edge of a knife a crease is made to one side of the center of the dough round. The roll is brushed lightly with melted butter or margarine and the larger half is folded over so that the edges just meet. The edges are sealed together.

Pan Rolls

To make pan rolls the dough is formed into a roll approximately 12 inches long and cut into 12 equal pieces. Each piece is formed into a smooth ball and placed in a shallow, greased square or round baking pan, as shown in Figure 17-11. If pan rolls are placed 1/4 inch apart they will have soft sides; if they are placed 1 inch or more apart, they will have a crusty surface.

Cloverleaf

To form a cloverleaf a roll of dough is formed approximately 9 inches long and the roll is cut into 9 equal pieces. Each piece of dough is cut into three equal pieces from which three

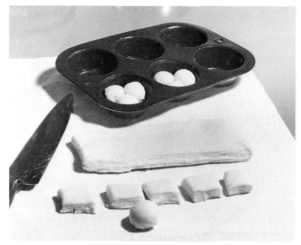

Figure 17-12.
Cloverleaf rolls are three small balls of dough held together in a muffin tin.

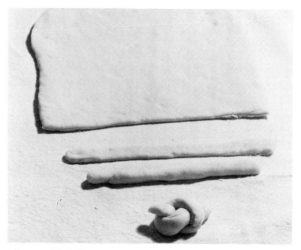

Figure 17-13.
Bow-knots are shaped from a long thin roll of dough that is tied in a loose knot.

balls are shaped. Each ball is dipped into melted butter or margarine and three balls are placed in each section of a greased muffin tin, as depicted in Figure 17-12.

Bow Knots

To form bow knots the dough is shaped into a roll 10 inches long and cut into 1-inch pieces. Each piece is rolled in the hands as a pencil is rolled until it is approximately 6 inches long. Each piece is then tied in a loose knot and placed on a greased cookie sheet 2 inches apart, as shown in Figure 17-13.

Baking Bread

After loaves and rolls are shaped, they are again covered and allowed to rise in a warm place until they are nearly doubled in bulk, or a slight indentation remains when the dough is lightly pressed with a finger. A loaf is ready to bake when it has risen slightly over the edge of the pan. Loaves and rolls that rise too much will collapse or have a coarse, open texture.

Approximately 15 minutes before the baking time, the oven should be turned on to preheat. If bread or rolls are rising in the oven, they must be removed before the oven is turned on. Depending on the recipe, bread is usually baked between 350° and 400° F (175° and 205° C).

Rolls that are brushed with melted butter or margarine before baking will have a tender crust. Brushing rolls with milk or egg diluted with milk will produce a crisp crust.

It is difficult to tell when a loaf has completed baking. Removing the loaf from the pan and checking for a firm, compact, and not soggy feeling is a sign that the bread is done. Bread that browns too quickly before the cooking time is completed may be loosely covered with foil. Table 17-2 gives the quality characteristics of yeast breads.

Brown-and-serve rolls can also be prepared from a home-prepared yeast roll dough. The rolls are shaped and placed in greased muffin tins and allowed to rise until they reach three-quarters of their final size. They are then baked at 300° F (150° C) for about 40 minutes. The rolls should not brown. After baking, the rolls

Table 17-2
Quality Characteristics of Yeast Breads

Quality	Characteristic
Appearance	Well-shaped, same size
	Smooth crust, batter bread may
	have pebbly surface
	Golden brown color
Crumb	Moist and tender
Grain	Even grain with air cells of same
	size and shape
	(Note: Batter breads may have less
	uniform cells)
Texture	Fine texture with no crumbliness
Flavor	Nutty flavor

should stand in the pan for about 20 minutes, and then they are removed from the pan, cooled, wrapped in an airtight package, and frozen. When they are ready to use, the rolls are thawed at room temperature in their wrapper and baked at 400° F (205° C) for 5 to 7 minutes.

Immediately after bread and rolls are taken from the oven, they should be removed from the baking pan and placed on a wire rack to cool. A shiny surface and a tender crust are achieved by brushing hot bread with melted butter or margarine immediately after the bread or rolls are removed from the oven.

Microwave Cooking

Baked breads can be heated very quickly in a microwave oven because the heat passes quickly through the porous structure of the dough. Three to four rolls or slices of bread can be heated in a microwave oven in about 30 seconds. Breads should not be covered while being heated as they will become too moist, but they should be heated on a paper towel or napkin to absorb moisture.

Breads cook very quickly in a microwave oven because of their structure. The resulting product does not brown as in conventional cooking and the texture is likely to be tough, rubbery, and dry if it is even slightly over-cooked. Most yeast breads are better when they are baked in a conventional oven.

When quick breads are cooked in a microwave oven, they will cook more evenly in a circular pattern. For example, a quick bread batter is best put into a glass baking dish that contains a small custard cup in the center of the baking dish, and muffins are best cooked in either paper baking cups placed in custard cups, or in one of the nonmetallic muffin pans designed for microwave oven use.

RECIPES

Biscuits

	Standard	Metric
Sifted, all-purpose flour	2 cups	500 mL
Baking powder	1 Tbsp.	15 mL
Salt	1/2 tsp.	2 mL
Shortening	1/4 cup	60 mL
Milk	3/4 cup	175 mL

1. Preheat the oven to 450° F (230° C).
2. Sift dry ingredients together into a mixing bowl.
3. Cut the shortening into the dry ingredients with a pastry blender or two table knives until the mixture resembles coarse crumbs.
4. Add the milk all at once and mix with a fork until a soft dough is formed.
5. Turn the dough out onto a lightly floured surface and knead lightly for 30 seconds.
6. Roll the dough out to a 1/2-inch thickness and cut with a floured biscuit cutter.
7. Place the dough on an ungreased baking sheet and bake for 12 minutes or until it is a light golden brown.

Yield: 14 to 16 biscuits

Crepes

All-purpose flour,	Standard	Metric
sifted	1-1/2 cups	375 mL
Sugar	1 tsp.	5 mL
Salt	1/8 tsp.	0.5 mL
Eggs	3	3
Milk	1-1/2 cup	375 mL
Butter or margarine,		
melted and cooled	2 Tbsp.	30 mL

1. Sift the flour, sugar, and salt together into a bowl.
2. Beat the eggs in another bowl until well blended.
3. Add the eggs and 1/2 cup of milk to the dry ingredients and stir until well blended.
4. Stir in the remaining 1 cup of milk and then the melted butter or margarine.
5. Let the crepe batter rest for at least 1 hour before cooking. Crepe batter may be held for 3 hours at room temperature or refrigerated overnight.
6. Cooking Crepes

   (a) Use a 6-inch cast iron skillet or a special crepe pan for cooking crepes. The pan should be well-seasoned if it does not have a special nonstick finish. To season the pan melt a small amount of fat in the pan and wipe out the excess with a paper towel.

   (b) Fill a 1/4 cup measuring cup slightly less than 1/2 full of the crepe batter and pour it into the crepe pan, which should be slightly smoking hot. Tilt the pan so that the batter swirls around and covers the bottom of the pan.

   (c) Return the pan to the heat; the crepe will cook in 1 minute or less. Using a table knife, lift the edges of the crepe and flip to cook the other side, which will take 1/2 to 1 minute. Continue cooking until all the crepe batter is used.

   (d) As crepes are cooked they may be stacked on a plate and kept warm in a warm oven if they are to be used immediately. If they are to be used at a later time the crepes may be stacked between layers of waxed paper and refrigerated for up to 2 days or they may be wrapped in foil and frozen.

Variations to Mixing:

1. Beat the eggs in the mixer until well blended; add half the dry ingredients and mix until the batter is smooth; add the remaining dry ingredients and then the liquid. Add the melted butter or margarine and allow the batter to rest before cooking, as in the basic instructions.
2. In the blender mix the eggs, milk, and salt, and then the remaining ingredients; blend for 1 minute. Push down the unblended ingredients and blend for 1 more minute. Allow the batter to rest before cooking.

Yield: 16 crepes

Muffins

	Standard	Metric
Sifted, all-purpose flour	2 cups	500 mL
Baking powder	4 tsp.	20 mL
Salt	3/4 tsp.	4 mL
Sugar	1/4 cup	60 mL
Egg, beaten	1	1
Shortening, melted	1/4 cup	60 mL
Milk	1 cup	250 mL

1. Preheat the oven to 400° F (205° C).
2. Melt the shortening and let it cool.
3. Sift the flour, baking powder, salt, and sugar together into mixing bowl.
4. Combine the egg, cooled shortening, and milk. Add all at once to the dry ingredients.
5. Stir the mixture until the dry ingredients are just moistened.
6. Fill the greased muffin tins two-thirds full.
7. Bake for 25 minutes. Serve immediately.

Variations

1. Add 3/4 cup of fresh blueberries to the dry ingredients.
2. Add 1/3 cup of chopped nuts.
3. Add 1/3 cup of raisins.
4. Sift only 1 cup of white flour with the dry ingredients and stir into the dry ingredients 1 cup of whole wheat flour.

5. Dip the baked muffins into melted butter or margarine and then into a mixture of cinnamon and sugar.

Yield: 12 muffins

——————— Pancakes ———————

	Standard	Metric
Melted shortening or vegetable oil	2 Tbsp.	30 mL
Sifted, all-purpose flour	1-3/4 cups	425 mL
Baking powder	1 Tbsp.	15 mL
Sugar	1 Tbsp.	15 mL
Salt	1/2 tsp.	2 mL
Egg, beaten	1	1
Milk	1 cup	250 mL

1. Melt the shortening and let it cool slightly.
2. Sift the flour, baking powder, sugar, and salt together into a mixing bowl.
3. Combine the egg, melted shortening, and milk and add all at once to the dry ingredients. Mix only until all the ingredients are moistened.
4. Cook the pancakes on a lightly greased griddle.

Variations:
1. Sprinkle 1 Tbsp. of washed blueberries on top of pancake before turning.
2. Add 3/4 cup chopped walnuts to pancake batter.

Yield: 8 pancakes

——————— Waffles ———————

	Standard	Metric
Shortening, melted	1/2 cup	125 mL
Sifted, all-purpose flour	1-3/4 cups	425 mL
Baking powder	1 Tbsp.	15 mL
Salt	1/2 tsp.	2 mL
Egg yolks, beaten	2	2
Milk	1-1/4 cups	310 mL
Egg whites, stiffly beaten	2	2

1. Preheat the iron.
2. Melt the shortening and cool it slightly.
3. Sift the flour, baking powder, and salt together into a mixing bowl.
4. Combine the egg yolks, melted shortening, and milk; add all at once to the dry ingredients.
5. Fold in the stiffly beaten egg whites.
6. Bake in the hot waffle iron.

Yield: 7 to 8 waffles

——————— Popovers ———————

	Standard	Metric
Eggs	2	2
Sifted, all-purpose flour	1 cup	250 mL
Salt	1/2 tsp.	2 mL
Milk	1 cup	250 mL
Shortening or salad oil, melted	1 Tbsp.	15 mL

1. Preheat the oven to 450° F (230° C).
2. Sift the flour and salt together.
3. Beat the eggs with a rotary or electric mixer and add the milk.
4. Beat in the dry ingredients to make a smooth batter.
5. Fill greased custard cups or muffin tins 2/3 full.
6. Bake at 450° F (230° C) for 15 minutes; reduce the heat to 350° F (175° C) and continue baking for another 20 to 25 minutes or until the crust is brown and firm.

Yield: 8 to 10 popovers

——————— Tea Nut Bread ———————

	Standard	Metric
Sifted, all-purpose flour	3 cups	750 mL
Sugar	1 cup	250 mL
Salt	1-1/2 tsp.	17 mL
Baking powder	4 tsp.	20 mL
Shortening, melted	1/4 cup	60 mL
Milk	1-1/2 cups	310 mL

Egg, slightly beaten	1	1
Nuts, coarsely chopped	1 cup	250 mL

1. Preheat the oven to 350° F (175° C).
2. Sift together into a mixing bowl the flour, sugar, salt, and baking powder.
3. Combine the egg, milk, and melted cooled shortening and add to the dry ingredients; add the nuts. Mix only until the ingredients are well moistened.
4. Pour the batter into a well-greased loaf pan and bake for 60 to 70 minutes.

Yield: 1 loaf

———————— Basic Quick Bread Mix ————————

	Standard	Metric
Sifted, all-purpose flour	9 cups	2250 mL
Baking powder, double-acting	1/3 cup	75 mL
Nonfat dry milk	1 cup plus 2 Tbsp.	280 mL
Salt	4 tsp.	20 mL
Shortening	1-3/4 cup	425 mL

1. Sift the baking powder, salt, and flour together into a large bowl.
2. Stir the nonfat dry milk into the flour mixture until well blended.
3. Cut the fat into the flour mixture until the mixture resembles coarse meal.
4. Store in a tightly covered container. The mix may be stored at room temperature for 6 weeks.
5. To use the mix, stir lightly before measuring; do not sift; spoon lightly into a measuring cup and level.

Note: Because the standard flour sifter will hold only about 4-1/2 cups of flour, it is wise to sift half the baking powder and half the salt with each 4-1/2 cups of flour to assure adequate mixing of the ingredients.

Yield: 13 cups

Basic Quick Bread Mix Recipes

———————— Basic Biscuits ————————

	Standard	Metric
Basic quick bread mix	2 cups	500 mL
Water	1/2 cup	125 mL

1. Add liquid to the mix.
2. Stir 20 to 25 times.
3. Turn onto a lightly floured board and knead about 15 times.
4. Roll to 1/3-inch thick. Cut with a floured biscuit cutter or in squares, using a floured knife.
5. Place on an ungreased baking sheet.
6. Bake in a hot oven at 425° F (220° C) for 10 minutes.

Yield: 12 to 14 biscuits

Variations:

Bacon Biscuits

Add 1/4 cup of minced crisp cooked bacon to mix. Follow the recipe for basic biscuits.

Cheese Biscuits

Add 1/3 cup of grated sharp cheese to mix. Follow the recipe for basic biscuits.

———————— Basic Muffins ————————

	Standard	Metric
Basic quick bread mix	2 cups	500 mL
Sugar	4 tsp.	20 mL
Egg	1	1
Water	2/3 cup	150 mL

1. Stir sugar into the mix. Beat the egg and add to the liquid.
2. Add the liquids to the dry ingredients. Stir about 15 strokes or just enough to blend.
3. Bake in well-greased muffin pans in a hot oven, 400° F (205° C) about 20 minutes.

Yield: 12 medium muffins

Variations:

Apple Muffins

Add 3/4 cup of finely diced peeled apples, 1/4 teaspoon of cinnamon, and a dash of nutmeg to the mix. If the apples are very tart, sugar may be increased to 2 Tbsp.

Blueberry Muffins

Add 1/3 cup of canned, fresh, or frozen blueberries to the muffin batter. Canned blueberries should be drained and rinsed before using.

Cranberry Muffins

Add 1/2 cup of finely chopped cranberries to the mix. Increase the sugar to 2 Tbsp.

──────── Basic Coffee Cake ────────

	Standard	Metric
Basic quick bread mix	2 cups	500 mL
Sugar	1/3 cup	75 mL
Egg	1	1
Water	1/2 cup	125 mL

1. Stir sugar into the mix. Beat the egg and add to the liquid. Add the liquid to the mix. Stir until the ingredients are thoroughly blended (about 25 strokes). Do not beat.
2. Spread half of the batter in a greased pan (8 × 8 × 2). Sprinkle one half of the topping evenly over the batter. Spread the remaining batter in the pan and cover with the rest of the topping.
3. Bake at 375° F (190° C) for about 20 minutes.

Yield: 4 servings

──────── Basic Cinnamon Sugar Topping ────────

	Standard	Metric
White sugar*	1/4 cup	60 mL
Brown sugar*	1/4 cup	60 mL
Mix	2 Tbsp.	30 mL

Cinnamon	1 tsp.	5 mL
Margarine	3 Tbsp.	45 mL

1. Combine the dry ingredients. Cut the fat into the dry ingredients with a pastry blender.
2. Use half of the mixture in the center of the coffee cake and the rest on the top, or all may be used on the top.

* All-brown or all-white sugar may be used.

──────── White Bread—Straight-Dough Method ────────

	Standard	Metric
Milk, warmed	2 cups	500 mL
Sugar	2 Tbsp.	30 mL
Salt	2 tsp.	10 mL
Shortening	1 Tbsp.	15 mL
Active dry yeast or	1 package	1
compressed yeast	1 cake	1 cake
Water	1/4 cup	60 mL
Sifted, all-purpose	6 to 6–1/4 cups	1,500–
flour		1,560 mL

1. Pour the warmed milk into a large mixing bowl. Add the sugar, salt, and shortening and stir to dissolve.
2. Sprinkle the yeast over the 1/4 cup water of proper temperature and stir to dissolve.
3. Add 1 cup of flour to the milk mixture and beat until smooth. Check the temperature to determine if the mixture has cooled to lukewarm.
4. Stir in the yeast.
5. Add the remaining flour to make a stiff dough, 1 cup at a time, beating after each addition until it is smooth.
6. Turn out onto a lightly floured surface and knead until smooth and satiny.
7. Place the dough in a lightly greased bowl, turning to grease all surfaces of the dough. Cover and let rise until doubled in bulk, approximately 1-1/2 hours.
8. Punch the dough down; turn over in the bowl; cover and let rise again until double in bulk.
9. Cut the dough into two pieces and shape each

piece into a smooth ball. Cover and let rest 10 minutes.

10. Shape into two loaves and place in two greased loaf pans, 8-1/2 × 4-1/2 × 2-1/2 inches.

11. Cover and let rise until double in bulk, about 1 hour.

12. Bake at 400° F (205° C) for about 35 minutes.

Yield: two loaves

———— White Bread—Cool-Rise Method ————

	Standard	Metric
Sifted, all-purpose flour	5-1/2 to 6-1/2 cups	1,375– 1,625 mL
Yeast, active dry	2 packages	2
Sugar	2 Tbsp.	30 mL
Salt	1 Tbsp.	15 mL
Shortening, softened	1/4 cup	60 mL
Water, very hot	2-1/4 cups	560 mL
Vegetable oil	2 tsp.	10 mL

1. In a large mixing bowl combine 2 cups of flour, the yeast, sugar, and salt. Add the soft shortening.

2. Add the hot water and beat with an electric mixer for 2 minutes.

3. Add 1 cup of flour and beat with the mixer for 1 minute, or until the dough is thick and elastic.

4. Gradually stir in by hand enough of the remaining flour to make a soft dough.

5. Turn the dough onto a lightly floured surface and knead until the dough is smooth and elastic.

6. Cover with a plastic wrap and a towel and allow to rest for 15 minutes on the working surface. Punch down.

7. Divide the dough in half and shape each portion into a loaf. Place in two greased 8-1/2 × 4-1/2 × 2-1/2-inch pans. Brush the surface of the dough with the vegetable oil.

8. Cover the pans loosely with waxed paper that has been lightly brushed with vegetable oil and then with plastic wrap. Place in the refrigerator for 2 to 48 hours.

9. When ready to bake, remove from the refrigerator, uncover, and let stand for 10 minutes.

10. Bake at 400° F (205° C) for 35 to 40 minutes.

Yield: two loaves

———— Raisin Bread—Sponge Method ————

	Standard	Metric
Potato water, warm	1 cup	250 mL
Yeast, active dry *or*	2 packages	2
compressed yeast	2 cakes	2
Potatoes, mashed	1/4 cup	60 mL
Sugar	1/2 cup	125 mL
Sifted, all-purpose flour	4 to 4-1/2 cups	1,000– 1,125 mL
Salt	1 tsp.	5 mL
Eggs, beaten	2	2
Shortening, melted	1/2 cup	125 mL
Raisins	1 cup	250 mL

1. Sprinkle the active dry yeast over warm potato water or crumble in compressed yeast. Stir to dissolve.

2. Add mashed potatoes, 2 Tbsp. of the sugar, and 1 cup of flour. Beat until smooth. Cover and allow to rise until bubbly. Stir down.

3. Add 6 Tbsp. sugar, 1 tsp. salt, and 1 cup of flour. Beat until smooth.

4. Stir in the eggs, cooled melted shortening, and raisins.

5. Stir in 1-1/2 cups of flour.

6. Turn dough onto a floured surface and knead until smooth.

7. Place the dough in a lightly greased bowl, turning to grease all surfaces. Cover and let rise until doubled in bulk; about 1 hour.

8. Punch down; divide into 2 equal parts; cover and let rest 5 minutes.

9. Shape each piece into a loaf and place in a greased 8-3/4 × 4-3/4 × 2-3/4-inch loaf pan. Cover and let rise until double, about 1 hour.

10. Bake at 350° F (175° C) for 1 hour.

Yield: two loaves

Refrigerator Roll Dough

	Standard	Metric
Milk, warmed	1 cup	250 mL
Sugar	1/4 cup	60 mL
Shortening	1/4 cup	60 mL
Salt	1 tsp.	5 mL
Yeast, active dry	1 package	1
Water, warm	1/4 cup	60 mL
Egg, slightly beaten	1	1
Sifted, all-purpose flour	3-1/2 cups	875 mL

1. Pour the warm milk in a large mixing bowl. Add the sugar, salt, and shortening and stir to dissolve.

2. Sprinkle the yeast over 1/4 cup of warm water and stir to dissolve.

3. Add 1 cup of flour to the milk mixture and beat until smooth. Check the temperature to determine if it has cooled to lukewarm.

4. Stir in the yeast and egg.

5. Add the remaining flour, 1 cup at a time, beating after each addition until smooth.

6. Place the dough in a greased bowl; brush a small amount of melted fat over the surface; cover and refrigerate for a minimum of 4 hours or up to 4 or 5 days.

7. To make rolls, turn the dough onto a lightly floured surface and shape as desired.

8. Cover and let rise until doubled in bulk, about 1 hour.

9. Bake at 400° F (205° C) for 12 to 15 minutes.

Yield: 2 dozen rolls

Sweet Roll Dough

	Standard	Metric
Sifted, all-purpose flour	3-1/2 to 4 cups	875–1,000 mL
Yeast, active dry	1 package	1
Milk, warmed	1 cup	250 mL
Sugar	3/4 cup	185 mL
Shortening	1/4 cup	60 mL
Salt	1 tsp.	5 mL
Eggs, beaten	2	2

1. In a large mixing bowl combine 2 cups of flour and the yeast.

2. Add the sugar, shortening, and salt to the warm milk and stir to dissolve. Add the flour and yeast mixture; add the eggs.

3. Beat at the low speed of an electric mixer for 1/2 minute. Beat for 3 minutes at a high speed.

4. Stir in enough remaining flour to make a stiff dough.

5. Turn the dough onto a lightly floured surface and knead until smooth, 8 to 10 minutes.

6. Place the dough in a greased bowl, turning to grease all surfaces; cover and let rise until doubled in bulk.

7. Punch down; divide dough in half; cover and let rest 10 minutes.

8. Shape as for cinnamon rolls.

9. Cover and allow to rise until doubled, approximately 30 minutes.

10. Bake at 375° F (190° C) for 20 minutes.

Yield: 1-1/2 to 2 dozen

Batter Bread

	Standard	Metric
Milk, warmed	3/4 cup	185 mL
Sugar	2 Tbsp.	30 mL
Salt	1 tsp.	5 mL
Shortening	2 Tbsp.	30 mL
Yeast, active dry *or*	1 package	1
compressed yeast	1 cake	1
Water	1/4 cup	60 mL
Sifted, all-purpose flour	2-3/4 cups	685 mL
Egg	1	1

1. Pour the warmed milk into a mixing bowl. Add the sugar, salt, and shortening and stir to dissolve.

2. Sprinkle the dry yeast over warm water or crumble compressed yeast into lukewarm water. Stir to dissolve.

3. To the milk mixture add 2 cups of flour and beat until smooth.

4. Stir in the dissolved yeast and egg. Beat 1 minute.

5. Add the remaining flour and beat until smooth, about 2 minutes.

6. Scrape the batter down from the sides of the bowl; cover and let rise until doubled in bulk, about 1 hour.

7. Stir the batter down and turn into a greased 9-inch round cake pan, 1-1/2 inches deep, or a loaf pan 9 X 4-1/2 X 2-3/4 inches.

8. Bake at 350° F (175° C) for 45 minutes. Turn out on a rack and cool slightly. Serve warm with butter or margarine.

Yield: 1 loaf

——————— Pizza Dough ———————

	Standard	Metric
Yeast, active dry	1 package	1
Water, warm	1/2 cup	125 mL
Sugar, brown	1 Tbsp.	15 mL
Sifted, all-purpose flour	2 cups	500 mL
Salt	3/4 tsp.	4 mL
Egg, beaten	1	1
Vegetable oil	2 Tbsp.	30 mL

1. Sprinkle the dry yeast over the warm water and stir to dissolve. Sprinkle the brown sugar over the yeast mixture. Let sit until the mixture is frothy, 2 to 5 minutes.

2. Sift the salt and flour together into a large mixing bowl. Add the yeast, egg, and vegetable oil. Beat 3 or 4 minutes or until the dough is elastic.

3. Cover and allow to rise until doubled in bulk, about 1 hour.

4. Punch the dough down and divide into two pieces or into smaller pieces to make individual pizzas.

5. Sprinkle the work surface with about 1/2 cup flour. Knead the dough briefly. Roll each piece into a circle that is less than 1/3-inch thick. Keep the working surface well floured and turn the dough often.

6. Spread the dough with pizza filling; sprinkle with grated mozarella cheese, parmesan cheese, and a small amount of vegetable oil. Condiments, such as cooked hamburger, bacon, or sausage, mushrooms, seafood, chicken, or Canadian bacon, may be added.

7. Bake the pizzas on a cookie sheet or in a pizza pan on the bottom shelf of the oven for 10 minutes or until bubbly at 500° F (260° C).

Yield: Two 9-inch pizzas or 4 smaller ones

——————— Pizza Sauce ———————

	Standard	Metric
Vegetable oil	1-1/2 Tbsp.	22 mL
Finely chopped onions	1/2 cup	125 mL
Finely chopped garlic	1-1/2 tsp.	7 mL
Coarsely chopped canned tomatoes	2 cups	500 mL
Tomato paste	1/2 of 1 6-oz. can	80 gm
Oregano	1-1/2 tsp.	7 mL
Basil	1/2 tsp.	2 mL
Bay leaf, small	1	1
Sugar	1 tsp.	5 mL
Salt	1 tsp.	5 mL
Pepper	1/4 tsp.	1 mL

1. In a heavy fry pan sauté the onions in the vegetable oil, stirring frequently, for 7 to 8 minutes.

2. Add the garlic and cook for 2 minutes longer.

3. Stir in the tomatoes, tomato paste, oregano, basil, bay leaf, sugar, salt, and pepper. Bring the sauce to a boil, lower the heat to simmer, and cook for 45 minutes to 1 hour, stirring occasionally. Sauce may be cooked in microwave for 20 minutes, stirring every 5 minutes.

4. Remove the bay leaf from the sauce and spoon over pizzas.

Yield: 1 pint of sauce

LEARNING ACTIVITIES

1. Do a survey of five males and five females to learn how much bread they consume in 7 days. Make a list of reasons why these people do or do not eat bread. Report your findings to the class.

2. If you do not know, write to your state Department of Agriculture to find out if your state has a mandatory enrichment program for breads and other products made from flour.

3. Plan three separate menus in which bread is the main contributor of shape in one, texture in another, and flavor in a third.

4. Plan a dinner menu that includes a quick bread. Work out a time schedule so that the quick bread will be ready to serve with the other food.

5. Plan a dinner menu that includes yeast rolls. Work out a time schedule so that the rolls will be fresh, warm, and ready to serve with the other foods.

6. Check the labels at a local supermarket to determine what, if any, chemical preservatives have been added to the bread. If preservatives have been added, do research to find out their function and report to the class.

7. Make a list of herbs and spices that would change the flavor of breads.

8. Using 1 cup of flour, add water to it to determine how much water the flour will absorb.

9. Make muffins by using a mixer to thoroughly mix the ingredients; make another batch and mix only until all the ingredients are moistened. Analyze the muffins made by both procedures for differences in volume, shape, texture, grain, and eating quality.

10. Make one muffin batter using all-purpose flour and another using cake flour. Bake the muffins and evaluate the differences in volume, shape, texture, grain, and eating quality of the muffins made from each batter.

11. Make a rolled biscuit dough, and divide the dough in half. Knead one-half of the dough for 30 seconds and the other half for 2 minutes. Bake the biscuits and analyze them for tenderness and flakiness.

12. Make up a yeast dough by the straight-dough method and divide the dough in half. Let half of the dough rise by one of the suggested methods in this chapter and let the other half rise in a cool, drafty area. Compare the difference in the time for rising.

13. Dissolve one packet of activated dry yeast in 1/2 cup of warm water. Add 1 tsp. of sugar. Record and analyze what happens over a 5-minute period.

14. Prepare muffins from a conventional recipe, a commercially prepared mix, and a home-prepared mix. Chart the differences in the muffins in terms of volume, shape, texture, grain, eating quality, cost, and time of preparation.

15. Prepare a yeast bread from a conventional recipe, a commercially prepared mix, and a frozen, ready-to-bake bread. Compare the differences in cost, time of preparation, grain, flavor, and texture. Decide which bread you would serve to guests.

16. Store a slice of bread with a chemical preservative added and a slice of bread without a chemical preservative added for 1 week. Note what changes take place in the appearance and taste of the two slices.

17. Make a batter yeast bread and note the difference in textural quality 15 minutes; 1 hour; and 24 hours after removal from the oven.

1. Which ingredients in most breads help to make bread a more complete protein food?
2. Of which vitamins and minerals are breads a major contributor?
3. Why should bread not be considered a fattening food?
4. How can bread add flavor variation to a meal?
5. What kind of bread is an economical purchase at the supermarket?
6. How is the staling of bread best prevented?
7. How can stale bread be used for other food-preparation purposes?
8. What two basic ingredients do all breads contain?
9. Why is wheat flour the most desirable flour to use in bread making?
10. What is gluten?
11. How does a bread made from rye flour differ from a bread made from wheat flour?
12. Why is cake flour not suitable for making breads?
13. What six ingredients do eggs give to bread?
14. What are the three leavening agents?
15. When does baking soda produce carbon dioxide?
16. Why is starch used as an ingredient in baking powder?
17. How does a double-acting baking powder react?
18. Why is a double-acting baking powder more desirable to use in home cooking than a single-acting baking powder?
19. What is meant by fermentation?
20. What is food for yeast?
21. What is meant by the "raising" period of bread?
22. In what two forms is yeast available?
23. How do air and steam always serve as a leavening agent in breads and other baked products?
24. What are the principal functions of a liquid in a baked product containing flour?
25. Why is salt an important ingredient in yeast-leavened products?
26. What is a quick bread?
27. What are the four steps involved in combining ingredients for pour and drop batters?
28. What does overmixing do to a quick bread?
29. Why is the fat cut into the flour mixture when making rolled biscuits?
30. Why do most quick breads need to be baked immediately after mixing?
31. Why are popovers started to cook in a very hot oven?
32. What are the two major causes for failure in making a yeast bread?
33. Why are some yeast breads kneaded?
34. What signs tell that the dough has been kneaded sufficiently?
35. What three methods can create the proper atmosphere for dough to rise?
36. What test can show that dough has completed its rising?
37. How does the sponge method differ

from the straight-dough method in ingredient mixing?

38. What is the advantage of using a refrigerator yeast dough?

39. What are the five ways in which rolls can be shaped?

40. What characteristic will rolls have when they are placed close together in a baking pan?

41. After bread and rolls are baked, how should they be cared for?

18

Cakes

Cakes have long been favorite desserts that add festivity to many occasions. With little time and effort a beautiful cake can be created for a party, picnic, or special birthday celebration. Many recipes for preparing cakes, frostings, and fillings are available, and some of the best convenience mixes on the market today are cakes.

Angel food, *sponge*, *chiffon*, and *shortened* are all terms relating to cakes. Each is a batter-flour mixture, and as with any flour mixture, it must be handled with a delicate touch to achieve a high-quality product. The reader may do well to review the chapter on eggs before working with cakes.

Nutritional Factors to Consider

Carbohydrate and Fat

Since all cakes contain some form of sugar and a high proportion of flour, they are always high in carbohydrate.

Protein, Vitamins, and Minerals

Cakes contain a minimal amount of protein. Although most varieties contain milk and eggs, a single serving of cake does not meet the human requirement for protein.

Practically no vitamins and minerals are provided by cake because the serving portions are usually small.

Calories

Because of the high sugar and fat content of cakes, they are high in calories. Plain cakes contain fewer calories than frosted ones, and angel food and sponge cakes are lower in calories than the shortened and chiffon types. For example, a plain 3-inch square of cake contains approximately 315 calories, whereas the same square with chocolate frosting contains approximately 450 calories. A 2-1/2-inch section of angel food cake prepared from a commercial mix contains approximately 140 calories.

311

Balance. A menu that includes cake as the dessert should be light in carbohydrate and fat, and still provide the necessary nutrients not offered by a serving of cake. For example, a cream soup with vegetable relishes plus rolls, or a vegetable salad with a high-protein food as the main ingredient, accompanied by rolls, can include cake as the dessert portion if other meals during the day have met additional human nutrient requirements.

Color and Shape. The color of a cake is achieved by the selection of ingredients. For example, a chocolate cake is made by adding cocoa or melted chocolate to the basic recipe, a white cake is made from egg whites, and a yellow cake is colored by the whole egg or the egg yolk.

Many different shapes of cakes for festive occasions can be created by cutting a single layer into various forms, such as a bunny, train, or heart, or by baking a cake in a specially shaped pan. Layer cakes that are cut into small portions and individually frosted are called "petit fours." Cupcakes provide additional shape variety.

Texture and Flavor. The flavor and texture of a cake are both varied by the method of mixing and the variation of flavor ingredients. Shortened cakes have a light and feathery texture, whereas angel food, sponge, and chiffon cakes have a more elastic and spongy texture. Added textural change in cakes is created by using such ingredients as nuts, fruits, vegetables, and coconut.

Changing the flavoring extract or adding the grated peel of citrus fruits can vary the taste of cakes that were previously flavored only with vanilla extract. Many different spices may also be added to cakes to give them a more pungent flavor.

Inherent Factors

Age and Culture. Cake is a popular dessert with people of all ages. The cake as it is known today is basically an American tradition. Tortes, the first cousin to American cakes, originated in Europe. They have a heavier texture and are usually served in several layers with a filling in between each layer.

Economics, Space and Equipment, and Time Scheduling. Cakes are often purchased in the bakery because of time factors. If cakes are baked at home from a basic recipe or a convenience mix, it is important to have the proper-sized pans called for in the recipe. Cakes are easier to prepare if an electric mixer is used, and some cakes can be made in the blender. Since cakes are best when eaten the day they are baked, time schedule allotments must be adjusted. If time is short, the cake may be frozen, and then thawed and served. Caked are best frozen unfrosted.

Ingredients and Their Functions

The principal ingredients of a cake are flour, eggs, a leavening agent, liquid, sugar, and sometimes fat. Other ingredients may be added to change the flavor, add more texture, or increase the moistness of the cake. Because a cake is most dependent on the correct proportions and manipulation of ingredients, it is difficult to alter ingredients within a specific cake recipe and still achieve a high-quality product. A better cake results from having all the ingredients at room temperature before preparation begins and being accurate in all measurements.

Flour

Cake flour is the principal flour used in cakes because it is finely ground and made from soft wheats that contain less gluten-forming properties. Although a high amount of gluten development is not desirable in cake, as it is in yeast breads, a small amount of gluten is needed to develop the cake's cell structure. All-purpose flour may be substituted for cake flour in a recipe by using 2 tablespoons less per cup; some recipes specify all-purpose flour. However, cakes made in this manner will not have as fine a texture.

Eggs

It is important to use large-sized eggs because these are the sizes used when cake recipes are developed. Depending on the type of cake being prepared, either the whole egg, the egg yolk, or the egg white is used. Eggs give a cake both flavor and color, but the amount will vary depending on which portion of the egg is included. The emulsifying property of eggs helps to disperse the fat evenly throughout the batter, and eggs contribute to the leavening of a cake by trapping air as they are beaten. During baking, the eggs coagulate and give a permanence to the cell structure; they also add liquid.

Fats

The presence of fat accounts for the tender texture of a cake, and as a fat is manipulated to become softer, air is trapped in the mixture. The fats, butter and margarine, contribute a rich flavor and color to the cake, but because these fats are difficult to make creamy, they do not incorporate as much air into the mixture. Whipped margarine should not be substituted for regular margarine, since whipped margarine does not contain as high a percentage of fat. The most desirable fat to use in cakes is hydrogenated shortening. Cooking oils should be used only when cakes are made by the muffin or chiffon method; they should not be interchanged with the solid fat in a cake recipe,

because they do not trap air. Lard is rarely used as a fat for cakes because of its flavor and its inability to become creamy when it is manipulated.

Leavening Agents

All cakes use air and/or steam as a leavening agent; some types of cakes use baking powder or soda with the needed acidic ingredient.

Liquid

Most cakes use liquid as an ingredient, and most often the liquid is milk. Reconstituted dried milk and diluted evaporated milk may be substituted for fresh milk in cake recipes and some recipes specify the use of buttermilk or sour milk. Fruit juices and fruit purees, such as that attained from mashing bananas, may be used as the liquid. A cake that does not have enough liquid will have a dry texture, whereas a cake with too much liquid will lack good volume. With the exception of water, liquids also add flavor to a cake.

Sugar

Sugar accounts for most of a cake's sweetness. It also contributes to tenderness by competing with the gluten for water, and thus preventing a strong gluten development. Most cakes use granulated sugar, but recipe variations may use brown sugar, a sugar syrup, or honey.

Other Ingredients

Other ingredients used in making cakes include various flavoring extracts such as almond, peppermint, and vanilla, or spices such as cinnamon, nutmeg, and cloves. Pureed vegetables, such as carrots and zucchini, pureed fruits, such as bananas and pumpkin, and some cereals, such as oatmeal, produce moist and more nutritious cakes with a heavier texture.

Types of Cakes

Cakes are classified into two groups: shortened cakes and foam cakes. Each type of cake differs in the proportion of ingredients and in the method of manipulation.

Shortened Cakes

Shortened cakes contain fat as a principal ingredient. Some shortened cakes, called pound cakes, are leavened by air and steam; although they may also contain a small amount of a chemical leavening agent. These cakes have a heavier and more compact texture than other types of cakes. Some pound-cake recipes use all-purpose flour rather than cake flour; they are baked in a loaf pan or in a tube pan.

Other shortened cakes use baking powder or soda with an acidic ingredient as the leavening agent, in addition to the air incorporated in the mixing of ingredients. These cakes have a feathery texture with more volume than a pound cake.

Foam Cakes

Foam cakes are of three types: angel food, sponge, and chiffon. Foam cakes have a moist and elastic texture. The major ingredients of these cakes are eggs, sugar, and flour; the leavening agents are air and steam. A chiffon cake is not a true foam cake because it does contain fat.

Angel Food Cake. The principal ingredients of an angel food cake are egg whites, granulated sugar, and cake flour. Salt, cream of tartar, and an additional flavoring agent are also used. Cream of tartar stabilizes the egg white foam so that as the cake is baked the foam does not collapse before the heat coagulates the egg white. Whether angel food cakes are made from a basic recipe or a convenience mix, it is essential that no fat be present on any of the mixing utensils or on the baking pan, as fat interferes with foam formation, and thus, coagulation.

Sponge Cake. A sponge cake contains the whole egg, sugar, flour, and an acidic ingredient such as lemon juice or cream of tartar. Some recipes for sponge cake may include an additional amount of liquid.

Chiffon Cake. The chiffon cake is similar to the sponge cake except that a fat, namely a cooking oil, is used with the ingredients. This cake has the rich flavor of a shortened cake.

Basic Methods of Preparation

Each type of cake has one or two methods by which the ingredients are mixed. With each method it is important that the ingredients be thoroughly blended, and that they be mixed and baked as quickly as possible so as not to lose the air that has been incorporated as a leavening agent. In all cake mixing it is important to keep the bowl continuously scraped down to assure uniform blending of the ingredients.

One-Bowl Method

The one-bowl method is used to prepare shortened cakes that contain a chemical leavening agent. The quickness of the one-bowl technique has made this method very popular and the cake produced by the method has a fine, soft texture. The recipes for one-bowl cakes contain a higher proportion of sugar and liquid than recipes for shortened cakes mixed by the conventional method. Therefore, methods cannot be interchanged for a given recipe. Either an electric mixer at medium speed or a hand mixer may be used. If mixing is done by hand, the time allowance is 150 strokes per minute.

In the one-bowl method, the dry ingredients are sifted together into the bowl, the fat and part or all of the liquid are added, and the mixture is beaten for 2 minutes, or 300 strokes by hand. The unbeaten eggs, egg yolks, or whites are added together with any remaining liquid; this mixture is beaten for an additional 2 minutes.

Conventional Method

The conventional method for mixing shortened cakes has been used for several centuries and many cake recipes today still follow this prescribed method. Although it takes more time than the one-bowl method, the light-airy texture of the cakes made by this method is worth the effort.

The mixing may be done with an electric mixer or by hand. With the conventional method a solid fat is placed in the mixing bowl and creamed until it is light and fluffy. To cream a fat means to work it with the electric beaters or the back of a wooden spoon until it reaches a fluffy consistency. Sugar is added to the softened fat and the sugar-fat mixture is creamed together until it is light and fluffy and forms a mass away from the sides of the bowl, as illustrated in Figure 18-1. Flavoring is added to the sugar-fat mixture during the creaming process.

If mixing is done by hand, the eggs are beaten first and then added to the creamed mixture. If an electric mixer is used, unbeaten eggs are added, one at a time, to the creamed mixture, and the mixture is beaten well after each addition. The dry ingredients are sifted together onto a piece of waxed paper and divided into four portions, and the liquid is divided into thirds. For example, if 1 cup of liquid is used in the recipe, each portion would be 1/3 of a cup. The flour mixture is added alternately with the liquid mixture, always beginning and ending with the flour. After each addition, the

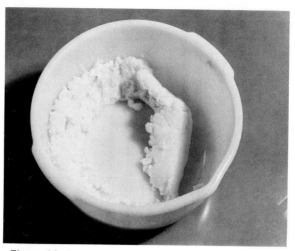

Figure 18-1.
When sugar and fat are thoroughly creamed, they form a light and fluffy mass that does not cling to the sides of the bowl.

ingredients are mixed only until they are well blended. However, a very rich cake will require more manipulation. If an electric mixer is used, the ingredients are blended at low speed until they are just mixed.

Muffin Method

Some cake recipes may call for ingredients to be mixed by the muffin method that is described in the chapter on breads. Cakes mixed by this method may not have as great a volume and may be more compact than cakes mixed by the conventional or one-bowl method.

Sponge Cakes

In making a sponge cake the whole egg may be used, or the egg yolks and whites may be beaten separately and used. The first step in making a sponge cake is to sift the dry ingredients, except sugar, together. These ingredients are set aside and the whole egg or egg yolk,

Table 18-1
Poor-Quality Cakes

Fault	Caused By:
Coarse texture	Undermixing or not enough creaming
	Too much leavening or underbeaten eggs
	Too low a baking temperature
Heavy texture	Too much liquid
	Underbeating eggs or undermixing
	Not baking promptly
Hard, humped crust	Baking temperature too high or baked too long
	Excess of flour or sugar
Sticky crust	Underbaked or too much sugar
Uneven top	Uneven heat or too hot
Fallen	Excess of ingredients
	Undermixing
	Baked too slowly
Undersized	Too little leavening
	Baking temperature too high
	Pan too large
Crumbling	Excess of leavening, sugar, or fat
	Undermixing

the liquid, and the flavoring are then beaten to a stiff consistency. Sugar is gradually added, and the mixture is beaten until it is thick and lemon-colored. If the egg whites are separate, the beaters are washed and the egg whites are beaten to the stiff peak stage. The sifted dry ingredients are folded into the egg-yolk mixture and if egg whites are separate, the mixture is folded into the stiffly beaten egg whites.

Chiffon Cakes

A chiffon cake is mixed by first sifting the dry ingredients into a bowl and then beating the egg whites to the stiff peak stage. Part of the sugar may or may not be beaten into the egg whites. The cooking oil, egg yolks, liquid, and flavoring agent are added to the dry ingredients all at once and mixed until blended. This mixture is then folded into the stiffly beaten egg whites. Table 18-1 lists the characteristics of a poor-quality cake and Table 18-2 gives the characteristics of a good quality cake.

Table 18-2
Good-Quality Cakes

Quality	Characteristics
Texture	Light, tender crumb
	Slightly moist, not soggy or dry
Crust	Tender
	Dry, not sticky to the touch
Appearance	Slightly rounded on the top
Size	Adhere to size of baking pan
	Maintain size upon cooling
Slicing	Maintain form, not crumble, when sliced

Baking Cakes

Cakes should be baked in pans that are as close to the size called for in the recipe as possible. Pans used for baking cakes may be round, square, or oblong. Loaf pans may be used to make pound cakes, and tube pans are used for pound, angel food, sponge, and chiffon cakes. Muffin tins are used for baking small cakes, called cupcakes. Cupcakes are easier to remove and serve if the batter is poured into a paper baking cup that has been placed inside the tin. A thin sponge cake, called a cake roll, is baked in a jelly-roll pan.

The pans for shortened cake batters are greased on the bottom and floured. To flour a pan, it is first greased, and about 1 tablespoon of flour is then added per one 9-inch cake pan, as shown in Figure 18-2. The flour is shaken around to coat the grease and the excess is tapped out. The sides of the pan are not greased so the batter can cling to the non-coated sides while it is baking. Angel food, sponge, and chiffon cakes are baked in non-greased pans. Nongreasing allows the mixture to cling to the sides while baking and helps prevent the egg mass from falling until the heat coagulates the egg. An exception to this rule is a sponge cake that is made into a cake roll. In this procedure, the bottom of the pan is greased, and heavy paper is cut to the size of the bottom of the pan and is also heavily greased. This facilitates the easy removal of the thin cake from the pan. A cake batter should fill a pan to 1/2 or 2/3 of its depth.

Temperatures for baking cakes vary with the recipe. Most cakes are baked between a temperature of 325° F to 375° F (165° C to 190° C). If glass pans are used, the temperature is reduced 25° F (4° C). The oven should always be preheated and the oven rack should be in the center of the oven. If one cake pan is used in baking, it should be evenly centered on the rack; if more than one pan is used, the pans should be evenly spaced as shown in Figure 18-3. The cake pans should not touch one another or the sides of the oven so as to enable the heat to be evenly distributed.

A cake is completely baked when the top springs back when it is lightly touched with the finger, or when a wooden pick is inserted and comes out clean, as shown in Figure 18-4. Another test for doneness of a cake is to check if the cake shrinks slightly back from the edges of the pan. After a cake is baked, it is placed on a cooling rack. Layer cakes that are to be removed from the pan need to cool in the pan on the rack for approximately 10 to 15 minutes before they are removed from the pan.

Angel food and sponge cakes need to be inverted on a cake rack. The tube of the cake pan is inverted over a funnel in a bottle, or propped up on another base to completely cool. If these cakes are removed from the pan before they are completely cool, they will sink because of

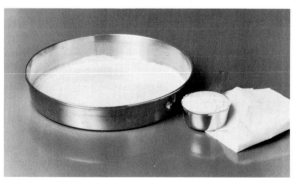

Figure 18-2.
The bottom of a cake pan is greased lightly and floured so that the cake is easy to remove after baking.

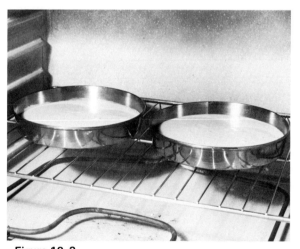

Figure 18-3.
Baking pans should be evenly spaced to allow proper heat circulation.

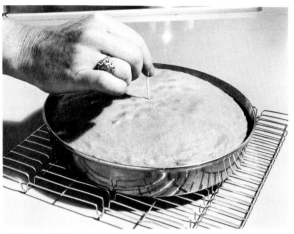

Figure 18-4.

One method for testing if a cake is done is to insert a wooden pick. If the pick comes out clean, it is done.

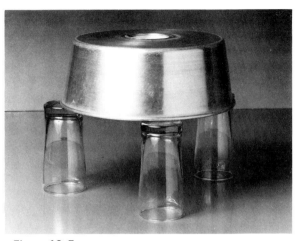

Figure 18-5.

Angel food and sponge cakes are cooled by placing over a funnel or setting the edge of the pan on upside down glasses.

the incomplete coagulation of the egg that binds the cell structure. One method for cooling angel food and sponge cakes is shown in Figure 18-5.

To remove a cake from the pan, a knife is slid around the edge to loosen any clinging cake. A cake rack is placed on top of the pan, and the cake is turned over to fall out onto the rack. A cake that has not cooled properly will leave portions clinging to the pan.

Frostings and Fillings

A cake is often covered with a frosting to increase the flavor and to make it more decorative. In layer cakes a special filling or a frosting is spread between the layers before the outside of the cake is frosted. Angel food, sponge, and chiffon cakes are often glazed with a thin icing. Some cake batters are poured over a topping and they are baked together. These are called "upside down cakes." A baked upside down cake is shown in Figure 18-6.

Other cakes are served with a fruit topping, such as fresh strawberries or with whipped cream. Angel food and sponge cakes can be cut in half and a portion of the center is removed. The central section is filled with ice cream, and the top is then replaced and the cake frozen until it is ready to serve. Cakes may also be covered with ice cream. The cake and the ice cream is sealed with a soft meringue, and then baked in a hot oven until the meringue is lightly browned. This cake is called a "Baked Alaska."

There are many recipes for different types of frosting, but the two most often used are a boiled frosting and a butter-cream frosting. A boiled frosting is made with a sugar syrup that is cooked to the firm ball stage and then poured over stiffly beaten egg whites, beating continuously until the frosting forms peaks that hold their shape.

A butter-cream frosting is prepared by blending butter or margarine until creamy, then adding sifted powdered sugar and a small amount of cream or milk, blending until thoroughly mixed and of the proper spreading consistency.

The filling of the cake may be frosting or it may be specially prepared. Some fillings are

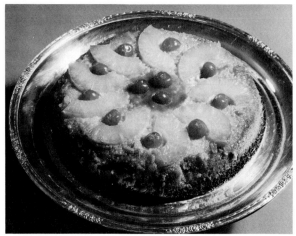

Figure 18-6.

A pineapple upside-down cake is a delectable dessert.

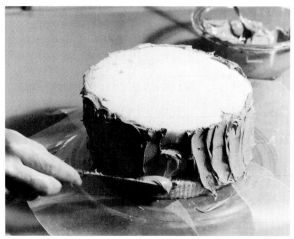

Figure 18-7.

The sides of a cake are frosted before the top. Wax paper placed under the edge of the cake makes cleanup easier. Frosting is easier to spread with a small metal spatula.

similar to cream pie fillings; fruit and jam fillings are also flavorful. If a filling or frosting is whipped cream or a cream filling, the cake must be refrigerated until it is served. An attractive cake is made by splitting cake layers in half and spreading filling between four layers.

It is important to remember that all fillings and frostings, no matter how good they taste, add additional calories.

Once a cake has completely cooled, it is ready to frost, since a warm cake will melt the frosting. All loose crumbs are brushed from the cake. Four strips of waxed paper are arranged around the edge of the serving plate and a cake layer is placed upside down on the plate. Approximately 1/4 of the frosting is spread on the layer, and the second layer is placed right side up on the filling. The sides of the cake are frosted first with a thin layer of frosting to coat any remaining crumbs; a second layer is then spread over the sides and the top of the cake. Frosting a cake is shown in Figure 18-7.

Microwave Cooking

Cakes baked in a microwave oven will be both light and tender if allowance is made for carry-

over cooking and if the cake pan is filled no more than 1/2 full. Cake pans used in microwave oven cooking may be either lightly greased, sprayed with a nonstick coating, or lined with a paper towel. Pans should not be filled more than 1/2 full because of the expansion that occurs during baking. Cakes need to be rotated 1/4 turn during baking; if a high proportion of liquid is used in the recipe, a better product will result by reducing the liquid by 1/4. For example, if 1-3/4 cup of liquid is called for, 1-1/2 cup of liquid should be used. Cupcakes may be baked in paper-lined custard cups.

Storage

Unless cakes contain ingredients that give them a high degree of moisture, they will begin to stale in 1 to 2 days. Cakes are always best when they are eaten the day they are baked. As noted, cakes and frosting that contain ingredients such as whipping cream need to be refrigerated to prevent the danger of microorganism growth. Other cakes can be stored in a cake tin or with a glass bowl inverted over the cake.

Cakes freeze well and are best when they are frozen without an icing. However, a buttercream frosting does freeze satisfactorily. To freeze a cake, the cake should be wrapped in moisture-proof wrapping and frozen for not longer than 6 months, if unfrosted, and 2 to 3 months if frosted. Cakes are thawed in their wrapping at room temperature.

Convenience Forms

Many convenience forms of cakes, frostings, and fillings are available on the market. Packaged mixes offer a wide variety of shortened, angel food, sponge, pound and chiffon cakes. The quality of the product is good and the cost, for the time saved, is not exorbitant. Frostings come ready-to-mix or ready-to-spread. Bakery cakes and frozen cakes are also available.

RECIPES

Pound Cake

	Standard	Metric
Sifted, all-purpose flour	2 cups	500 mL
Baking powder	3/4 tsp.	4 mL
Salt	1/4 tsp.	1 mL
Butter or margarine	1 cup	250 mL
Grated lemon peel	2 tsp.	10 mL
Vanilla extract	1-1/2 tsp.	7 mL
Almond extract	1/4 tsp.	1 mL
Sugar	1 cup + 2 Tbsp.	280 mL
Eggs	4	4

1. Preheat the oven to 325° F (165° C) and grease the bottom of a 9-1/2 × 5-1/4 × 2-3/4-inch loaf pan. Cut a piece of waxed paper to fit the bottom of the pan; place in the pan and grease.
2. Sift together the flour, baking powder, and salt onto a piece of waxed paper and set aside.
3. In a mixing bowl, cream the butter or margarine, grated lemon peel, vanilla, and almond extracts until the butter or margarine is very soft.
4. Gradually add the sugar and cream until light and fluffy.
5. Add the eggs, one at a time, and beat well after each addition.
6. Divide the dry ingredients into four portions. After each portion is added, beat the mixture only until smooth.
7. Pour the batter into a prepared cake pan and bake for 1 hour, 10 minutes or until the cake tests done. Cool on a rack and remove from the pan.

Yield: 1 loaf cake

Plain Layer Cake

	Standard	Metric
Cake flour, sifted	2-2/3 cups	650 mL
Baking powder	4 tsp.	20 mL
Shortening	3/4 cup	175 mL
Sugar	1-1/4 cup	310 mL
Vanilla extract	1-1/2 tsp.	7 mL
Eggs	3	3
Milk	3/4 cup	175 mL

1. Preheat the oven to 375° F (190° C) and grease and lightly flour the bottoms of two 9-inch round cake pans.
2. Sift the flour and baking powder together onto a piece of waxed paper and set aside.
3. Cream the shortening; gradually add the sugar and continue creaming until the mixture is light and fluffy. Add the vanilla.
4. Add the eggs, one at a time, beating well after each addition.
5. Divide the flour mixture into four portions; add alternately with three portions of milk, beating until the mixture is smooth after each addition.

6. Divide the batter evenly as it is poured into the prepared cake pans. Bake for 25 to 30 minutes or until cake tests done.

Yield: Two 9-inch layers

——————— Lemon Sponge Cake ———————

	Standard	Metric
Cake flour, sifted	1 cup	250 mL
Egg yolks	5	5
Sugar	1/2 cup	125 mL
Lemon juice	2 Tbsp.	30 mL
Grated lemon peel	1 tsp.	5 mL
Vanilla extract	1 tsp.	5 mL
Egg whites	5	5
Salt	1/2 tsp.	2 mL
Sugar	1/2 cup	125 mL

1. Preheat the oven to 325° F (165° C) and have ready a 9-inch tube pan.
2. Measure and set aside 1 cup of sifted cake flour.
3. Combine the egg yolks, sugar, lemon juice, grated lemon peel, and vanilla extract and beat until the mixture is very thick and lemon-colored.
4. Wash the beaters.
5. Beat the egg whites and salt together until frothy. Continue while gradually adding the sugar and beat until soft, rounded peaks are formed.
6. Gently fold the egg-yolk mixture into the beaten egg whites.
7. Sift 1/4 cup of the flour over the surface and gently fold into the mixture. Repeat until all the flour is used.
8. Turn the batter into an ungreased tube pan and bake for 1 hour or until the cake tests done. Cool completely before removing from the pan.

Yield: one tube cake

——————— One-Bowl Spice Cake ———————

	Standard	Metric
Cake flour, sifted	2 cups	500 mL
Sugar	1-1/4 cups	310 mL
Baking powder	2-1/2 tsp.	12 mL
Salt	1/2 tsp.	2 mL
Cinnamon	1 tsp.	5 mL
Nutmeg	1/2 tsp.	2 mL
Cloves	1/4 tsp.	1 mL
Milk	2/3 cup	150 mL
Shortening	1/2 cup	125 mL
Milk	1/3 cup	75 mL
Eggs	2	2

1. Preheat the oven to 350° F (175° C) and grease and flour the bottoms of two 8-inch round cake pans.
2. Sift the flour, sugar, baking powder, salt, cinnamon, nutmeg, and cloves into a mixing bowl.
3. Add 2/3 cup of milk and shortening and stir to blend. Beat 2 minutes on medium speed of an electric mixer or 300 strokes by hand.
4. Add 1/3 cup of milk and two eggs and beat 2 minutes on medium speed of an electric mixer or 300 strokes by hand.
5. Divide the batter evenly as it is poured into the prepared pans. Bake for 25 to 30 minutes or until the cake tests done.

Yield: two 8-inch layers

——————— Muffin-Method Cake ———————

	Standard	Metric
Cake flour, sifted	1-1/2 cups	375 mL
Sugar	3/4 cup	175 mL
Salt	1/4 tsp.	1 mL
Baking powder	2 tsp.	10 mL
Milk	3/4 cup	175 mL
Vanilla extract	1 tsp.	5 mL
Shortening melted or oil	1/4 cup	60 mL
Egg, beaten	1	1

1. Preheat the oven to 350° F (175° C) and grease and flour the bottom of one 8 × 8-inch square cake pan.
2. Sift the flour, sugar, salt, and baking powder together into a mixing bowl.

3. Combine the milk, vanilla extract, melted shortening or oil, and beaten egg. Add all at once to the dry ingredients.
4. Beat the mixture for 2 minutes at medium speed of the mixer or 300 strokes by hand.
5. Pour into a prepared pan and bake for 30 minutes or until the cake tests done.

Yield: one 8-inch layer

Pineapple Chiffon Cake

	Standard	Metric
Cake flour, sifted	2-1/4 cups	560 mL
Sugar	1-1/2 cups	375 mL
Baking powder	1 Tbsp.	15 mL
Salt	1 tsp.	5 mL
Cooking oil	1/2 cup	125 mL
Egg yolks, unbeaten	5	5
Unsweetened pineapple juice	3/4 cup	175 mL
Vanilla	2 tsp.	10 mL
Cream of tartar	1/2 tsp.	2 mL

1. Preheat the oven to 325° F (165° C) and set aside a 13 × 9-inch oblong pan.
2. Sift together the flour, sugar, baking powder, and salt into a mixing bowl.
3. Make a well in the center of the dry ingredients and add the cooking oil, egg yolks, unsweetened pineapple juice, and vanilla. Beat until smooth.
4. Wash the beaters.
5. Beat the egg whites until frothy; add the cream of tartar and continue beating until stiff peaks form.
6. Pour the egg yolk mixture over the egg whites in a thin stream, covering the entire surface of the egg whites, and gently fold until the ingredients are just blended.
7. Turn the batter into a pan and bake for 60 to 65 minutes or until the cake tests done. Cool completely before removing from the pan.

Yield: one 13 × 9-inch cake

Blueberry Upside-Down Cake

	Standard	Metric
Butter or margarine	1/4 cup	60 mL
Sugar	1/2 cup	125 mL
Blueberries, fresh or frozen	2 cups	500 mL
Grated lemon peel	1 tsp.	5 mL
Yellow cake mix	1 (8-1/2 oz.) pkg.	1 (250 gm)
Lemon peel, grated	1 tsp.	5 mL

1. Preheat the oven to 375° F (190° C) and set out an 8-inch square baking pan.
2. Melt the butter in a baking pan and evenly sprinkle sugar over the melted butter.
3. Mix together the blueberries and 1 tsp. grated lemon peel. Add the berries to the sugar-butter mixture.
4. Prepare the cake mix according to the package directions, stirring in 1 tsp. grated lemon peel at the end of the mixing time.
5. Spread the batter evenly over the berries.
6. Bake for 30 minutes or until the cake tests done. Let cool on a cake rack for 10 minutes and then turn out onto a serving plate. Serve warm.

Yield: one 8-inch layer

Chocolate Cake Roll

	Standard	Metric
Powdered sugar	1/3 cup	75 mL
Egg yolks	4	4
Sugar	3/4 cup	175 mL
Vanilla extract	1 tsp.	5 mL
Cake flour, sifted	3/4 cup	175 mL
Cocoa	1/4 cup	60 mL
Baking powder	3/4 tsp.	4 mL
Salt	1/2 tsp.	2 mL
Egg whites	4	4

1. Preheat the oven to 375° F (190° C). Grease the bottom of a 10 × 15-inch jelly roll pan. Cut a piece of heavy paper to fit the bottom of the pan. Place the paper in the pan and grease heavily. Lay

out a clean towel and sprinkle with 1/3 cup of powdered sugar.

2. Beat the egg yolks until thick and lemon-colored. Add the sugar to the egg yolks gradually and beat until smooth.

3. Sift together the flour, cocoa, baking powder, and salt and gradually add to the egg-sugar mixture. Mix just until the ingredients are blended.

4. Beat the egg whites until stiff, but not dry, peaks form.

5. Fold the egg-sugar-flour mixture into the egg whites gently until blended.

6. Spread the batter in the prepared pan and bake for 15 minutes or until done.

7. Immediately after the cake roll has completed baking, turn out onto a towel; remove the paper; cut off any hard edges that may have formed; roll up in a towel. Let cool.

8. Unroll the cake and spread with 2 cups of sweetened whipped cream. Refrigerate or freeze.

Yield: one cake roll

————— Poppy Seed Pudding Cake —————

	Standard	Metric
Yellow cake mix (8-1/2 oz.)	1 pkg.	1 (524 gm)
Butterscotch pudding (3-5/8 oz.)	1-1/2 pkgs.	1-1/2 (99 gm)
Poppy seeds (2 oz.)	1 pkg.	1 (57 gm)
Eggs	4	4
Cooking oil	1/2 cup	125 mL
Water	1 cup	250 mL

1. Preheat the oven to 350° F (175° C) and grease and flour the bottom of a 9 × 13-inch pan.

2. Mix together the cake mix and pudding mix until well blended.

3. Add the eggs, cooking oil, and water and beat for 3 minutes on medium speed of the electric mixer or 450 strokes by hand.

4. Pour into the prepared pan and bake for 25

minutes or until the cake tests done. Lightly dust top of cake with powdered sugar.

Yield: one 13 × 9 × 2-inch cake

————————— Carrot Cake —————————

	Standard	Metric
All-purpose flour	2 cups	500 mL
Soda	2 tsp.	10 mL
Salt	1/8 tsp.	0.5 mL
Brown sugar	2 cups	500 mL
Eggs	3	3
Cooking oil	1-1/2 cups	375 mL
Vanilla extract	1 tsp.	5 mL
Shredded coconut	1-1/2 cups	375 mL
Grated carrots	2 cups	500 mL
Chopped nuts	1 cup	250 mL
Pineapple, crushed and undrained	1 (6-1/2 oz.) can	1 (193 gm)

1. Preheat the oven to 350° F (175° C) and grease and flour one 13 × 9-inch oblong pan.

2. Sift together the flour, soda, and salt in a mixing bowl.

3. Add the brown sugar, oil, eggs, and vanilla to the dry ingredients and mix until thoroughly blended.

4. Stir in the coconut, carrots, nuts, and pineapple until well blended.

5. Pour into the prepared pan and bake at 350° F (175° C) for 50 to 60 minutes or until the cake tests done.

——————— Carrot Cake Icing ———————

	Standard	Metric
Powdered sugar	2 cups	500 mL
Butter	1/4 cup	60 mL
Cream cheese	1 (3 oz.) pkg.	1 (85 gm)
Vanilla	1 tsp.	5 mL

1. Mix together the powdered sugar, butter, cream cheese, and vanilla until thoroughly blended.

2. Spread on the cooled cake.

Yield: one 13 × 9-inch cake

——————— Easy Oatmeal Cake ———————

	Standard	Metric
Boiling water	1-1/4 cups	310 mL
Oats, uncooked	1 cup	250 mL
Butter or margarine	1/2 cup	125 mL
Sugar	1 cup	250 mL
Brown sugar, packed	1 cup	250 mL
Eggs	2	2
Vanilla	1 tsp.	5 mL
Flour, sifted	1-1/2 cups	375 mL
Baking soda	1 tsp.	5 mL
Salt	1/2 tsp.	2 mL
Cinnamon	3/4 tsp.	4 mL
Nutmeg	1/4 tsp.	1 mL

1. Preheat the oven to 350° F (175° C) and grease and flour a 9 × 9-inch pan.
2. Pour the boiling water over the oats, cover, and let stand for 20 minutes.
3. Beat the butter or margarine until creamy and gradually beat in the sugars. Continue beating until light and fluffy.
4. Blend the eggs and vanilla into the creamed mixture. Stir in the oat mixture.
5. Sift together the flour, soda, salt, cinnamon, and nutmeg and add to the creamed mixture. Blend well.
6. Pour into the prepared pan and bake for 50 to 55 minutes or until the cake tests done.

Yield: one 9 × 9-inch layer

——————— Broiled Oatmeal Cake Topping ———————

	Standard	Metric
Butter, melted	1/4 cup	60 mL
Brown sugar, packed	1/2 cup	125 mL
Light cream	3 Tbsp.	45 mL
Chopped nuts	1/2 cup	125 mL
Coconut	3/4 cup	175 mL

1. Preheat the oven to broil.
2. Combine the butter, brown sugar, light cream, chopped nuts, and coconut and spread over the top of the baked cake.
3. Place under a broiler and cook until the topping is bubbly.

Yield: frosting for one 9 × 9-inch layer

——————— Butter Frosting ———————

	Standard	Metric
Butter or margarine	1/4 cup	60 mL
Vanilla extract	1 tsp.	5 mL
Powdered sugar, sifted	2 cups	500 mL
Milk or cream	1-1/2 Tbsp.	22 mL

1. Cream the butter or margarine and vanilla extract together until the butter is softened.
2. Gradually add the sugar, beating after each addition.
3. Add enough milk or cream to beat the frosting to spreading consistency.

Yield: frosting for tops and sides of two 8-inch layers

Variation:
1. Chocolate butter frosting. Blend in two squares of melted chocolate after the sugar has been added.
2. Lemon-orange butter frosting. Substitute 1 teaspoon of grated orange peel and 1/2 tsp. of grated lemon peel for vanilla extract. Use 1 Tbsp. of orange juice and 1-1/2 tsp. of lemon juice for the milk or cream.

——————— Boiled Frosting ———————

	Standard	Metric
Sugar	2 cups	500 mL
Water	3/4 cup	175 mL

Light corn syrup *or*	1 Tbsp. *or*	15 mL *or*
cream of tartar	1/4 tsp.	1 mL
Salt	1/8 tsp.	0.5 mL
Egg whites, stiffly beaten	2	2
Vanilla extract	1 tsp.	5 mL

1. Combine the sugar, water, corn syrup or cream of tartar, and salt in a saucepan. Cook over low heat, stirring until the sugar dissolves.
2. Put a cover on the pan and cook 2 to 3 minutes to dissolve the sugar crystals. Continue cooking until the sugar mixture reaches the soft-ball stage, 236° F (113° C).
3. Gradually pour the hot syrup over the stiffly beaten egg whites, beating constantly, until the frosting holds soft peaks and is of spreading consistency. Add the vanilla and continue beating.

Yield: frosting for the top and sides of two 9-inch layers

─────────── Chocolate Glaze ───────────

	Standard	Metric
Semisweet chocolate	3 oz.	85 gm
Butter or margarine	3 Tbsp.	45 mL

1. Partially melt the chocolate and butter together over hot, not boiling water. Remove from the hot water and stir until completely melted.

2. Spoon over the cake and let drizzle down the sides of the cake.

Yield: Glaze for one angel food, sponge, or chiffon cake

─────────── Individual Baked Alaska ───────────

	Standard	Metric
Egg whites, stiffly beaten	4	4
Sugar	3/4 cup	175 mL
Oblong layer cake	4, 3-in. squares	4, 3-in.
Ice-cream	4 scoops	4 scoops

1. Preheat the oven to 450° F (230° C).
2. Gradually beat the sugar into the egg whites and continue beating until the meringue is stiff.
3. Place the cake squares on a cutting board and put one scoop of ice cream on each square.
4. Cover each square with a one-quarter portion of the meringue, being careful to seal in all edges of the cake and ice cream.
5. Bake in the oven until the meringue is a golden brown. Immediately remove to serving plates and serve.

Yield: 4 servings

LEARNING ACTIVITIES

1. Investigate cake recipes and make a list of cakes that would be suitable to take to an all-day picnic.
2. Plan three dinner menus that could include cake being served as the dessert because one third of the human requirement for nutrients is met in other foods served at the meal.
3. Plan a party at which the cake is the entrée and design a method to cut and decorate a cake that is in keeping with the theme of the party.
4. Compare the cost of purchasing a bakery cake and a ready-made frozen cake with the cost of purchasing a convenience mix and making it.
5. Prepare a convenience mix and compare it in flavor and texture with a bakery cake.
6. Prepare three shortened cakes by the

same recipe but use hydrogenated shortening in one, lard as the fat in a second, and butter or margarine as the fat in the third. Compare the difference in taste, texture, and volume between the three and explain to the class the reasons why the results are different.

7. Prepare a cake that calls for cake flour in a recipe and prepare the same cake again but substitute all-purpose flour for the cake flour. Compare the difference in texture and volume between the two.

8. Prepare a sponge cake and divide the batter equally between two loaf pans. After baking is completed, let one cake cool completely in the proper method for a foam cake and remove the second after only 10 minutes of cooling and note the change in volume that occurs. Explain the results to the class.

9. Prepare three cakes of similar ingredients but with each separate recipe using the one-bowl method, the conventional method, and the muffin method. Compare the difference in texture, volume, flavor, and time of preparation with each of the three methods and determine which type of recipe you would select to use in the future.

10. Prepare a sponge-cake batter that uses the egg whites separately to the point of folding the egg-flour mixture into the egg whites. Divide the egg-flour mixture and the egg whites in half. To one half of the beaten egg whites, rapidly stir in the egg-flour mixture; to the second portion of egg whites, fold in the egg-flour mixture. Bake the two cake mixtures in separate loaf pans, and after they have properly cooled, compare the two cakes for volume, texture, and flavor. Evaluate why differences occurred and report to the class.

11. Compare the cost of ingredients in a basic home-prepared boiled icing with a convenience boiled icing mix. Prepare each form of icing and determine which you would use, based on cost, taste, and time of preparation.

12. Prepare a two-layer shortened cake. Let one layer stand at room temperature for 3 days. Wrap and freeze the second layer immediately after it has cooled. On the third day thaw the frozen layer and compare in quality with the layer that was not frozen.

REVIEW QUESTIONS

1. What kind of a flour mixture are cakes?
2. Why are cakes a concentrated form of carbohydrates?
3. Why do cakes contribute a minimal amount of nutrients and a high number of calories to the human diet?
4. What types of cakes contain the least number of calories?
5. At what kind of meals could a cake be served that would not interfere with the human requirement of nutrients? What else must be considered in making this decision?
6. What types of cakes are the most economical to prepare and serve?
7. Why is it not considered good practice to alter the major ingredient proportions of a cake?

8. What is the formula for substituting all-purpose cake flour for cake flour in a recipe?
9. What size eggs should be used in preparing a cake?
10. What does the emulsifying property of egg have to do with the tenderness of a cake?
11. What is the most desirable fat to use in cake? Why?
12. What is the characteristic of a cake without enough liquid?
13. How does sugar help to make a cake tender?
14. What are the distinguishing characteristics of the two types of cakes?
15. What is the difference between a chiffon cake and a sponge and angel food cake in ingredients, texture, and flavor?
16. Why is the one-bowl method of cake preparation less time-consuming than the conventional method?
17. What is meant by "creaming" a fat?
18. How are flour and liquid added to the creamed mixture in a conventional method of cake preparation?
19. Why should the beaters be washed after beating egg yolks and before beating egg whites?
20. In what type of pan is a cake roll baked?
21. How is the pan preparation for a cake roll different from that for a shortened cake and for an angel food cake?
22. Why should an angel food cake be cooled completely before being removed from the pan?
23. How long should a shortened cake be cooled before being removed from the pan?
24. What is the basic procedure for making a boiled frosting?
25. What is the basic method for frosting a cake?
26. Why should cakes that contain whipped cream be refrigerated?
27. How should a cake be frozen? Should a cake to be frozen be frosted?
28. How much should the liquid be reduced if a cake is being baked in a microwave oven?

19
Pastry and Pies

The words *pastry* and *pie* bring to most minds pictures of tempting desserts. Generally speaking, pastry includes all forms of sweets, such as cakes, pies, tarts, and sweet, yeast-leavened rolls. As it does in this chapter, pastry can also mean the dough from which a pie crust is made.

A flaky and tender pastry crust combined with a sweetened filling makes a pie, which is one of the most popular desserts in the United States. Pies can also be filled with a food such as meat, poultry, fish, or cheese, and be the entrée of a meal. Entrée pies are not discussed in this chapter; however, the procedure to make the pie crust is the same for dessert pies and entrée pies.

Many individuals have a difficult time making a pie crust that is tender and flaky. The proper procedure to make a pie crust is not difficult, and, if followed, will produce quality pie crusts every time.

Nutritional Factors to Consider

Carbohydrate and Fat

Pastry has a high carbohydrate and fat content because its two main ingredients are flour, a carbohydrate, and fat. Pie fillings vary in their carbohydrate content, depending on the amount of sugar or fruit used, and usually have only a minimal amount of fat. When pies are served with whipped cream or a sugar-sweetened syrup, their fat and carbohydrate content is increased.

Protein

The protein content of pie crust is minimal, but a filling containing milk and eggs, such as a custard pie, does contribute some protein to the diet.

Vitamins and Minerals

Only a minimal amount of vitamins and minerals is found in a pie crust. The vitamin and mineral content of a filling will vary with the ingredients used. For example, a cream filling made with whole milk provides some vitamin A, calcium, and phosphorus, and fruit pies have small amounts of the B vitamins, plus iron. However, serving portions of pies are sometimes so small that their nutrient contribution is not great.

Calories

Because of the high fat and carbohydrate content of pies, their calorie content is high. A 1/8th section of a 9-inch pie averages between 250 and 300 calories. The calorie content of a pie can be somewhat reduced by using a minimal amount of sugar in the preparation of the filling, and by serving one-crust pies whenever possible.

Menu-Planning Points

Inherent Factors

Balance. The type of pie filling chosen can help to balance a menu. For example, a meal that did not contain fruit in another course is complemented with a fruit filling. A meal in which a creamed meat is the entrée would not be balanced by serving a pie with a cream filling as the dessert.

Color. Because desserts are usually served alone, they are more attractive when served with some type of garnish. Shaved chocolate, toasted coconut, or cookie crumbs are attractive garnishes on cream fillings. Pastry cutouts and lattice pastry are attractive on fruit fillings, as they allow the color of the fruit to show and eliminate some of the calories. Fresh fruits, such as sliced bananas or sectioned oranges, canned drained fruits, such as mandarin oranges or sliced peaches, and dehydrated fruits, such as raisins or chopped dates, all add attractiveness and color to pies.

Shape, Texture, and Flavor. Most pies are cut into wedges to be served, but a variation called a *tart*, which is a small, individual pie, can add a contrast in shape.

The texture of most pies is soft, but a variation in texture can be achieved by adding nuts or by combining fruits in a cream filling.

Most pies have a sweet flavor, but this can be varied somewhat by the choice of ingredients. The flavor of the piecrust can be altered both by the choice of fat in the crust and by the use of other ingredients, such as cookie crumbs or crushed cereal flakes. Pie fillings can be varied both by the ingredients and flavoring agents used. For example, a chocolate or butterscotch cream filling can be made by changing some ingredients and flavoring agents, and a fruit filling can be made to differ in flavor by using strawberries or cranberries as the main ingredient.

External Factors

Age and Culture. It is rare to find a person of any age who does not like pie. Our forefathers created many of the favorite pie recipes that are used today, including those two long-standing favorites, apple pie and pumpkin pie.

Space and Equipment. The making of a pie requires only a small amount of space. The essential equipment for making the crust includes a pastry cloth and stockinet for the rolling pin. A pastry blender is also an aid in making a flaky crust.

Time Scheduling. Pies can be made ahead of time. Fresh pies are easier to cut into serving portions if they are allowed to stand until they are cooled, and some pies require thorough chilling or freezing before being served. Many pies and pie crusts can be made ahead of time and frozen.

Ingredients and Their Functions

The ingredients used in making a piecrust are flour, fat, salt, and liquid. The proper proportions and mixing of these ingredients will yield the desirable characteristics of flakiness and tenderness. A flaky pie crust is one in which the fat is dispersed between layers of flour and a tender pie crust means a crumb that is tender, not tough, to the bite.

Flour

Enriched all-purpose flour is preferred in making a pie crust. Pastry flour, made from soft wheat, is used mainly by the commercial baking industry. Whole wheat flour and instant-blending flour do not yield satisfactory piecrusts.

Fat

The flakiness, tenderness, flavor, and color of a pie crust are determined by the type of fat used. Tenderness is dependent on the shortening power of the fat, that is, the ability of the fat to cover the gluten strands of flour and thereby prevent them from absorbing water.

A tender crust is achieved by preventing gluten development. This is best achieved by having the proper proportion of fat, evenly distributed before adding the water, and not overmixing or rolling the dough out in too much flour.

A flaky crust is dependent on having clumps of fat in the dough mixture. When the dough is baked these clumps of fat melt. The resulting characteristic of a flaky crust is a crust that peels in thin layers when it is broken.

Because of its shortening power and moldability, lard produces a pie crust that is both tender and flaky. A crust made from lard is also lighter in color and has a stronger flavor than one made from other fats. Pie crusts made with hydrogenated shortening are also flaky and tender, but have a slightly darker color when baked and a blander flavor. A mixture of half-lard and half-hydrogenated shortening yields a pie crust with a pleasing flavor that is both tender and flaky.

A pie crust made with a liquid fat will be tender, but have a mealy, less flaky crumb, and butter or margarine will make a piecrust that has a rich flavor and color. However, unless these fats are used in exact proportions with the flour, the crust may be so crumbly that it will be difficult to remove from the pan.

The flakiness and tenderness of a piecrust are also affected by the amount of fat that is used, the temperature of the fat when it is mixed into the flour, and the amount of liquid used. The usual proportion is 1/3 cup of lard or hydrogenated shortening to 1 cup of flour. With a liquid fat, the proportion is 1/4 cup of fat to 1 cup of flour. Since butter or margarine are only 80 per cent fat and thus have less shortening power, 1/3 cup plus 1 tablespoon of butter or margarine is used with 1 cup of flour.

Chilling the fat before adding it to the flour will produce a more flaky piecrust, because the flour will absorb less water and develop less gluten at a lower temperature. Fats used at room temperature will produce a more tender crust.

Liquid

Water is most often used as the liquid in making pie crust. Ice water helps to achieve a more flaky crust, but cold tap water may also be used. The amount of water will vary with the kinds and proportions of fat and flour, but a usable guide is 2 to 3 tablespoons of water per 1 cup of flour. A citrus juice may sometimes be used for part of the liquid.

Salt

Salt is used as the flavoring agent in pie crust.

Basic Method of Pastry Preparation

It is most important to work quickly and to handle the dough gently when making pastry. The principal aim is not to overwork the dough, thereby to avoid long gluten strands from developing.

Mixing Ingredients

The ingredients for a pie crust can be mixed by several methods. Four of these methods are discussed here. The first method, called "the pastry method," is based on the same mixing procedure as for rolled biscuits, except for kneading. Pastry dough is never kneaded.

The flour is sifted, measured, and returned to the sifter with the salt, and the ingredients are sifted into a mixing bowl. A fat, other than a liquid fat, is cut into the flour mixture with a pastry blender or two table knives, until some of the fat is the size of small peas and some of the fat is more thoroughly blended in the flour mixture. When mixing dough for several pie

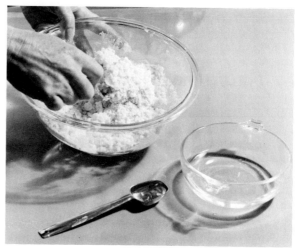

Figure 19–1.

The flour-fat portion of a pie crust is sprinkled with a portion of the water and the ingredients are quickly tossed with a fork.

crusts at one time, an electric mixer at low speed may be used to blend the fat into the flour.

The cold water is then sprinkled evenly, a little at a time, over the flour-fat mixture. After adding a portion of water, the flour-fat mixture is quickly mixed with a fork in a tossing motion, as illustrated in Figure 19–1. More water is added and quickly mixed in. The water is not added all at once or all in one area, because the object is to dampen slightly all of the flour particles so they will cling together. It is important, when mixing the water into the flour, to reach to the bottom of the bowl to make sure that all of the flour becomes dampened. As soon as the flour-fat particles tend to cling together when pressed gently, the mixture is shaped into a ball with the hands. Too much water will make a tough crust, and too little water will produce a crumbly mass that will not hold together.

A second method for mixing the ingredients is called "the paste method." After sifting the flour, 2 tablespoons are removed for each cup of flour used in the recipe. The remaining flour and salt are sifted into a mixing bowl and the fat is cut in. The reserved portion of flour and the water are stirred together to form a paste. The paste is then quickly stirred into the flour-fat mixture to dampen the ingredients, and the mixture is formed into a ball.

In the hot water method, the water is heated to the boiling point and poured over the fat in a small mixing bowl. The fat and water are beaten together until creamy and added all at once to the sifted dry ingredients. The mixture is stirred to dampen the ingredients, and the dough is then shaped into a ball.

When using a liquid fat, it is best first to mix the oil and water by rapidly stirring or shaking them together, and then to add the mixed oil and water to the sifted dry ingredients. The ingredients are tossed together until they are all dampened and the dough is shaped into a ball.

In each of these methods the dough will be easier to roll out if it is wrapped in waxed paper and allowed to chill. After the dough is chilled, it is brought to room temperature before the rolling is begun. However, if time is short, this is not a necessary procedure. Simply allowing the dough to rest a few minutes on the work surface before rolling it will make the dough easier to handle.

Rolling Dough

Only one piecrust should be rolled at a time. The ball of dough is placed on a lightly floured surface and flattened with the hand. At this stage of pastry making several more factors can inhibit the formation of a tender and flaky piecrust. Only enough flour should be spread on the working surface as is needed to prevent the dough from sticking to the working surface as the dough is rolled. Additional flour will make a tough piecrust. A canvas cover, called a pastry cloth, and a cover for the rolling pin, called a stockinet, aid in rolling out the dough

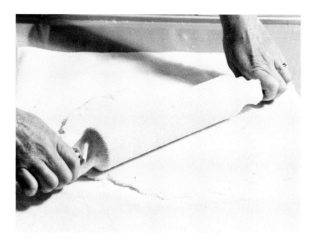

Figure 19–2.
Pie crust dough is placed on a lightly floured surface and rolled from the center to the outer edge. This is repeated along each section of dough.

without too much of the dough sticking to the working surface or to the rolling pin. Both covers are lightly floured before rolling of the dough is begun. If these materials are not available, the rolling pin should be lightly floured, and any dough that may cling to the rolling pin should be scraped off. Dough made with a liquid fat is more easily rolled between two pieces of waxed paper.

The dough is rolled from the center to the outer edge with short, light strokes, to a thickness of 1/8-inch. Care needs to be taken to avoid rerolling over areas of the dough that have already been rolled. Proper rolling of dough is illustrated in Figure 19-2. The dough should be turned over only if it appears to be sticking excessively.

Dough for a bottom crust is rolled into a circle that is approximately 1-1/2 inches larger than the top diameter of the pie pan. A top pie crust is rolled slightly larger to allow for the filling and to finish the edge.

The easiest way to place the rolled piecrust into the pie pan, or on top of the pie filling, is to place the rolling pin on the center of the pie dough, flip one half of the dough over the

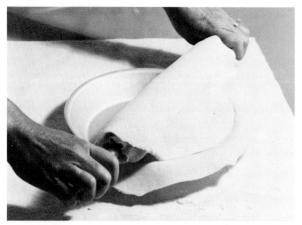

Figure 19-3.
The rolled dough is placed in the pie pan by placing the rolling pin on the center of the rolled dough; flipping one half of the dough over the rolling pin; lifting the dough on the rolling pin to the center of the pie pan.

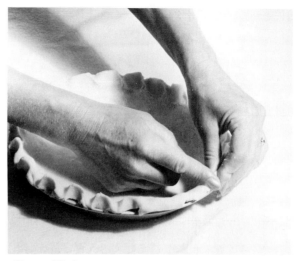

Figure 19-4.
Fluting the edge of a pie crust is done with the forefinger.

rolling pin, and with the pie pan in back of the rolling pin, lift the rolling pin with the dough to the center of the pie pan. The rolling pin is then removed, as shown in Figure 19-3. The dough is gently eased into the pie pan by lifting a portion of the dough and letting it fall to the side of the pan. Care must be taken not to stretch the dough in fitting it into the pie pan, as this will cause shrinkage during baking.

Several methods are available to finish the edge of pastry. One method for a single pie-crust is to trim the dough so that 1/2-inch overhangs the edge of the pie pan. Trimming is easily done with a pair of kitchen shears. This edge is folded underneath to form an edge that is even with the edge of the pie pan. Fluting is done by pinching the lapped edge together with the forefingers, as shown in Figure 19-4. A double-crusted pie is fluted in the same manner except that the bottom crust is trimmed even with the edge of the pan and moistened with water. The top crust is trimmed to a 1-inch overhang and folded under the bottom edge.

Top crusts must have some kind of venting to allow the steam to escape and to help prevent juices from boiling over into the oven. This can be done by cutting out a design while the dough is still on the working surface, or by pricking the surface with a fork after the top crust has been placed over the filling.

Some top crusts are made by a lattice topping. The rolled top crust is cut into 1/2-to 1-inch strips while the top crust is on the work surface. The lattice is made by laying some of the strips one way across the filling and folding them back to the center of the pie. The remaining strips are woven in and out from the center between the first-placed strips. Another type of top crust is made by cutting out large shapes from the dough and placing them on top of the filling.

Tart Shells

Tart shells are small, individual piecrusts made by rolling the dough out to a 1/8-inch thickness and cutting circles that fit into muffin tins. The usual size of muffin tins is 4 to 5

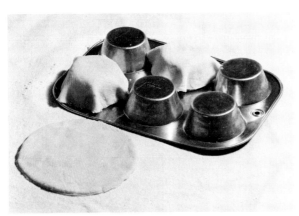

Figure 19-5.
Tart shells may be shaped on the back side of a muffin tin and baked. If they are to be filled with an uncooked filling, they are shaped on the inside of the tin.

inches in diameter. The dough is shaped in the muffin tin, a filling is added, and the tart is baked. If the tarts are to contain a cooked filling, the dough is shaped on the back side of the muffin tin, pricked with a fork, and baked. Special tart pans are also available on the market. Methods for baking tart shells are shown in Figure 19-5.

Baking Piecrusts

The best kinds of pie pans are those made of dull-finished aluminum or of glass. However, lightweight foil pans are a convenience if more pies are being made than there are available pans. When using shiny, lightweight pans, it is important to place the pie pans on a baking sheet so that the pies cook thoroughly. A shiny pan reflects heat, causing the bottom crust not to bake thoroughly when the pan is placed directly on a rack in the oven. The most common sizes of pie pans used are the 8-inch, 9-inch, and 10-inch. It is important always to

check the recipe to determine which size pan the recipe requires.

Single Crusts. Depending on the pie filling, single-crust pie shells may be baked before the filling is added or may be baked with the filling. Single-crust pie shells baked without a filling must be pricked generously with a fork on the bottom and the sides to allow the steam to escape and to prevent shrinkage. Piecrusts baked with a filling are not pricked.

Another method to bake a shell without a filling is to line the shell with waxed paper and partially fill the shell with uncooked rice or dried beans. The waxed paper and the rice or beans are removed after the first 10 minutes of baking. A third method is to set a second pan of the same size on top of the dough for the first 10 minutes of baking.

Single piecrusts without a filling are baked for approximately 15 minutes at 450° F (230° C) or until the crusts are delicately browned. For single-crust pies baked with a filling, the baking temperature of the recipe needs to be followed.

Double Crusts. Double-crusted pies are usually baked at a temperature of between 400° F to 450° F (205° C to 230° C) for the entire cooking time, or they are baked at 450° F (230° C) for the first 10 minutes of cooking time and then the temperature is lowered to 350° F (175° C) for the completion of baking. Raw fillings will take longer to cook than fillings that have been partially or completely precooked. It is advisable to follow the baking temperature recommended on the filling recipe.

To make a more browned top crust, the crust may be brushed with melted butter or margarine before baking. A shiny top crust is made by brushing the crust first with milk and then sprinkling it with granulated sugar. To achieve a glazed top crust, the crust is coated with a mixture of one egg yolk and 1–1/2 teaspoons water.

Characteristics of Successful Pastry

A successful pastry is tender and/or flaky, depending on its ingredients, and it has a blistered rather than a smooth appearance. The color of the pastry crust should be a delicate golden brown.

Other Types of Crusts

In addition to pastry crusts, other types of piecrusts may be made for single-crust pies having a cooked filling. These include crusts made from graham cracker crumbs, vanilla or chocolate wafer crumbs, bread crumbs, crushed cereal flakes, and coconut. The crumbs can be made either in a blender or rolled between two pieces of waxed paper to a crumb consistency. A portion of melted butter or margarine is added to make the crumbs mold together, and a small amount of sugar may be added to give the crust a sweeter flavor. Other ingredients used in crumb crusts include chocolate, nuts, and special flavorings. When the ingredients have been mixed together, they are pressed into a pie pan. A second pie pan set atop the crumbs helps to mold the crumbs to the pie pan. Crumb shells are baked at 375° F (190° C) for 6 to 8 minutes to set the crust Chocolate crumb crusts need not be baked.

Hard meringues (discussed in the chapter on eggs) can be shaped into a pie pan and used as a delicate crust for certain cream and fruit fillings.

A pastry pie crust may be varied in both flavor and texture by adding seasonings such as cinnamon or nutmeg, grated cheese, or chopped nuts.

Types of Pie Fillings

There are several types of pie fillings and, of these, many different ingredients are combined to make delectable pies. Some pie fillings are cooked and put into a previously prepared crust. For example, a cream pie filling is cooked on top of the range and put into a baked piecrust. These kinds of pies may be topped with a soft meringue (discussed in the chapter on eggs) and the meringue-topped pie is further cooked in the oven. These pies are sometimes served with a whipped topping.

Other pie fillings are added uncooked, or partially cooked, to an unbaked piecrust and the cooking is completed in the oven. For example, a custard filling is baked in an unbaked or partially baked pie shell, and a raw fruit pie filling is baked in an unbaked shell with a top crust. Two-crusted pies are often served with a whipped topping, sauce, or ice cream.

Cream Fillings

Cream fillings, similar to milk puddings (discussed in the chapter on milk) are composed of milk, a starch, egg yolks, sugar, salt, and additional flavorings. The basic procedure for cooking a cream filling is to combine the sugar, starch, and salt together in a saucepan and then to gradually add the scalded milk. The filling is stirred constantly over medium heat until it thickens. Stirring prevents the milk from scorching. A small amount of the thickened filling is stirred into slightly beaten egg yolks, and then the heated egg yolk mixture is stirred rapidly into the filling mixture.

The mixture is cooked for an additional 2 to 4 minutes and removed from the heat. The flavoring and sometimes additional fat are stirred in, and the filling is cooled to room temperature before being put into the baked pie crust. The pie is then refrigerated until serving time.

Many different cream fillings may be prepared by adding additional ingredients such as coconut, chocolate, different fruits, and nuts. A lemon pie filling is prepared on the same principle as a cream pie filling except that water is used in place of milk as the liquid, and the lemon juice is added after the eggs have been cooked in the filling mixture.

Chiffon Fillings

A chiffon filling is made by heating a liquid, salt, and sometimes egg yolks, and dissolving the gelatin in the heated mixture. The mixture must not boil, as this would coagulate the egg. The mixture is then cooled until it begins to thicken. At this point, egg whites beaten stiffly with some sugar, and usually an additional ingredient such as fruit, chocolate, nuts, or coconut, are folded into the mixture. Some recipes call for the gelatin to be whipped to a foamy mass after it begins to thicken, and other recipes use whipped cream or ice cream in place of the egg whites. The chiffon filling is poured into a baked pie shell and chilled or frozen until firm. This usually takes from 2 to 4 hours.

Custard Fillings

A custard pie filling is a baked custard (discussed in the chapter on eggs) cooked in an unbaked or partially baked piecrust and is composed of eggs, milk, sugar, and flavorings. The crust of a custard pie will become less soggy if the pie is baked on the bottom rack of the oven to help set the crust more rapidly. A pumpkin pie is a variation of a custard pie.

Fruit Fillings

A fruit filling is made from fresh, frozen, canned, or dehydrated fruit. Most fruit fillings require some type of thickener such as flour, tapioca, or cornstarch to be added to the fruit and/or juices before cooking, and some fruits require an additional amount of sugar. Canned fruits and fruits frozen with sugar usually do not need additional sugar.

Most fruit fillings are baked in an unbaked pie shell with the fruit, thickener, and sugar being mixed together before they are added to the pie shell. However, some recipes call for the fruit, thickener, and sugar to be partially cooked before they are added to the pie shell, and other recipes require that the juice and thickener be precooked.

A fruit pie with a top crust must have adequate venting of the top crust to allow the steam to escape and to keep the juices from boiling over into the oven. A lattice crust is not only attractive but helps to prevent the juices from spilling over.

Other Pie Fillings

Some pie fillings use melted marshmallows as the thickening and sweetening agent, whereas others may use whipped cream. Simple and nutritious pie fillings can be made by spreading different layers of ice cream in a baked pie crust and freezing the filling until serving time.

A variation to fruit fillings is done by spreading a layer of softened cream cheese on the bottom of a baked pie shell and then covering the cheese with a cooked and cooled fruit filling. Frozen fruits, such as strawberries or raspberries, may be beaten with egg whites and sugar for an extended period of time, and a whipped topping is then folded in and the entire mixture is frozen in a baked pie shell. Another variation to fruit fillings is to crush some of the fruit or use a fruit liquid, and to make a sauce thickened with cornstarch and sugar as an additional ingredient. After the sauce is cooked, it is poured over fresh fruit arranged in a baked piecrust.

Microwave Cooking

Pastry and crumb crusts can both be successfully baked in a microwave oven. A single-pastry piecrust may be baked by pricking the dough with a fork and baking, or a paper towel may be placed over the pie shell and a smaller pie pan placed on top of the paper towel for the first 3 minutes of cooking. The paper towel and top pie pan are then removed, and the pie shell is baked for an additional 3 minutes. Better results are attained by this method. Crumb crusts are cooked for 1 minute. Better browning of the top crust on a two-crusted pie is attained by baking the pie in a microwave oven for approximately 7 minutes, or until the filling is bubbling, and then completing the baking in a conventional oven at 450° F (230° C) for 10 to 15 minutes.

Many pie fillings can be made in a microwave oven and then put into a baked crust, including cream pie fillings, fillings made from commercial mixes, and those recipes using marshmallows as a thickening agent. Pies topped with meringues can also be successfully cooked in a microwave oven. Frozen pies need to be transferred to glass baking dishes before being cooked in a microwave oven.

Storage

All pies, except for frozen pies, should be eaten when they are freshly baked. The longer a pie is stored, the soggier the crust will become. Some pies are more flavorful when they are eaten warm and some are better served cold. Any pies that contain dairy products or eggs need to be refrigerated until serving time because of the danger of microorganism growth. For example, cream pies and custard and chiffon pies need to be continuously refrigerated.

Pastry mixtures that contain flour, salt, and cut-in fat can be stored in a tightly covered container in the refrigerator for 2 to 3 weeks. Balls of pastry dough may be tightly wrapped and frozen. When ready to use, the ball of pastry dough is thawed and then rolled and used as freshly made pastry. Freshly made pastry may be rolled, put in pie pans, and frozen. Frozen pie shells are baked without thawing at 450° F (230° C) for a baked pie shell. To save freezer space, pastry may be rolled to the given top diameter of a pie pan, placed on a square of cardboard covered with plastic wrap, wrapped tightly, and frozen. To use, the pastry is thawed and baked in the correct-sized pie pan.

Pies may be frozen, both baked and unbaked. Both kinds of pies need to be well wrapped for freezer storage. When an unbaked frozen pie is baked it is baked at the recommended temperature for 10 to 20 minutes longer than the recommended baking times. Frozen baked pies are partially thawed at room temperature and then baked for 30 minutes at 350° F (175° C) or until warm.

Fruit fillings can also be mixed, freezer wrapped, and frozen in a pie pan. After the filling is frozen, it is removed from the pie pan and frozen separately. When ready to use, the fruit filling is unwrapped, placed in a pie shell, topped with a crust, and baked for 10 to 20 minutes longer than an unfrozen filling. The ingredients for a pumpkin pie filling can be mixed together and frozen in a freezer container. When it is ready to use, the mixture is partially thawed and poured into an unbaked pie crust and baked. An additional 10 to 15 minutes of baking time is required for frozen fillings.

Convenience Forms

Piecrust mixes containing the flour, fat, and salt are available on the market. These mixes need only the addition of a liquid to make a pie crust. Some commercial mixes contain both the ingredients for a crumb crust and a cream filling. Both frozen pastry and crumb crusts are also available. Several canned fruit fillings for pies are available, and frozen ready-to-eat and frozen ready-to-bake pies are sold.

Plain Pastry

	Standard	Metric
All-purpose flour, sifted	2 cups	500 mL
Salt	1 tsp.	5 mL
Shortening or lard or half and half	2/3 cup	150 mL
Water, cold	4 to 6 Tbsp.	60 to 70 mL

1. Sift the flour and salt together into a mixing bowl.
2. Cut in the shortening with a pastry blender or two table knives until shortening is size of small peas.
3. Sprinkle 1 Tbsp. of water over the flour mixture and toss lightly with a fork. Keep adding water, 1 Tbsp. at a time, and tossing with a fork to mix until the dough clings together when gently pressed.
4. Form the dough into two balls and wrap in waxed paper and chill thoroughly, or let the dough stand several minutes before rolling.

Yield: one 9-inch crust or one 2-crust, 8-inch pie

Hot-Water Pastry

	Standard	Metric
Shortening	2/3 cup	150 mL
Water, boiling	1/3 cup	75 mL
All-purpose flour, sifted	2 cups	500 mL
Salt	3/4 tsp.	4 mL

1. Place the shortening in a small mixing bowl, and pour over it the boiling water. Beat the water and shortening together until creamy.
2. Sift the flour and salt into a mixing bowl. Add the shortening-water mixture and mix with a fork until all the ingredients are dampened.
3. Form the dough into a ball; wrap in wax paper and chill before rolling.

Yield: one 9-inch crust or one 2-crust, 8-inch pie

Liquid Fat Pastry

	Standard	Metric
All-purpose flour, sifted	2 cups	500 mL
Salt	1 tsp.	5 mL
Salad oil	1/2 cup	125 mL
Water, ice cold	4 to 5 Tbsp.	60 to 75 mL

1. Sift the flour and salt together into a mixing bowl.
2. Shake, stir, or beat together the oil and water and pour over the flour mixture immediately. Mix with a fork until all the ingredients are dampened.
3. Form the dough into a ball, wrap in waxed paper, and let chill, or allow to stand several minutes before rolling.

Yield: one 9-inch crust or one 2-crust, 8-inch pie

Paste Method

	Standard	Metric
All-purpose flour, sifted	2 cups	500 mL
Salt	1 tsp.	5 mL
Water	1/4 cup	60 mL
Shortening	2/3 cup	150 mL

1. Sift the flour and salt into a mixing bowl. Remove 1/4 cup of this mixture and set aside.
2. Cut the shortening into the flour-salt mixture in the mixing bowl, until the shortening is the size of small peas.
3. Mix together the 1/4 cup of remaining flour with the water to form a paste, and add to the flour-fat mixture. Mix with a fork until all the ingredients are dampened.
4. Form the dough into two balls, wrap in wax paper, and let chill, or allow to stand several minutes before rolling.

Yield: one 9-inch crust or one 2-crust, 8-inch pie

Crumb Crust

	Standard	Metric
Butter or margarine, melted	1/4 cup	60 mL
Graham crackers, cookie crumbs, bread crumbs, or cereal flakes	1-1/2 cup	310 mL
Sugar	1/4 cup	60 mL

1. Preheat the oven to 375° F (175° C)
2. Combine the crumbs, melted butter or margarine, and sugar in a mixing bowl. Mix until well-blended.
3. Press onto the bottom and sides of a 9-inch pie pan.
4. Bake for 6 to 8 minutes. If chocolate crumbs are used, bake at 350° F (175° C)

Yield: one 9-inch crumb crust

Super Cereal Crust

	Standard	Metric
Butter or margarine, melted	1/2 cup	125 mL
Brown sugar, packed	1 cup	250 mL
Corn flakes	3 cups	750 mL
Chopped nuts	1 cup	250 mL
Coconut, shredded	1 cup	250 mL

1. Blend together the butter or margarine and sugar in a mixing bowl. Blend in the corn flakes, nuts, and coconut.
2. Press 2 cups of the mixture into a 9-inch pie pan.
3. Use the remaining mixture as a topping for a cream-filled or ice cream pie.

Yield: one 9-inch corn-flake crust

Apple Pie with Crumb Topping

	Standard	Metric
Pastry shell, 9-inch, unbaked	1	1
Tart apples, peeled, cored, and cut into 1/8 inch slices	6 to 7	6 to 7
Sugar	2/3 cup	150 mL
Cinnamon	1 tsp.	5 mL
Butter or margarine	2 Tbsp.	30 mL

1. Preheat the oven to 400° F (205° C).
2. Mix together the sugar and cinnamon. Place the apple slices in a mixing bowl and mix lightly with sugar-cinnamon mixture.
3. Arrange the apple slices in the pastry shell, and dot with the butter or margarine.

Crumb Topping

	Standard	Metric
Butter or margarine	1/2 cup	125 mL
Brown sugar, packed	1/2 cup	125 mL
All-purpose flour, sifted	1 cup	250 mL

4. Cream the butter or margarine and brown sugar together. With a pastry blender or two table knives, cut in the flour.
5. Cover the top of the apples in the pie shell with the crumb topping.
6. Bake for 50 to 60 minutes.

Yield: one 9-inch pie

Cherry Lattice Pie

	Standard	Metric
Tart red cherries	1 (16 oz.) can	1
Granulated tapioca	2-1/2 Tbsp.	37 mL
Salt	1/4 tsp.	1 mL
Butter or margarine, melted	1 Tbsp.	15 mL
Sugar	1/2 cup	125 mL
Flour	1 tsp.	5 mL
Red food coloring	2 to 3 drops	2 to 3 drops
Pastry recipe for a 2-crust, 9-inch pie	1	1

1. Preheat the oven to 450° F (230° C).

2. Mix the undrained cherries with the tapioca, salt, melted butter or margarine, sugar, flour, and food coloring in a mixing bowl. Let the mixture stand for 15 minutes.

3. Stir the cherry mixture well and pour into a pastry shell. Cut the top crust into 3/4 inch strips and make a lattice topping over the cherry filling.

4. Bake the pie at 450° F (230° C) for 10 minutes; reduce the heat to 350° F (175° C) and continue baking for 20 to 25 minutes.

Yield: one 9-inch pie

—————————— Strawberry Glaze Pie ——————————

	Standard	Metric
Strawberries, washed and hulled	5 cups	1250 mL
Powdered sugar	1/2 cup	125 mL
Water	1 cup	250 mL
Cornstarch	1-1/2 Tbsp.	22 mL
Granulated sugar	1/2 cup	125 mL
Pastry shell, 9-inch, baked	1	1

1. Mix together 4 cups of strawberries with the 1/2 cup of powdered sugar.

2. Crush the remaining 1 cup of strawberries; combine in a saucepan with the water and cook for 2 minutes.

3. Mix together the cornstarch and granulated sugar and stir into the berry juice. Cook over a low heat, stirring constantly until the mixture cooks clear.

4. Arrange the 4 cups of berries in the pie crust and cover with the hot berry sauce. Chill.

Yield: one 9-inch pie

—————————— Raisin Pie ——————————

	Standard	Metric
Seedless raisins	2 cups	500 mL
Boiling water	2 cups	500 mL
Sugar	1/2 cup	125 mL

Flour	3 Tbsp.	45 mL
Chopped nuts	3/4 cup	175 mL
Grated lemon rind	1 Tbsp.	15 mL
Lemon juice	3 Tbsp.	45 mL
Pastry for 9-inch, 2-crust, unbaked pie	1	1

1. Preheat the oven to 425° F (220° C).

2. Pour the boiling water over the raisins in a saucepan and cook 3 to 5 minutes or until tender.

3. Blend the sugar and flour together, add to the raisin mixture, and cook over low heat until thickened, stirring constantly.

4. Add the nuts, lemon rind, and lemon juice and stir to blend all the ingredients. Cool to room temperature.

5. Pour into a pastry-lined pie pan; add the top crust.

6. Bake for 40 to 50 minutes.

Yield: one 9-inch pie

—————————— Mile-High Frozen Fruit Pie ——————————

	Standard	Metric
Egg whites	2	2
Raspberries, frozen, blackberries, or sliced strawberries, partially thawed	1 (10 oz.) pkg.	1 (284 gm)
Sugar	1 cup	250 mL
Lemon juice	1 Tbsp.	15 mL
Heavy cream, whipped	1 cup	250 mL
Pastry for 9-inch, baked, pie crust	1	1

1. Beat the egg whites until very soft peaks form.

2. Add the berries, sugar, and lemon juice to the egg whites and beat at the high speed of an electric mixer for 15 minutes.

3. Fold in the whipped cream and pour into the baked pastry shell. Cover and freeze for several hours. Remove from the freezer and cut and serve at once.

Yield: one 9-inch pie

Lemon Orange Chiffon Pie

	Standard	Metric
Gelatin, unflavored	1 Tbsp.	15 mL
Water, cold	1/4 cup	60 mL
Egg yolks	4	4
Orange juice	1/2 cup	125 mL
Lemon juice	1 Tbsp.	15 mL
Salt	1/2 tsp.	2 mL
Grated orange rind	1 Tbsp.	15 mL
Grated lemon rind	1 tsp.	5 mL
Pastry shell, 9-inch, baked	1	1

1. Sprinkle the gelatin on top of the cold water and let soften for 5 minutes.
2. Beat the egg yolks, add the orange juice, lemon juice, and salt.
3. Cook the egg yolk mixture in the top of a double boiler over boiling water until the mixture coats a wooden spoon. Add the gelatin, orange rind, and lemon rind. Stir thoroughly to dissolve the gelatin.
4. Cool the mixture until it thickens.
5. Beat the egg whites to the soft peak stage; gradually add the sugar and continue beating until the egg whites are stiff.
6. Fold the egg whites into the egg yolk-gelatin mixture. Pour into a pie shell and chill until firm. The pie may be served with a whipped topping.

Yield: one 9-inch pie

Custard Pie

	Standard	Metric
Eggs, slightly beaten	4	4
Salt	1/4 tsp.	1 mL
Sugar	1/2 cup	125 mL
Milk, scalded	3 cups	750 mL
Vanilla	3/4 tsp.	4 mL
Pastry shell, 9-inch, unbaked	1	1

1. Preheat the oven to 450° F (230° C).
2. Combine the eggs, salt, sugar, and vanilla; add the milk gradually.

3. Pour the mixture into the unbaked pastry shell and bake on the lower rack of the oven, at 450° F (230° C) for 10 minutes. Reduce the heat to 325° F (165° C) and continue baking for 30 to 40 minutes or until a knife inserted in the center comes out clean.

Yield: one 9-inch pie

Cream Pie

	Standard	Metric
All-purpose flour, sifted	1/3 cup	75 mL
Sugar	2/3 cup	150 mL
Salt	1/4 tsp.	1 mL
Milk, scalded	2 cups	500 mL
Egg yolks, slightly beaten	3	3
Vanilla	3/4 tsp.	4 mL
Pastry shell, 9-inch, baked	1	1
Egg whites	3	3
Cream of tartar	1/4 tsp.	1 mL
Sugar	6 Tbsp.	90 mL

1. Combine the flour, sugar, and salt in a saucepan. Gradually stir in the milk. Bring the mixture to a boil, stirring constantly, and continue cooking for 2 minutes.
2. Remove from heat and stir a small amount of the mixture into the egg yolks. Rapidly stir the heated egg yolks into the mixture in the saucepan; return to medium heat and cook 1 minute, stirring constantly.
3. Stir in the butter and vanilla; let the filling cool to room temperature. Pour into a baked pastry shell.
4. Preheat the oven to 350° F (175° C).
5. Beat the egg whites until frothy; add the cream of tartar and gradually add the sugar. Continue beating until stiff.
6. Top the filling with the meringue, being careful to seal in the edges.
7. Bake for 12 to 15 minutes or until the meringue is golden brown.

Yield: one 9-inch pie

──────── Lemon Meringue Pie ────────

	Standard	Metric
Sugar	1-1/2 cups	375 mL
Cornstarch	1/4 cup plus 3 Tbsp.	105 mL
Salt	1/4 tsp.	1 mL
Water	1-1/2 cups	375 mL
Egg yolks, slightly beaten	3	3
Grated lemon peel	1 tsp.	5 mL
Butter or margarine	2 Tbsp.	30 mL
Lemon juice	1/2 cup	125 mL
Pastry shell, 9-inch, baked	1	1
Egg whites	3	3
Cream of tartar	1/4 tsp.	1 mL
Sugar	6 Tbsp.	90 mL

1. Combine the sugar, cornstarch, and salt in a saucepan. Add the water and stir until blended. Bring the mixture to a boil over medium heat and continue cooking 4 minutes, stirring constantly.

2. Remove from the heat and stir a small amount of the mixture into the egg yolks. Rapidly stir the heated egg yolks into the mixture in the saucepan; return to medium heat, stirring constantly, and bring to boil. Boil 1 minute. Remove from heat.

3. Slowly stir in the lemon peel, butter, and lemon juice.

4. Cool the filling to room temperature and pour into the baked pie shell.

5. Preheat the oven to 350° F (175° C).

6. Beat the egg whites until frothy; add the cream of tartar and gradually add the sugar and continue beating until stiff.

7. Top the filling with the meringue, being careful to seal in the edges.

8. Bake for 12 to 15 minutes or until the meringue is golden brown at 350° F (175° C).

Yield: one 9-inch pie

LABORATORY ACTIVITIES

1. Plan a dinner menu that would be complemented by the inclusion of a cream pie for dessert.

2. Prepare a time schedule for the menu planned in number 1 that includes time to prepare the pie.

3. Investigate at a local market the kinds of fresh fruits and frozen fruits that are available and select a pie recipe that could be used with these fruits.

4. Prepare a piecrust from a commercial mix and one using the paste method. Evaluate the difference in cost, time of preparation, and eating quality.

5. Prepare a cream pie with a crumb crust, purchase a frozen pie of the same kind, and analyze the difference in eating quality.

6. Prepare a cream pie filling using a basic recipe and one using a commercial mix. Evaluate the difference in cost, time of preparation, and eating quality.

7. Prepare four pie crusts using one of the four different kinds of fats and a different method of preparation for each pie crust. Compare the piecrusts for taste, tenderness, and flakiness. Make a comparison chart and present it to the class.

8. Prepare a pie dough using the pastry method. After the fat has been cut in, divide the mixture into three parts. To the first flour mixture add the liquid all at once, and then stir the mixture with a spoon and roll. To the second mixture add the liquid in the proper manner and toss lightly with a fork to dampen the ingredients. Knead the

dough for 1 minute before rolling. Add the liquid to the third portion in the same manner as the second flour mixture and roll the dough. Label each portion of dough as to the method used, and bake at 450° F (230° C) for 12 minutes. Evaluate each portion of dough for flakiness and tenderness.

9. Using 2 saucepans, blend the following ingredients:

Saucepan number 1	Saucepan number 2
1 Tbsp. cornstarch	2 Tbsp. flour
1-1/2 Tbsp. sugar	1-1/2 Tbsp. sugar
1/2 cup cherry juice	1/2 cup cherry juice
1 cup cherries	1 cup cherries

a. In each saucepan blend the dry ingredients together and gradually stir in the juice. Cook over medium heat, stirring constantly, until smooth and thickened. Add the cherries.
b. Evaluate the two mixtures for their clearness or opaqueness. Determine which thickener would be suitable for different kinds of fruit fillings.

10. Bake a single unfilled piecrust in the oven without pricking with a fork. Bake another piecrust that has been pricked. Evaluate what happened during the baking of each piecrust.

REVIEW QUESTIONS

1. Why does a pie contain an excessive amount of carbohydrate and fat?
2. How can a pie be made more attractive when it is served?
3. What are the major ingredients used in making a piecrust?
4. How does the type of fat affect a piecrust's flakiness?
5. How does the type of fat affect a piecrust's tenderness?
6. What different characteristics are found in a piecrust made from a liquid fat and one made from a hydrogenated shortening?
7. What is the disadvantage in using butter or margarine as the fat in a piecrust?
8. What is the advantage of chilling a fat when making a piecrust?
9. What is the usual amount of water used with 1 cup of flour in making piecrust?
10. Why is it important not to overwork a pastry dough?
11. What are four basic methods for mixing pastry dough?
12. Why is the water not added to the flour mixture all at once in the pastry method?
13. What are three important factors to remember about rolling out dough?
14. What procedure for baking should be followed if a shiny, lightweight pie pan is used? Why?
15. What are two ways to vent a piecrust?
16. What are three different ways to bake a single, unfilled piecrust?
17. What are four characteristics of a successful pastry?
18. What ingredients are used in a crumb crust?
19. What is the difference in the cooking procedure used in making a cream filling and a custard filling?
20. What kinds of thickeners are used in fruit fillings?

21. What are four types of crust toppings that may be used on fruit-filled pies?
22. What are three ways that pastry dough can be frozen?
23. What happens to a pie if it is stored for an extended period of time?
24. What are two disadvantages to using convenience forms of pie crusts and pie fillings?

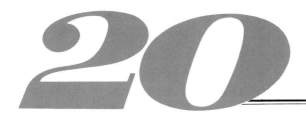

Frozen Desserts

Cool and refreshing, smooth-textured, and flavorful, frozen desserts are a welcome addition to any meal and are always a crowd pleaser at a party. Frozen desserts include such popular foods as ice cream, ice milk, and sherbet. Many frozen desserts are combinations of these foods, and others are mixtures of fruits, juices, and whipped dairy products.

A high-quality frozen dessert is characterized by tiny ice crystals that form during the freezing process. Some mixtures, such as ice cream and sherbet, are stirred during the freezing process; others are frozen without stirring. Many frozen desserts are purchased in ready-to-serve form, whereas others are made in the home.

Nutritional Factors to Consider

Carbohydrate and Fat

The carbohydrate content of a frozen dessert is dependent upon the sugar and fruit content of the mixture. If a frozen dessert contains a high proportion of fruit or juice to the other ingredients, then the carbohydrate content is not only higher but the other nutrients are also increased. This condition is most often found in fruit mousses and ices.

The fat content is high in those desserts that include cream. Many frozen desserts contain a large amount of heavy cream; ice cream is particularly high in fat.

Protein, Vitamins, and Minerals

Frozen desserts made from dairy products and eggs are excellent sources of protein. However, since servings of desserts are usually small, desserts are generally not a major source of protein in the diet. In commercially made ice cream, as the percentage of fat increases, the protein level decreases.

The vitamin and mineral content of a frozen dessert is dependent on the ingredients used. Fortified and whole milk are good sources of vitamins A and D and riboflavin, and the minerals calcium and phosphorus. Cream products are a rich source of vitamin A.

Calories

Frozen desserts made with heavy cream and a large amount of sugar are high in calories. Both evaporated milk and nonfat dried milk can be whipped and substituted for the heavy cream in a recipe, if desired. There is little advantage to choosing ice milk or sherbet over ice cream for a dessert, because the increased sugar in these two products makes up for the decreased milk fat content. Fruit ices are the least caloric of all frozen desserts.

Menu-Planning Points

Inherent Factors

Balance. Because frozen desserts have a delicate flavor and texture, they are a good balance to a meal that has a strongly flavored or spicy food as the entrée. For example, halibut steak or sweet and sour pork is complemented by a frozen dessert. An entrée that has a heavy concentration of a dairy food, such as a cheese soufflé, is not balanced when a frozen dessert containing similar ingredients is served. When planning frozen desserts, or any dessert, calorie balance must always be considered.

Color and Shape. The color of a frozen dessert is determined by the choice of ingredients. Many flavorful ice creams, sherbets, and ice milks come in a variety of colors. For example, strawberry ice cream or lime sherbet adds brightness to a dessert serving. Desserts can be frozen in a variety of molds for individual and group servings, and these molds add a contrast of shape to a meal. Additional shape and color variety is achieved by serving frozen desserts in hollowed-out orange, lemon, or pineapple shells, or by serving a frozen dessert atop a melon wedge or a hollowed-out pear. Shape and color are also enhanced by using fresh berries, nuts, or chocolate shavings as a garnish.

Texture and Flavor. The texture of a high-quality frozen dessert is smooth and creamy. Although some frozen desserts are very rich, they all have a lightness that makes them desirable desserts. One type of frozen dessert, called a fruit ice, can add both texture and flavor contrast to the main portion of a meal. For example, a cranberry or lemon ice is a nice accompaniment to a poultry or pork entrée.

A wide range of flavors is achieved in frozen desserts by varying the ingredients. A bland-flavored frozen dessert might be a vanilla mousse, a fruit-flavored dessert could be a raspberry sherbet, or a strongly flavored frozen dessert might use coffee as part of the liquid for a more pungent flavor.

External Factors

Age and Culture. Because frozen desserts are easy to eat, most people enjoy them. However, the richness of frozen desserts made with heavy cream cannot be tolerated by some individuals.

Economics. When the cost per serving is figured, commercially made ice cream is a good buy if the extra-fancy and richer products are avoided. Frozen desserts that call for heavy cream are expensive to make, but the ingredients can be altered.

Space and Equipment. Frozen desserts require a freezer at 0° F (–18° C) to be made and held successfully. Metal refrigerator trays or shallow metal pans are important to make some frozen desserts. Decorative molds also enhance the serving of some frozen desserts.

Time Scheduling. The main advantage to time scheduling in making a frozen dessert is that it must be made ahead of time. Some frozen desserts require several steps in the freezing process, and a time allowance for preparation must be included in a time schedule.

Types of Frozen Desserts

All frozen desserts are similar in that they contain ice crystals and a sweetener. Ingredients that are common to frozen desserts include fat, egg, some form of milk and/or fruit or fruit juices, a stabilizer, an emulsifier, and flavoring. A stabilizer helps to prevent large crystals from forming in the dessert, and an emulsifier aids in the blending of ingredients, thereby improving the texture. Some frozen desserts are made by freezing while stirring, whereas others are frozen without stirring or are made from products that were previously frozen while stirring.

Ice Cream

Because of its nutrient content, acceptable flavor, and texture and the many ways it can be eaten, ice cream is the most popular of the frozen desserts. Ice cream is eaten alone as a snack or as the dessert portion of a meal. It can also be used as a filling or topping for other desserts and in making such popular food items as milkshakes, sodas, and sundaes. Commercially made ice cream is the form most often

chosen, but ice cream can also be made at home in the freezing section of the refrigerator or in a specially designed piece of equipment called an ice cream freezer.

The major ingredients of commercially made ice cream are milk fat, milk solids-not-fat, a sweetener, and a flavoring such as vanilla, fruit, or nuts. A stabilizer and an emulsifier are used, and the ingredients are mixed, pasteurized, and homogenized to make the ice cream safe, improve the texture, and improve the keeping quality.

Milk fat and milk solids-not-fat contribute the creamy flavor, body, and texture to ice cream. Sugar accounts for the ice cream's sweetness, and the addition of sugar also lowers the freezing point of the mixture, which helps to create small, rather than large and coarse, ice crystals to form.

Federal standards of identity have been established for ice cream sold in interstate commerce; each state has standards for ice cream that are similar to the federal standards. These regulations specify that ice cream must contain not less than 10 per cent milk fat and less than 2.7 per cent protein. However, as the milk fat content increases, the percentage of protein required decreases. When ice cream is made, it is agitated in some manner to incorporate air and to prevent the ingredients from forming a hard mass; this increases the volume of the mixture. This increased volume is called the *overrun*, and federal regulations state the amount of overrun an ice cream may have.

If ice cream contains an excess of 1.4 per cent egg yolk solids, it is called frozen custard, French ice cream, or French custard ice cream. These products have a much richer flavor than regular ice cream.

Ice Milk

Ice milk contains the same basic ingredients as ice cream, but the fat content is lower and the sugar content is higher. Federal standards require that the milk fat content not be less than 2 per cent nor more than 7 per cent. The protein content is to be not less than 1.75 per cent. Most soft-frozen products, commonly known as "soft ice cream," are made from ice milk.

Sherbet

Sherbet is made from milk and nonfat milk solids, a sweetener, and either a fruit or fruit juice, or an ingredient such as spices, chocolate, or cocoa. More sugar is used in sherbet than in ice cream. The tart flavor of a fruit sherbet is obtained from both the fruit or fruit juice used and the addition of a fruit acid, such as citric.

Federal standards for sherbet are that it contain not less than 1 per cent nor more than 2 per cent milk fat.

Mellorine

Mellorine is a product similar to ice cream except that it contains fat from another animal or vegetable source rather than milk fat. Mellorine does contain nonfat milk solids, and the fat content according to federal regulations must be not less than 2 per cent nor more than 7 per cent, with a protein content of not less than 1.75 per cent.

Water Ices

Water ices contain no milk ingredients and no egg except for the egg white. They have a high sugar content and a high percentage of fruit juice, and they are characterized by their tart flavor.

Other Frozen Desserts

There are many other types of frozen desserts. Some are combinations of ice cream, ice milk, sherbet, or water ices; others are combinations of various ingredients mixed with a whipped cream or milk. They further differ from the frozen desserts just discussed in that they are not stirred during the freezing process.

Basic Methods of Preparation

This section discusses basic preparation methods for desserts that are frozen without stirring during the freezing process with the exception of ice cream, fruit ices, and sherbets. All frozen desserts require a freezer setting of $0°$ F $(-18° $ C), and because rapid freezing is important for a high-quality product, other foods should not be frozen at the same time nor should the freezer door be opened unnecessarily. It is important to use pasteurized milk and milk products, because dairy products are highly susceptible to bacterial growth.

If fruit is used to make frozen desserts, it is bettter to use it in the pureed form because there is less chance of developing a coarse crystalline texture. Pieces of fruit tend to become icy. Desserts that have a high proportion of sugar will take longer to freeze, as sugar slows the freezing process.

Refrigerator Ice Cream

Several different methods can be used to make refrigerator ice cream and there are many ingredient variations, but all ice creams will use some form of milk, sugar, and flavoring. Fresh milk, evaporated milk, condensed milk, nonfat dried milk, or cream can all be used. Because it is difficult to prevent the formation of large crystals in a nonstirred product, another ingredient such as marshmallows or gelatin, beaten eggs, or whipped cream or evaporated milk is used to inhibit large crystal formation.

Since the mixture is not stirred during the freezing process, air must be incorporated into the mixture prior to freezing to help eliminate the formation of large, coarse ice crystals. This is done by beating the egg or egg white; whipping the cream, evaporated milk, or nonfat dried milk; or whipping the entire product. A mixture should not be whipped after whipped cream or milk has been folded into the product, because this would cause it to lose air.

Some refrigerator ice creams are made with a custard base. Another variation is to use a pudding mix.

Mousse

A mousse is prepared by folding some type of flavoring base into whipped cream or whipped milk. Some bases are gelatin-thickened fruits, others are of the custard type, and still others include beaten egg white. If the base has been warmed or cooked, it is important that it be cooled before it is folded into the whipped product. After the base is folded into the whipped ingredient, the mousse is frozen in a refrigerator tray, in individual or large molds, or in paper cups.

Parfait

A parfait is composed of a sugar syrup, whole eggs or egg whites, and whipped cream. The sugar-water mixture is cooked to 230° F (110° C) or until a thin thread spins from a spoon that has been dipped into the mixture. The syrup is then poured over stiffly beaten egg whites, and the mixture is beaten until it cools. Additional ingredients such as fruits, nuts, and flavorings may be added to the mixture at this point. The mixture is then folded into whipped cream, spooned into refrigerator trays or individual molds or serving dishes, and frozen until firm.

A variation of the parfait is made by layering portions of ice cream, fruit or a fruit-flavored sauce or liquor, and whipped cream in individual serving dishes and freezing until firm.

Bombe

A bombe is a combination of two or more layers of different ice creams, sherbets, or ices. It is made by placing a layer of a softened frozen product in a melon-shaped mold, freezing until firm, and then adding another layer and freezing.

Neapolitan

A Neapolitan is similar to a bombe except that the ice cream, ice milk, sherbet, or water ice is layered in a lengthwise mold.

Fruit Ices

Fruit ices are made from a sugar syrup to which a fruit juice or pureed fruit is added. This mixture is placed in refrigerator trays and stirred several times during the freezing process.

Sherbet

The basic method for making a sherbet is to combine a sugar syrup with softened gelatin and fold the mixture into stiffly beaten egg whites. Some recipes use a whipped cream or milk in place of the egg whites, and the mixture is stirred during the freezing process.

Storage

All frozen desserts should be stored at 0° F (–18° C). If ice cream is not stored in a separate freezer section, it should be used within 3 to 4 days. Home-prepared frozen desserts have their best quality if eaten 1 to 2 days after preparation.

Because foods containing dairy products are

highly susceptible to bacterial contamination, it is most important that the equipment used in the preparation of frozen desserts as well as the area of storage are clean.

RECIPES

Vanilla Custard Ice Cream

	Standard	Metric
Sugar	1/2 cup	125 mL
Cornstarch	2 Tbsp.	30 mL
Salt	1/2 tsp.	2 mL
Egg, beaten	1	1
Milk	2 cups	500 mL
Vanilla	1-3/4 tsp.	9 mL
Evaporated milk, chilled	1 cup	250 mL

1. Combine the sugar, cornstarch, and salt in a heavy saucepan. Stir in the egg. Gradually add the milk.
2. Cook over a medium heat, stirring constantly, until the mixture is slightly thickened or coats a wooden spoon.
3. Remove from the heat; stir in the vanilla; cool.
4. Pour into a refrigerator tray and freeze until just firm.
5. Place the chilled mixture in a bowl and beat with a rotary beater or electric mixer until the mixture is smooth.
6. Beat the chilled evaporated milk with the lemon juice until it holds soft peaks. Fold the beaten custard mixture into the whipped milk. Pour into a refrigerator tray and freeze until firm. This will take approximately 3 hours.

Yield: 1 quart

Chocolate Ice Cream

	Standard	Metric
Evaporated milk	1 cup	250 mL
Heavy cream	1/2 cup	125 mL
Chocolate instant pudding	1 (4-1/2 oz.) pkg.	1 (136 gm)
Milk	2 cups	500 mL
Sugar	1/4 cup	60 mL
Gelatin	2 tsp.	10 mL
Cocoa	1/4 cup	60 mL
Salt	1/8 tsp.	0.5 mL
Milk, hot	1/2 cup	125 mL
Vanilla	1/4 tsp.	1 mL

1. Chill the evaporated milk in a refrigerator tray in the freezer section until fine crystals form around the outer edges.
2. Chill the heavy cream, bowl, and beaters in the refrigerator.
3. Prepare the chocolate pudding with the 2 cups of milk according to the package directions.
4. Mix together the sugar, gelatin, cocoa, and salt, and add the hot milk. Combine with the prepared pudding and 1/4 teaspoon of vanilla.
5. Beat the chilled evaporated milk and heavy cream in the chilled bowl until soft peaks form. Fold in the pudding mixture. Pour into two refrigerator trays and freeze until firm around the edges.
6. Place the chilled mixture in a bowl and beat with a spoon until smooth. Put the mixture back in the refrigerator trays and freeze until firm.

Yield: 1-1/2 quarts

Raspberry Ice Cream

	Standard	Metric
Marshmallows	24	24
Lemon juice	3 Tbsp.	45 mL
Evaporated milk, chilled	1 cup	250 mL
Grated lemon peel	1 tsp.	5 mL
Frozen raspberries, partially thawed	1 cup	250 mL
Heavy cream	1 cup	250 mL

1. Cut the marshmallows in quarters with kitchen shears. Place in the top of a double boiler with the lemon juice. Melt over simmering water, stirring occasionally. Remove from heat and cool slightly.
2. To the cooled marshmallow mixture, add the chilled evaporated milk, grated lemon peel, and raspberries.
3. Whip the heavy cream until it holds soft peaks; fold into the raspberry mixture. Pour into two refrigerator trays and freeze until ice crystals form around the edges.
4. Pour the mixture into a large chilled bowl and beat until smooth. Return to the refrigerator trays and freeze until firm.

Yield: 1 quart

Cranberry Sherbet

	Standard	Metric
Gelatin	1 Tbsp.	15 mL
Water	1/4 cup	60 mL
Sugar	1 cup	250 mL
Water	1/2 cup	125 mL
Cranberry juice	2 cups	500 mL
Orange juice	1/2 cup	125 mL
Grated orange peel	1 tsp.	5 mL
Egg whites	2	2
Salt	1/8 tsp.	0.5 mL

1. Sprinkle the gelatin over 1/4 cup of water to soften.
2. Combine the sugar and 1/2 cup of water in a saucepan and bring to a boil. Boil 5 minutes. Remove from heat; add the gelatin and stir to dissolve. Let the mixture cool.
3. To the cooled mixture add the cranberry juice, orange juice, and grated orange peel. Pour into two refrigerator trays and let freeze until ice crystals begin to form around the edges.
4. Turn the mixture into a chilled bowl and beat until the mixture is fluffy.
5. Beat the egg whites with salt until stiff peaks form. Fold the cranberry mixture into the egg whites, return the mixture to the trays, and freeze until

firm. Stir the mixture occasionally during the freezing process.

Yield: 1 quart

Orange Ice

	Standard	Metric
Gelatin	2 tsp.	10 mL
Water	1/4 cup	60 mL
Water	2 cups	500 mL
Sugar	1-1/4 cups	310 mL
Orange juice	2 cups	500 mL
Lemon juice	2 Tbsp.	30 mL
Grated orange peel	2 tsp.	10 mL
Orange food coloring	2-3 drops	2-3 drops

1. In a small bowl, sprinkle the gelatin over 1/4 cup of water to soften.
2. Heat the 2 cups of water to boiling. Remove from heat and stir in the gelatin to dissolve. Add the sugar and stir until dissolved.
3. To the sugar mixture add the orange juice, lemon juice, and grated orange peel, and stir to blend ingredients. Add the desired amount of food coloring.
4. Pour into two refrigerator trays and freeze until firm, stirring occasionally.

Yield: 1 quart

Chocolate Parfait

	Standard	Metric
Sugar	1/2 cup	125 mL
Water	1/2 cup	125 mL
Egg whites, stiffly beaten	2	2
Salt	1/8 tsp.	0.5 mL
Chocolate, melted	2 (1 oz.) squares	2 (57 gm)
Evaporated milk, chilled	1-2/3 cups	400 mL
Vanilla extract	2 tsp.	10 mL

1. Combine the sugar and water in a saucepan and

cook to 230° F (110° C) or until it spins a thin thread when the mixture is dropped from a spoon.

2. Pour the syrup over the beaten egg whites, beating constantly. Add the salt and continue beating until the mixture is cool.

3. Add the chocolate to the egg white mixture.

4. Whip the evaporated milk; add the vanilla. Fold the egg white mixture into the whipped milk; turn the mixture into a refrigerator tray and freeze.

Yield: 3 cups

Chocolate Mousse

	Standard	Metric
Chocolate	1 (1 oz.) square	1 (28 gm)
Evaporated milk	1/4 cup	60 mL
Water	1/4 cup	60 mL
Sugar	1/2 cup	125 mL
Egg yolks, beaten	2	2
Salt	1/8 tsp.	0.5 mL
Evaporated milk, chilled	1 cup	250 mL
Vanilla	1 tsp.	5 mL

1. Melt the chocolate over hot water.

2. Combine 1/4 cup of milk, water, sugar, egg yolks, and salt. Stir to blend the ingredients. Cook over medium heat, stirring constantly until the mixture thickens or coats a wooden spoon.

3. Remove from heat; stir in the melted chocolate and vanilla; cool.

4. Beat the 1 cup of evaporated milk until stiff peaks form. Fold the chocolate mixture into whipped milk and freeze until firm.

Yield: 4 to 6 servings

Strawberry Mousse

	Standard	Metric
Strawberries	2 cups	500 mL
Sugar	1/2 cup	125 mL
Egg white	1	1
Heavy cream	1 cup	250 mL

1. Clean and mash the strawberries. Add the sugar and stir to mix in the sugar.

2. Beat the strawberry mixture and egg white together until of a stiff consistency.

3. Whip the cream until stiff peaks form. Fold the strawberry mixture into the whipped cream; pour into a freezing container and freeze until firm.

Yield: 6 to 8 servings

Coffee Mousse

	Standard	Metric
Gelatin	2 tsp.	10 mL
Coffee, double strength and hot	2 cups	500 mL
Heavy cream	2 cups	500 mL
Powdered sugar	1/2 cup	125 mL
Vanilla extract	1 tsp.	5 mL

1. Add the gelatin to hot coffee and stir until dissolved.

2. Chill the coffee mixture in the refrigerator until it is the consistency of an unbeaten egg white.

3. Whip the cream with the powdered sugar until soft peaks form. Fold in the vanilla. Fold the coffee mixture into the whipped cream. Turn into a freezer container and freeze until firm.

Yield: 6 to 8 servings

Chocolate Peppermint Bombe

	Standard	Metric
Chocolate ice cream	1 pint	500 mL
Peppermint ice cream	1 pint	500 mL

1. Rinse a 1-quart melon-shaped mold with boiling water and place in freezer section to chill.

2. Have the ice cream slightly softened so it can be molded.

3. Spread the chocolate ice cream along the sides and bottom of the mold to a depth approximately 3/4 inch thick. Freeze until firm.

4. Fill the center of a mold with slightly softened

peppermint ice cream to within 3/4 inch of the top. Freeze until firm.

5. Spread the chocolate ice cream over the top of the mold to cover the first two layers. Freeze until firm.

6. To serve, place the mold on a serving platter and cover with a cloth that has been dipped in hot water and wrung out. After a few seconds, remove the mold.

Yield: 4 to 6 servings

Neapolitan

A Neapolitan is made in the same manner as a bombe except that the ice cream is molded in a loaf pan.

LEARNING ACTIVITIES

1. Plan a day's menu, including breakfast, lunch, and a dinner that includes a frozen dessert. Make sure that the day's calorie needs are not exceeded because of the inclusion of a frozen dessert.

2. At a local market, investigate the difference in cost between differently priced ice creams, and if a specialty ice cream store is in the area, compare the costs of the different ice creams. Make a list of the reasons why the costs may differ.

3. Analyze the nutrient content of a 1/2-cup serving of ice milk, ice cream, and sherbet. Determine how each of these servings can contribute to your daily calcium need.

4. Prepare a mousse requiring a whipped dairy product. Divide the basic mixture into three portions. To each third portion add (a) whipped heavy cream; (b) whipped evaporated milk; and (c) whipped nonfat dry milk. Freeze the mixture. Compare the frozen mixtures for flavor and texture.

5. Calculate the calorie value per 1/2 cup serving for each of the three mousses prepared in number 4.

6. Plan a party menu in which the frozen dessert is the highlight of the menu in color and shape, flavor and texture.

7. Take one dinner menu from number 1 and plan a time schedule that allows the frozen dessert to be made the previous day.

8. Prepare a fruit ice using gelatin as an ingredient. Prepare the same recipe, omitting the gelatin. Compare the difference in texture between the two products.

9. List the stabilizing ingredients in each recipe included in this chapter.

10. Make a list of six different combinations of frozen dessert products that could be used for making a bombe or a Neapolitan.

11. Develop three dinner menus in which a fruit ice could be an accompaniment to the main entrée.

12. Prepare a fruit ice and divide the mixture between two refrigerator trays. Stir one tray of ice two to three times during the freezing process. Do not stir the second tray. After the mixtures are frozen, compare the difference in texture and explain why there is a difference.

13. Plan a children's party in which ice cream cones or sundaes are the main food served. Design a way that the ice cream would be served.

1. What characteristics determine a high-quality frozen dessert?
2. What is the difference between a frozen dessert that contains just sugar and one that provides carbohydrate by its fruit content?
3. What ingredient accounts for the high amount of fat in some frozen desserts?
4. Why is a serving of a frozen dessert made with a high proportion of dairy product not considered adequate for meeting one third of the daily requirement for protein?
5. Why are ice cream, ice milk, and sherbet about the same in calorie count when the highest fat content is in ice cream?
6. What should be the basic consideration when planning a frozen dessert to complete a menu?
7. What are three different ways by which variety in shape in a menu can be created by different ways of serving a frozen dessert?
8. How are frozen desserts an asset to time scheduling when planning a meal? What special planning must be made with some types of frozen desserts?
9. What are the basic ingredients used in making a frozen dessert?
10. According to federal standards, what minimum percentage of milk fat and protein must be contained in a commercially made ice cream?
11. What is meant by the overrun of ice cream?
12. What is the difference between mellorine and ice cream?
13. Why is it important to use pasteurized dairy products when making frozen desserts?
14. What three ingredients are used to inhibit the formation of large crystals in a frozen dessert?
15. How is air incorporated into a refrigerator-made ice cream?
16. What is a mousse?
17. What are the two classifications of parfaits in relation to their preparation?
18. How do a bombe and a Neapolitan differ?
19. How can a bombe and a Neapolitan be successfully removed from their molds?
20. What is the difference between a fruit ice and ice cream?
21. How long should a home-prepared frozen dessert be stored in the freezer section before it is eaten?

21

Beverages: Coffee, Tea, Cocoa, and Wine

Most meals and social gatherings are considered incomplete unless some type of beverage is served. The beverage served may be water, milk, juice, coffee, tea, a chocolate or cocoa drink, an alcoholic or carbonated beverage, a punch, or a combination of these to complement the meal, to provide additional nutrition, or to fulfill social needs. This chapter discusses coffee, tea, chocolate, cocoa, and wine. Milk is discussed in Chapter 8 and juices are discussed in Chapter 11.

Coffee has been a popular beverage of Americans for several centuries. However, the consumption of coffee has declined in recent years. On a worldwide basis, tea can be considered the most popular beverage. Chocolate and cocoa, which are consumed not only as a beverage but are also used as an ingredient in other food products, have long been favorites of both children and adults. Nearly all coffee, tea, chocolate, and cocoa consumed in the United States are imported.

Nutritional Factors to Consider

The nutritive and calorie content of coffee and tea is negligible. Coffee does contain a small amount of the B-vitamin, niacin, with the average 6-ounce serving containing 1 milligram. Depending on the amount used, cream and sugar added to coffee and tea will increase the nutritive and calorie content of these beverages.

As shown in Table 21–1, chocolate, cocoa, and cocoa mixes that contain sugar and milk have a higher nutrient and calorie value.

Coffee, tea, chocolate, and cocoa all contain the stimulant, caffeine, whereas chocolate and cocoa contain caffeine and the stimulant

Table 21-1
Nutritive Value of Chocolate, Cocoa, and Cocoa Powder

Food	Amount	Calories gm	Protein gm	Fat gm	Carbohydrate gm	Calcium mg	Iron mg	Potassium mg	Vitamin A I.U.	Thiamine mg	Riboflavin mg	Niacin mg
Cocoa (High-medium fat)	1 Tbsp.	14	.9	1.0	2.8	7	.6	82	Trace	.01	.02	.1
Cocoa powder with nonfat milk	4 heaping tsps.	102	5.3	.8	20.1	167	.5	227	10	.04	.21	.2
Baking chocolate	1 oz. sq.	143	3.0	15.0	8.2	22	1.9	235	20	.01	.07	.4

Nutritive Value of American Foods. Agriculture Handbook No. 456. USDA, 1975.

theobromine. In consumption the greatest amount of caffeine is found in coffee. Because the caffeine that is present in chocolate and cocoa beverages is greatly diluted, it is not considered harmful to children.

Menu-Planning Points

Coffee, tea, chocolate, and cocoa can be served as either a hot or cold beverage and as shown in the recipe section of this chapter, the addition of other ingredients can create many flavorful beverages. Many different flavors of coffee and tea are now available on the market and these also add interesting variations to the beverage. The decision of whether to serve a hot or cold beverage is most often determined by climatic conditions or the type of social gathering at which the beverage is served.

Coffee

Coffee is grown on an evergreen plant in the tropical climates of Central and South America and Africa. At harvest time the coffee fruit, resembling a cherry, has a soft pulp that surrounds two coffee beans. The pulp is removed

by one of several processes and the green coffee beans are sized and graded. Most coffee beans imported to the United States are green.

The green coffee bean goes through a roasting process that develops the flavor and changes the color of the bean from tan to a darker brown, depending on the degree of roasting. Most American brands of coffee are made from beans that have been lightly roasted, whereas coffee made in other countries, such as Italy or France, uses the darker colored bean with a stronger flavor. After the bean is roasted, it is ground to the desired degree of fineness. Each coffee manufacturer uses several varieties of the coffee bean to develop the desired flavor of a particular brand.

Kinds of Coffee

There are several classifications for the kinds of coffee that are sold. Some coffees are sold according to the country in which the beans were grown, such as Columbian, Mocha, or Java coffees.

Other coffees are sold according to the grind. The coffee grind purchased is dependent on the type of coffee maker that is to be used. The finer the size of the coffee grind, the more surface area is exposed to water, and thus a better flavored coffee is obtained. A higher yield of coffee is obtained from finely ground coffee. Fine or vacuum grinds are used in a vacuum-type coffee maker, drip or all-purpose grind is used in the drip or drip-filter coffee maker, and a regular grind is used for a percolator. Coffee can also be purchased in flakes.

The coffee bean can be purchased at some markets and ground at the store or in a home coffee grinder.

Instant coffee is made by dehydrating or freeze-drying a freshly brewed coffee. The coffee crystals are a highly concentrated form of the coffee bean. Many flavor variations of instant coffee are available. Decaffeinated coffee, which is available in either instant or grind form, is coffee from which the caffeine has been removed from the green coffee bean before further processing. Acid-free coffee is coffee that has been processed to remove acids which are irritating to the digestive tract of some people. It is sold in both instant and granular forms.

Coffee substitutes are made from various dried cereals. Some coffee has chicory added. The addition of chicory gives coffee a darker color but lessens coffee flavor and aroma.

Purchasing and Storage of Coffee

Good coffee with full flavor and aroma is made from fresh coffee. Like many other food products, coffee will become stale when it is exposed to air and moisture and stored for long periods of time. Most coffee sold today is vacuum-packed to permit the least amount of flavor deterioration, but vacuum-packed coffee should be purchased only in amounts that can be used within 1 week. Therefore, the larger-sized containers of coffee are not always the better buy. Coffee should always be stored in a tightly sealed container. It may be stored in the refrigerator or freezer to help prevent flavor loss and staling.

Preparation of Coffee

The ability to brew a good cup of coffee is an asset to every individual's culinary skills. Knowledge of several factors will assure this success.

Coffee is best when it is brewed in a pot made from stainless steel, enamel, glass, or porcelain. Other metals such as tin or copper will impart a metallic taste to the coffee. Coffee will have its best flavor when it is made in a coffee maker that is at least three-fourths full. Therefore, the size of the coffee maker must be related to one's needs for coffee.

A clean coffee maker is essential. Because the interior of a coffee maker will build up an oily film, it should be washed in soapy water and rinsed thoroughly after each use.

The best flavor of coffee is achieved by using 2 level measuring tablespoons of coffee per 3/4 cup of water. If a weaker coffee is desired, the coffee may be diluted with water after it is brewed. Directions for the amount of instant coffee to use are found on the container. Most coffee cups hold 3/4 of a cup or 6 ounces of the beverage. Coffee is best made from fresh, cold tap water that is relatively soft. The brewing time for coffee should be kept to a minimum, since longer brewing times produce a beverage that is bitter and less flavorful. Boiling will also give coffee a bitter taste. The best temperature at which to boil coffee is 185° to 203° F (85° to 95° C).

Coffee should always be served freshly brewed and hot unless it is being served as an iced beverage. If it is necessary to hold coffee for a period of time, it may be kept warm over low heat. Some automatic coffee makers have a warming unit. The grounds should always be removed immediately after brewing and it is not advisable to hold coffee longer than 1 hour. Coffee should not be cooled and reheated.

Coffee is served black or with cream and sugar. Coffee served after dinner is often served

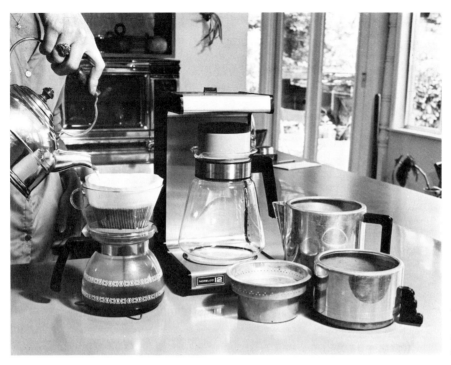

Figure 21-1.

*Automatic or stove top fil-
tered coffee makers and the
drip coffee maker with basket
are shown.*

in small cups called demitasse cups. This coffee is more strongly flavored and is made with 3 tablespoons of coffee per 3/4 cup of water. Additional coffee variations are found in the recipe section of this chapter.

Drip or Drip-Filtered Coffee. The construction of the drip coffee maker, consists of three parts. The upper section holds the hot water that drips through a basket containing the coffee into the lower section. Because the water passes over the coffee only once, a drip or finely ground coffee should be used to expose as much of the surface as possible. Drip-filtered coffee is the same as drip coffee except that a filter paper is placed in the basket before the coffee is added.

Drip or drip-filtered coffee is made by heating cold water to the boiling point in a pan and pouring the boiling water into the upper section of the pot. Drip coffee is made in approximately 4 to 6 minutes. The upper section and the basket are removed from the coffee maker, and the coffee is ready to serve.

The automatic drip-filter coffee maker operates on the same principle as the nonautomatic coffee maker except that cold water is poured into a reservoir which heats the water to the proper temperature. The heated water is then dispersed over the finely ground coffee which drips into the server. The coffee is kept at the serving temperature by a heating element at the base. Drip coffee makers are shown in Figure 21-1.

Percolated Coffee. Percolators are either automatic or nonautomatic but the basic construction is the same as shown in Figure 21-2. The percolator consists of the pot, a tube, and a basket that holds the ground coffee and sits on top of the tube. A lid covers the basket plus a lid that covers the pot. Regular grind coffee is used in the nonautomatic coffee maker and either regular grind or a special grind, as noted

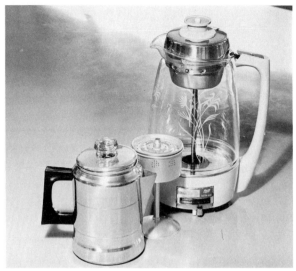

Figure 21-2
Both the automatic and stove-top percolators consist of the pot, a tube, basket, and lid.

on the label of some brands, is used for the automatic percolators.

In the nonautomatic type of percolator, coffee is made by first heating measured cold water in the pot until it boils. The pot is then removed from the heat and the basket containing the ground coffee and the tube are placed in the pot and covered. The percolator is placed over a low heat and the coffee is allowed to percolate for 6 to 8 minutes or until the coffee appears clear. Coffee is made in automatic percolators by adding the specified amount of cold water to the pot, inserting the stem and basket, and covering the pot. When the coffee reaches the desired strength, the percolation is automatically stopped. With this kind of coffee-maker the water level should always be below the basket.

Steeped Coffee. Steeped coffee is made by combining regular grind coffee with water that is just below the boiling point. Steeping time is approximately 6 to 8 minutes. The grounds may be removed by pouring the coffee into another container through a sieve lined with several layers of cheesecloth. Another method for clarifying steeped coffee is to mix the ground coffee with egg white and water and pour boiling water over the mixture. The steeping time is 3 minutes with this method.

Because steeped coffee can be made in any pan if a coffee pot is not available, this method is often used in preparing coffee for a large group or on recreational outings such as camping, back-packing, and boating.

Vacuum Coffee. One example of a vacuum coffee maker is shown in Figure 21-3. This coffee maker consists of a top section that resembles a funnel, a bottom bowl, and a filter of glass, metal, or fabric which closes the upper section.

Coffee is made by bringing cold water in the lower bowl to a boil. The filter is placed in the upper section and finely ground coffee is added. The boiling water is removed from the heat and the upper bowl is inserted with a slight twist to ensure a tight seal. The pot is then placed over low heat until most of the

Figure 21-3.
Vacuum-type coffee makers come in many different designs.

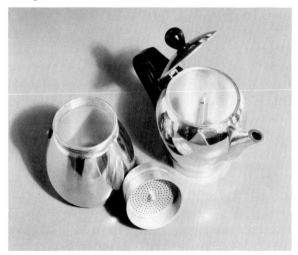

water rises to the upper bowl. The coffee is stirred several times and the pot is removed from the heat. As the lower bowl cools, a vacuum is created that pulls the coffee into the lower bowl.

Tea

Tea is grown on an evergreen bush that resembles the camellia bush. The principal tea producers are countries that have a rainy tropical climate, Africa, China, Japan, Indonesia, and Taiwan. The unopened leaf at the end of the shoot is the most prized tea leaf. Tea is graded on such factors as the size of the leaf, where the tea is grown, the plant variety, and the season when it is plucked.

Kinds of Tea

The principal kinds of tea are known as black, green, and oolong teas. Although these kinds of tea are made from the same leaves, it is the processing that gives them different coloring, flavor, and aroma.

Green tea is processed by steaming the leaves to inactivate enzymatic activity; then the leaves are rolled and dried. Green tea has a greenish-yellow color and has a more bitter taste with less flavor than black tea.

The terms Hysong, Young Hysong, Imperial, and Gunpowder denote the size of the leaves used in making green tea.

To make black tea the leaves are withered and rolled, causing the leaves to ferment. The fermented leaves are then heated and dried. Black tea has a golden color and is more flavorful than green tea.

Black teas are graded using the term *pekoe*, which describes the size of the leaf and may be seen on labels as Pekoe, Orange Pekoe, Broken Orange Pekoe, Broken Pekoe, Broken Pekoe Souchong, Fannings, and Dust. Black tea is often combined with spices or flavorings such as orange, jasmine, or mint.

Oolong tea has a shorter fermentation period than black tea and its characteristic flavor and aroma are between that of black and green tea.

Purchasing of Tea

Tea may be purchased in bulk form, in tea bags, or as an instant product. Bulk tea is used to prepare tea by the tea-ball method or as loose leaves in the pot or in a sieve. Tea bags contain crushed tea leaves and are popular for making tea in the United States. Instant tea is a pulverized form of tea made by spraying or drum drying the leaves; lemon flavoring and a sweetener may be added.

Preparation of Tea

Tea is best when it is made in a glass, ceramic ware, or porcelain tea pot. Metal will impart a metallic taste. The pot should be preheated before preparing the tea by adding boiling water to the pot and letting it stand for a few minutes to heat through. Soft water, freshly boiled, should be used for making tea. The longer that water is allowed to boil, the more oxygen is lost, which causes the tea to taste flat.

When using bulk tea, a small perforated, cylindrical-shaped container, called a tea ball, permits easy removal of the tea leaves. The tea ball should not be filled more than half full in order that the leaves may circulate in the water to permit the development of full flavor. Bulk tea can also be placed in a strainer or loose in the teapot. The usual proportion is 1/2 to 1 teaspoon of tea per cup. The number of tea bags to use to make more than 1 cup is dependent upon the amount and kind of tea in the bag.

Tea is prepared by pouring boiling water over the tea ball, loose tea, or tea bag. The tea is allowed to steep for 3 to 5 minutes and the tea ball or tea bag is removed. Loose tea can be removed by pouring the tea through a fine sieve or cheesecloth into a second container. Tea may be diluted by adding more boiling water. While the tea is steeping, it should be covered to retain the full aroma.

Tea may be served with milk or cream, sugar, or lemon or orange slices. Tea may also be made with additional spices such as whole cloves. Tea cups are smaller and deeper than regular cups so that the tea will stay hot but any cups may be satisfactorily used to serve tea.

Cocoa and Chocolate

Central and South America and Africa all have climates suitable to growing the cacao tree, which produces the seed pods from which chocolate and cocoa are made. Upon the removal of the seeds from the pod, the seeds are allowed to ferment to help eliminate the bitter taste. Following fermentation, the seeds are roasted, shelled, and cracked. The resulting meat of the seeds is called the nibs.

The nibs are then ground and the chocolate liquor produced is molded to produce cake or Baker's chocolate, which is sold in 1-ounce squares. Sweet chocolate is made by adding sugar and flavorings to the chocolate liquor, and milk chocolate is created by adding milk, sugar, and flavorings. These chocolates must contain not less than 50 per cent nor more than 58 per cent fat as ruled by the U.S. Food and Drug Administration for standard of identity purposes.

Cocoa is made by removing some of the fat, called cocoa butter, from the chocolate liquor. This accounts for the lesser richness in products made from cocoa. Breakfast cocoa must contain not less than 22 per cent fat; cocoas or medium-fat cocoas must contain 10 to 22 per cent fat; and low-fat cocoas must contain less than 10 per cent fat.

Cocoa that is treated with an alkali during processing, is called Dutch cocoa. It has a darker color and milder flavor than natural cocoa.

Chocolate and cocoa can be interchanged in food preparation, but because of the lesser amount of fat in cocoa, additional fat must be added. The proper substitution is 3 tablespoons of cocoa plus 1 tablespoon of fat for each 1-ounce (one square) of chocolate. Cocoa mixes cannot be used for this substitution.

In storage both chocolate and cocoa will show visual changes if they are exposed to excessive moisture or heat. Chocolate may develop a gray surface if it is stored in too warm an atmosphere, and cocoa will lump and lose its brownish color if it is stored in an area that is too warm or moist.

Method of Preparation

Both cocoa and chocolate contain starch. In preparing beverages with these foods, it is advisable to cook the starch before adding the milk. This is done by combining the cocoa or chocolate, sugar, and water in a saucepan and boiling for 2 or 3 minutes before adding the milk. Cooking the starch results in a product that has a better taste and one in which the cocoa or chocolate does not settle. After the milk is added, the mixture may be covered with a lid or beaten with a rotary beater to prevent scum formation. (See Chapter 8, "Milk.") The recipe section of this chapter provides further instructions.

In other cooking, cocoa is sifted with the dry ingredients or in making puddings it is combined with sugar and a small amount of liquid. Chocolate is usually melted before it is added to other ingredients or it may be grated.

Commercial cocoa mixes contain either sugar and flavorings or sugar, nonfat dry milk, and flavorings and a stabilizer or emulsifier. Commercial mixes may be readily prepared by stirring the mixture into water or milk because of the additions of a stabilizer or emulsifier to the mix.

Wine

In contrast to other countries, wine has not been a popular beverage in the United States until recently. It has now become increasingly popular as an aperitif or refreshment or as an accompaniment to meals. The study of wine is an immense and complex topic. This brief overview will discuss how wine is made, the most common types of wine and how they are served, and how wine should be stored.

Although wine is made in many countries of the world, certain European countries such as Germany, France, and Italy are best known for their fine wines. California and New York are the major wine-producing states of this country with California producing three-fourths of the wine made in the United States.

Method of Making Wine

At the desired stage of ripeness the grapes are picked. They are then pressed to extract the juice as in the making of white wines or crushed to a mixture of juice and pulp as in the making of red wines. The tannins in the skin of grape contribute both color and the puckerish taste of red wines. Grapes contain about 22 per cent sugar, and when the extracted juice or crushed mixture is allowed to ferment, the sugar changes to equal amounts of carbon dioxide and alcohol. The carbon dioxide escapes into the atmosphere and the remaining solution is approximately 14 per cent alcohol.

Dry wines are allowed to ferment until all the sugar is gone; for semi-sweet wines the fermentation is stopped by adding a small amount of sulfur dioxide or by pasteurization. Sweeter wines with an alcohol content of 14 per cent to 21 per cent are made by stopping fermentation earlier and adding a pure grape brandy. After fermentation, the pulp is separated from the juice and allowed to settle out before the wine is bottled. The length of time a wine is aged is dependent upon the type of wine being made.

Types of Wine and How It Is Served

The name of a wine may be a generic or "type" name, which is a general classification given to wines such as sherry, burgundy, port, rose, sauterne, and champagne. Other names are varietal and refer to the kind of grape which was used in the wine-making. Varietal names include Pinot Noir, Cabernet, Zinfandel, Riesling, and Chardonnay.

Cocktail or aperitif wines include the sherries and vermouths. Sherries have an alcohol content of 20 per cent by volume and vermouths an alcohol content of 16 to 20 per cent by volume. They are sold in varying degrees of dryness such as cocktail dry, very dry, or light. These wines need to be served chilled and may be served over ice. Vermouths are sometimes used as an ingredient in other mixed drinks.

Dessert and refreshment wines are sweet, full-bodied wines with an alcohol content of 20 per cent and include the ports, muscatel, cream sherry, and tokay. Sweet white wines, such as sauterne and sweet sauvignon blanc, having an alcohol content of 12 per cent, are also served as dessert and refreshment wines. These wines are particularly good when served with a dessert of fruit and cheese. Each of these wines should be served cool or chilled.

Table wines are all wines that have an alcohol content of 14 per cent or less by volume. The red dinner or table wines include the burgundies, clarets, chiantis, and "vino" reds. The term "vino" stands for many red wines bottled under different brands that are inexpensive. Red wines may be served with many kinds of food and should be served at a cool but not cold temperature. White dinner or table wines include the dry sauternes, rhine wines, and chablis. These are best when served chilled and particularly good when served with poultry and seafood.

Rosé is a pink, light-bodied wine that is good to serve with any meal. Rosé should be served chilled. Champagne is a light bubbling wine. The bubbles are created by a second fermentation process after which the bottle is corked. Pink champagne is less dry than champagne as is sparkling burgundy. Champagne should always be served chilled and is a pleasant compliment to any food and a special apertif to serve for festive occasions.

Storage of Wine

Wine should be stored in a cool place and away from direct light. If the bottle is corked, it should be stored on its side to keep the cork moist. Wine with a screw cap and those wines which have an alcohol content of 20 per cent or more should be stored in an upright position. Once a wine with an alcohol content of 12 per cent or less has been opened, it should be stored in the refrigerator and used within two or three days.

RECIPES

Cafe au Lait

	Standard	Metric
Freshly brewed coffee	4 6-ounce cups	710 mL
Hot milk	24 ounces	710 mL

1. Pour equal amounts of the coffee and hot milk from two separate containers into each cup.

Yield: 4 6-ounce cups

Cappuccino

	Standard	Metric
Instant espresso coffee or instant coffee	1/4 cup	60 mL
Boiling water	2 cups	500 mL
Whipping cream	1/2 cup	125 mL

1. Whip the cream until soft peaks form.

2. Dissolve the coffee in boiling water and pour into 6 small cups, holding approximately 3 ounces.
3. Top with a spoonful of whipped cream.
4. May be garnished with ground cinnamon or nutmeg.

Yield: 6 3-ounce servings

Coffee Demitasse

	Standard	Metric
Ground coffee	3/4 cup	180 mL
Water	3 cups	750 mL

1. Prepare the coffee as directed by any of the methods described in this chapter.
2. Serve hot.

Yield: 4 to 6 servings

Mocha Spiced Delight

	Standard	Metric
Water	3 cups	750 mL
Stick cinnamon	1	1
Cloves, whole	10	10
Allspice berries	8	8
Coffee	1/2 cup	125 mL
Cream, whipped	1/2 cup	125 mL

1. Combine the water and spices in a saucepan. Bring to a boil and simmer for 10 minutes.
2. Remove the spices from the liquid and measure the liquid. If necessary, add more water to equal 3 cups.
3. Using the spiced liquid, brew the coffee as usual.
4. Pour into coffee cups and top with a spoonful of whipped cream.

Yield: 4 servings

Coffee Butterscotch Frost

	Standard	Metric
Instant coffee	2 Tbsp.	30 mL
Boiling water	1 cup	250 mL
Cold water	3 cups	750 mL
Butterscotch topping	1/2 cup	125 mL
Vanilla ice cream	1 pint	500 mL

1. Dissolve the coffee in hot water; add the cold water.
2. Combine the coffee mixture with the butterscotch topping and ice cream in a large mixer bowl. Beat until frothy.
3. Pour into tall glasses and serve immediately.

Yield: 6 servings

Frosty Coffee Shake

	Standard	Metric
Strong, cold coffee	2-1/2 cups	625 mL
Chocolate syrup	5 Tbsp.	75 mL
Coffee ice cream	2 cups	500 mL

1. Combine the coffee, chocolate syrup, and ice cream in a large mixing bowl. Beat until smooth.
2. Pour immediately into tall glasses and serve.

Yield: 4 servings

Iced Coffee

	Standard	Metric
Coffee	8 Tbsp.	120 mL
Water	2 cups	500 mL
Ice cubes		

1. Prepare the coffee.
2. Fill glasses with ice cubes and pour the coffee over the ice cubes.

Yield: 4 servings

Variation:
1. Freeze the coffee into cubes in an ice tray.
2. Prepare regular-strength coffee and pour over the coffee ice cubes.

Iced Tea

	Standard	Metric
Tea leaves	2 Tbsp.	30 mL
Boiling water	4 cups	1000 mL

1. Pour the boiling water over the tea leaves and let steep for 3 minutes.
2. Fill tall glasses with ice cubes and pour in the tea.

Yield: 4 to 5 servings

Lemon Iced Tea

	Standard	Metric
Tea bags	6	6
Boiling water	2 cups	500 mL
Cold water	4 cups	1000 mL
Frozen lemonade concentrate	3 oz.	89 mL

1. Pour the boiling water over the tea bags and steep for 5 minutes.
2. Remove the tea bags.
3. Stir in the cold water and lemonade concentrate.
4. Fill tall glasses with ice cubes and pour in the tea.

Yield: 6 servings

--------- Hot Spiced Tea ---------

	Standard	Metric
Water	3 cups	750 mL
Whole cloves	1/2 tsp.	2 mL
Stick cinnamon	1/2 inch	1/2 inch
Black tea	1-1/2 Tbsp.	22 mL
Orange juice	1/3 cup	75 mL
Lemon juice	1 Tbsp.	15 mL
Sugar	1/4 cup	60 mL

1. Combine the water, cloves, and cinnamon. Bring to a boil and pour over the tea. Cover and steep for 5 minutes.
2. While the tea steeps, combine the orange juice, lemon juice, and sugar. Bring to a boil.
3. Strain the tea leaves. Stir the hot juice mixture into the tea. Serve at once.

Yield: 4 servings

--------- Instant Russian Tea ---------

	Standard	Metric
Tang	2 cups	500 mL
Sugar	1-1/2 cups	375 mL
Instant tea	1/2 cup	125 mL
Cinnamon	1 tsp.	5 mL
Cloves	1 tsp.	5 mL
Lemonade mix	1 package	1 package

1. Combine all ingredients in a mixing bowl and stir to thoroughly blend the ingredients.
2. To serve, mix 2 teaspoons of mixture with 3/4 cup of boiling water.

3. Store the mixture in a container with a tightly fitting lid.

Yield: 4 cups mixture

--------- Instant Mocha ---------

	Standard	Metric
Instant coffee	2 tsp.	10 mL
Instant cocoa mix	2 tsp.	10 mL
Milk	1 cup	250 mL

1. Combine the instant coffee and cocoa mix in a mug.
2. Heat the milk to just below the boiling point. Do not boil. Add to the coffee-cocoa mixture and stir to blend.

Yield: 1 8-oz. serving

--------- Instant Cocoa ---------

	Standard	Metric
Nonfat dry milk	1-1 lb. package	454 gm
Sugar	1 cup	250 mL
Cocoa	3/4 cup	180 mL
Salt	3/4 tsp.	3 mL

1. Sift the ingredients together three times.
2. Place in a tightly covered container. Store in a cool place.

Yield: 28 servings

To Use:

1. Combine 1/3 cup of mix with 1 cup (8 oz.) of hot water in a large cup or mug. Stir to blend.

Cocoa Syrup

	Standard	Metric
Cocoa, sifted	1/2 cup	125 mL
Sugar	1 cup	250 mL
Salt	1/8 tsp.	.05 mL
Boiling water	1 cup	250 mL
Vanilla	1 tsp.	5 mL

1. Combine the cocoa, sugar, and salt in a saucepan. Add boiling water gradually, stirring to form a smooth mixture.
2. Cook over medium heat, stirring until the mixture comes to a boil. Boil 1 minute without stirring.
3. Remove from heat and cool. Stir the vanilla into the cooled mixture.
4. Pour into a container with a lid. Cover and refrigerate.

Yield: 1–3/4 cups

Hot Cocoa

	Standard	Metric
Milk	2 cups	500 mL
Cocoa syrup	1/4 cup	60 mL

1. Heat the milk to just below the boiling point. Do not boil.
2. Stir the cocoa syrup into the hot milk until well blended.
3. May be garnished with a dollop of whipped cream or a marshmallow.

Yield: 2 8-oz. servings

Iced Cocoa

	Standard	Metric
Cocoa syrup	2 Tbsp.	30 mL
Milk	1 cup	250 mL

1. With a rotary beater, beat the cold milk and syrup to combine.
2. Pour over ice cubes in a tall glass.

Yield: 1 8-oz. serving

Hot Chocolate

	Standard	Metric
Baker's chocolate	2 (1-oz.) squares	57 gm
Water	1 cup	250 mL
Sugar	3 Tbsp.	45 mL
Salt	Dash	Dash
Milk	3 cups	750 mL

1. Cook the chocolate and water over low heat until the chocolate is melted.
2. Add the sugar and salt. Boil 5 minutes, stirring constantly.
3. Add the milk, stirring constantly. Heat over boiling water. Beat with a rotary beater until frothy just before serving.

Yield: 6 servings

LEARNING ACTIVITIES

1. Purchase a low-, medium-, and high-priced coffee and prepare them in one type of coffee maker. Determine which kind of coffee would be the best buy according to yield and flavor.
2. Prepare a party menu that would use an interesting variation of coffee or tea as the beverage.
3. If it is possible, grind some coffee beans. Prepare coffee with the freshly ground beans and with a coffee that has been vacuum-sealed and compare the flavor.

4. Prepare a black tea, green tea, and oolong tea and compare the difference in flavor and aroma to determine your preference.
5. Make and compare the flavor and cost of a regular coffee with an acid-free, decaffeinated, and cereal-substitute coffee.
6. Prepare a cup of tea using water that has boiled 15 minutes with a cup of tea that has been made with freshly boiled water. Determine the difference in flavor.
7. Compare the price of a breakfast cocoa and a commercial cocoa mix for making 4 cups. Prepare a cocoa beverage from the commercial mix and one from cocoa. Determine the best buy according to flavor, preparation time, and price.
8. Prepare a cocoa beverage using fresh milk and one made from nonfat dry milk to determine if there is a difference in flavor. Compare the costs.
9. Do a research paper on the reasons why coffee consumption in the United States appears to be on the decline.

REVIEW QUESTIONS

1. For what reasons do people consume coffee and tea when their nutrient content is so low?
2. Why is it not considered harmful to allow young children to consume chocolate and cocoa beverages when it is known that caffeine is a stimulant in these two foods?
3. In what countries are coffee and tea grown?
4. How is coffee imported into the United States?
5. From an economical standpoint, which grind of coffee is the best buy? Why?
6. What is meant by the terms *decaffeinated* and *acid-free* coffees?
7. Why is it usually not wise to purchase coffee in large amounts?
8. How can coffee be prevented from staling?
9. Why should coffee pots be thoroughly washed and rinsed?
10. What is the difference in processing green and black teas?
11. What is meant by the term *pekoe*?
12. Why should water be freshly boiled in making tea?
13. What is the difference in ingredients between cake chocolate and breakfast cocoa?
14. What are the proportions for interchanging cocoa and chocolate in a recipe?
15. Why should cocoa or chocolate, sugar, and water be cooked before milk is added.
16. How many tablespoons of coffee should be used per 3/4 cup of coffee?
17. How much loose tea should be used per cup?

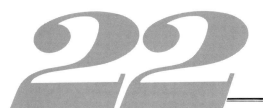

Food Preservation

Food preservation is the means by which the spoilage of food is deterred by eliminating the conditions under which microorganisms and enzymes can grow and act. By this preservation the eating quality of food is extended. Food is mainly preserved by adding heat (canning), lowering the heat (freezing), removing moisture (dehydration), or by the use of certain chemicals. Some chemicals preserve food by fermentation. Other more technical methods of food preservation are used by the food industry to preserve large quantities of food.

The sanitary handling of food is of great importance in all methods of food preservation and it is recommended that the causes of food spoilage and its prevention be reviewed in Chapter 3, "Food Safety." This chapter discusses the common methods of home food preservation including canning, freezing, and dehydration. Fruits are often preserved by

making them into jams, jellies, or other spreads. This is also discussed in this chapter.

Nutritional Factors to Consider

If foods are preserved by the proper methods, there will be little loss of nutrients, but all preserved foods do deteriorate and lose nutrients upon prolonged storage. Few, if any, preserved foods will keep longer than 12 months, and some preserved foods should be used in less time. It is advisable to always use foods within their recommended storage time.

Selection of Foods for Preservation

Economically, only those foods that are in abundance in a certain geographical area should be selected for preservation. In many instances there is little, if any, dollar savings derived from the home preservation of food because of the cost of purchasing equipment, the cost of heat and electricity, and the time consumed in food preservation. However, the sense of personal accomplishment and the feeling of family togetherness often outweigh these facts.

Fruits and vegetables that are to be home preserved are usually purchased in a quantity larger than the amount purchased for daily consumption at the market. Larger quantities can often be more economically purchased at a roadside stand or in rural areas where pick-your-own fields allow the consumer to obtain food at a reasonable price by using one's own labor. Some people grow their own food for preservation.

Meat, poultry, and fish may be a better purchase at certain times of the year, or store specials may offer a particular cut of meat at an economical price. In these instances home preservation can provide a substantial saving to the food budget.

All foods selected for preservation need to be at their peak of freshness. Fruits should be firm but well ripened without bruises or signs of decay. Vegetables are best for preservation when they are young and tender. Overly mature, bruised, and decayed fruits and vegetables can cause spoilage when they are preserved.

Canning

The canning of food in jars or tins is a means of preserving food by subjecting the food to heat to kill or inactivate the enzymes and microorganisms that are present. It is most important that foods be canned in sterilized containers or be sterilized in the processing and be sealed airtight to prevent any further contamination. Meats, poultry, fish, and vegetables, with the exception of tomatoes, are low-acid foods in which certain bacteria can grow if the foods are not processed at a temperature above 212° F (100° C). These foods must be processed in a pressure canner that reaches temperatures of 240° F (116° C). The most deadly bacterial growth that can occur in low-acid foods which are improperly processed is *Clostridium botulinum.*

Home-canned, low-acid foods should never be tasted without first being covered and boiled for 10 minutes. Meats, corn, and spinach must be boiled for 20 minutes. Any container with a bulging lid, leak, or off-odor must be discarded without tasting.

Depending on the variety and the soil and climate conditions under which they are grown, some tomatoes may have a low-acidity. It is best to consult with the local cooperative extension agent to determine what canning procedure should be followed for tomatoes in the area. To increase the acidity of tomatoes, 1/4 teaspoon per pint or 1/2 teaspoon per quart of citric acid may be added to the tomatoes.

Other microorganisms that grow on foods with a higher pH such as fruits and tomatoes have a lower resistance to heat and can be destroyed when these foods are processed in a boiling-water bath.

Equipment Needed for Canning

A pressure canner is used to process all meats and vegetables of low-acid content. It includes a rack that fits in the bottom of the pan on which the jars or cans are set; a steam-tight cover; and a petcock, safety valve, and steam gauge on top of the cover. Because the pressure gauge must be accurate to assure that the proper temperature is reached while processing food, it is important to have the pressure gauge checked for accuracy before the canning season begins. The method for checking the gauge's accuracy can be obtained from the dealer, manufacturer, or local county extension agent.

A pressure saucepan may be used for canning if it is equipped with a gauge or weight for showing and controlling pressure at 10 pounds. It is recommended that 20 minutes be added to the processing time to allow for the rapid rise in temperature at the beginning of the canning process and the rapid cooling at the end. The manufacturer's instructions for canning in the pressure saucepan must be followed exactly.

A large kettle called a water bath canner is used for the processing of fruits, tomatoes, and pickles. A water bath canner is equipped with a rack that holds the jars 1/2 inch above the surface of the pan and a lid. The water bath canner must be large enough to hold the jars with enough water to cover the jars by at least 1 inch.

Glass jars are the most common container used in home canning. They are available with either a narrow or a wide mouth, but the wide mouth is preferred because it is easier to place food in the jar. Jars with cracks or nicks must not be used. It is not advisable to use ordinary jars, such as mayonnaise or peanut butter jars, which are made of a thinner glass and may not withstand the high temperatures of processing nor may the canning lids that must be used in home canning, fit. Tin cans may also be used but a mechanical sealer must be available for sealing the lid.

Jars are available in 1/2-pint, pint, and quart sizes. The selection of the size of the jar is dependent upon the food being canned and the amount of food that will be used within the recommended storage time once the jar is opened.

Lids for jars are of two types. One consists of a screw band and a flat metal lid with a sealing compound that activates when it is covered with boiling water. These lids are kept in the water until they are ready to use but are not boiled. The second type is a porcelain-lined zinc lid with a separate rubber ring. Neither the rubber ring nor the flat metal lid can be used more than once.

Other equipment needed for home canning includes jar tongs that are used to remove the hot jars from the canner and a wide-mouth funnel for aiding the placement of small amounts of food into the jars and to aid in pouring liquid into the jars. Other items include a small brush for cleaning certain fruits and vegetables, a sharp knife, and a peeler. Figure 22-1 shows the types of equipment needed for home canning.

Preparation of Jars

Jars that are used in canning do not need to be sterilized because they, together with the food, are sterilized when they are subjected to the high temperature needed in processing. Jars must be washed in warm, soapy water; rinsed in hot water; and drained upside down on absorbent toweling until they are filled with food.

Preparation of Food for Canning

All fruits and vegetables must be washed, and root vegetables such as carrots may need to be scrubbed with a brush to remove all dirt. The fruits and vegetables should not be soaked as soaking removes valuable nutrients from the foods. Some fruits, such as tomatoes and peaches, are skinned prior to processing. Skinning is done by dipping the food in boiling water to loosen the skin, then dipping the food into cold water, and then removing the skin with a sharp knife.

Meats, poultry, and fish must be fresh before being canned. If it is not possible to process meat immediately, the meat can be frozen before it is processed. The frozen meat is cut or sawed into smaller pieces and placed in boiling water until it is soft enough to pack into the container.

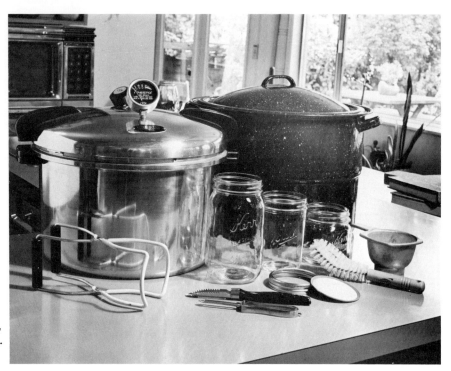

Figure 22-1.

Illustrated are the necessary pieces of equipment for canning.

Raw-Pack and Hot-Pack

Food is either canned by the hot-pack or raw-pack method. Foods canned by the raw-pack method are placed, uncooked into the container and then covered with hot water, syrup, or juice. The container is then sealed and the food is processed. Foods that are hot-packed are precooked in steam or in a boiling liquid for a short time and immediately packed into the container, which is then sealed and processed. With either method, fruits are usually packed in a thin sugar syrup to help the fruit maintain its shape, flavor, and color. A medium or thick syrup may be used for fruit that is to be served as a dessert. Fruit may also be packed in a fruit juice or in water.

If vegetables are hot-packed, the water in which they were precooked should be added to the container to preserve the nutrients. Additional boiling water may be needed to fill the jars. If salt is to be added, canning or pickling salt is best, since table salt leaves a sediment on the bottom of the jar. A mixture of two parts of sugar to one part of salt may be preferred for seasoning such vegetables as corn, peas, beets, and tomatoes.

Meat may be canned with or without the bone, but any excess fat should be trimmed away. Meat that is hot-packed is precooked and should be at a temperature of 170° F (77° C) before it is packed into the jars, covered with broth or hot water, and the lid adjusted. Liquid is not added to raw-packed meat, but the meat in the jars is heated to a temperature of 170° F (77° C) in a boiling water bath with the pan covered. This is done to remove any air in the jars and to prevent changes of flavor in the meat.

Corn, peas, lima beans, and meats are packed to within 1 inch of the top of the jar, and all other foods are packed to within 1/2 inch of the top. There will be less shrinkage of food when the food has been hot-packed. Air bubbles within the jar are removed by inserting a metal spatula along the inside of the jar.

Pressure Canning

All meats and vegetables, with the exception of acid varieties of tomatoes, are processed in a pressure canner. As discussed in the section of this chapter on equipment needed for canning, a pressure saucepan may be used. Either the raw- or hot-pack method may be used with the pressure canner. Foods are canned at 10 pounds pressure but the length of cooking time will vary with the food. Because processing times have been determined specifically for each food, the canning directions must be followed exactly.

The following steps are general procedures to be followed when pressure canning.

1. All equipment that will be needed should be set out prior to starting.

2. Jars need to be washed, rinsed, and drained.

3. The type of lid used will determine what preparation is necessary and the manufacturer's directions need to be followed.

4. When jars are ready to be filled, the canner is placed on the burner, with the rack inside, and filled with 1 to 2 inches of boiling water. After each jar is filled, the rim is wiped with a clean, damp cloth, and the lid is adjusted and the jar placed in the boiling water. Only enough jars are filled to fit the size of the rack. Figure 22-2 illustrates the procedure for preparing cut green beans for canning.

5. The manufacturer's instructions are then followed for the method of operating the canner and the cooling procedure.

6. After cooling, the jars are lifted from the canner and set on a rack or on several

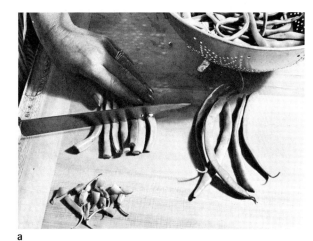

a

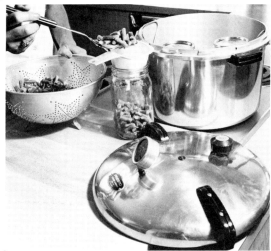

b

Figure 22-2.

(a) Green beans are washed, the ends trimmed, and cut into small pieces in preparation for pressure canning. (b) Cut green beans are placed in the jar to within 1/2 inch of the top and boiling water is added to within 1/2 inch of the top of the jar. The lid is placed on the jar. The jars are placed in the pressure canner and processed for the required length of time according to the size of the jar and the food at 10 pounds of pressure.

thicknesses of toweling. The porcelain-lined lid needs to be tightly screwed down after the jar is removed from the canner. The screw lid is not further tightened.

7. The next day the jars are checked to ensure a proper seal. Jars with porcelain-lined zinc closures are checked by laying the jar on its side and checking for leakage. Jars with the flat metal lid and screw band are checked by pressing the center of the lid. If the lid does not move, the jar is sealed. Another test for this lid is to tap the center of the lid with a metal spoon. If a clear ring is heard, the lid is sealed.

Boiling Water Bath

This method is used to process fruits, tomatoes with a high pH and pickles. These foods, which have a high-acid content, can be safely canned in boiling water at 212° F (100° C). The foods may be prepared by either the raw- or hot-pack method.

The following steps are general procedures to be followed with the boiling-water bath.

1. The equipment, jar, and food preparation are the same procedures used in pressure canning, as shown in Figure 22–3.

2. The water-bath canner is filled with enough water to cover the tops of the jars by at least 1 inch and heated to the boiling point.

3. The food is prepared according to the recipe and placed in the clean jars. The lid is adjusted and the jar placed on the rack. When the rack is filled, it is carefully lowered into the boiling water or individual jars may be individually lowered into the water when all are ready.

4. Additional water is added if needed, and the water is brought to a full rolling boil. This is when timing for the processing begins.

5. After processing is completed, the jars are removed from the kettle with jar tongs and set on a rack or padded surface to cool.

6. After the jars have thoroughly cooled, they are tested for proper seal following the procedure used in pressure canning.

If a jar has not sealed, the food must be immediately used, or the lid changed and the jar canned again, using the original process. Foods that have been reprocessed have a much poorer quality.

Jellies, Jams, and Preserves

One of the most popular ways to preserve fruit is to make jellies, jams, and preserves. These products may be either cooked or they may be an uncooked mixture that is frozen. The uncooked jams and jellies take less time to make, are simple to make, and will yield more jams or jellies than the cooked spreads, but they do require more sugar. Many prefer the flavor of the cooked products and freezer storage at 0° F (–18° C) may not be available.

Equipment Needed

A large, flat-bottomed pan, which will hold 8 to 12 quarts, is needed to make these products. The large pan is necessary to allow the fruit-sugar mixtures to boil rapidly without boiling over. To make jelly, a jelly bag or several layers of cheesecloth are needed. The cheesecloth is spread in a colander to retain the pulp while the juice is extracted. A fruit press may also be used. A timer is important for correct cooking, and a candy, jelly, or fat thermometer serves as a guide in determining the jellying point of jelly.

Other equipment that aids in the making of jams, jellies, and preserves includes liquid measures, a scoop ladle, and a funnel that can fit over the jars.

Since it is preferable to seal jars, small canning jars are preferably used. Glasses may be

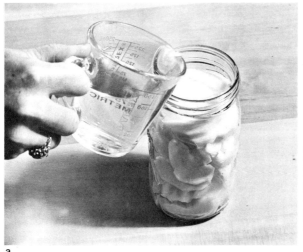

a

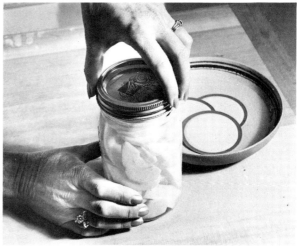

c

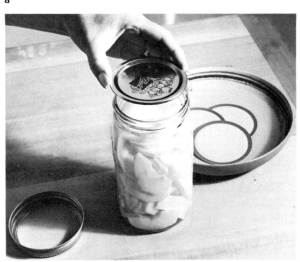

b

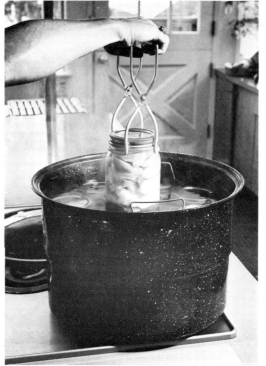

d

Figure 22-3.

(a) Fruits processed by the boiling water bath are placed in jars to within 1/2 inch of the top and a thin sugar syrup or water is poured over the fruit to within 1/2 inch of the top. (b) The top of the jar is wiped clean and the lid is placed on the jar. (c) The band is then screwed over the lid. (d) The jar is lowered into the boiling water with jar tongs, when all jars are ready to be processed. Additional water is added to cover the jars by 2 inches and the water is brought to boiling for processing.

used for jelly since they may be sealed with paraffin unless the climate is hot and humid. Jams and preserves are sealed with a lid, as in canning, to prevent the growth of mold. If paraffin is to be used for sealing, it is always melted in a container set in another pan of hot water. It is unsafe to melt paraffin over direct heat.

Preparation of Jars

Since many recipes do not require the sealed product to be further processed, and since jelly can be sealed with paraffin, the jars used must be sterilized. Jars are sterilized by washing them in soapy water, rinsing, and placing the jars on a rack in a pan. If a rack is not available, a folded cloth on the bottom of the pan will work. The jars are covered with water and boiled for 15 minutes. The jars need to remain in the hot water until they are used.

Jelly

Jelly is a gel made from the juice of fruit, sugar, acid, water, and pectin. Pectin is a carbohydrate-like substance found in fruit. The greatest amount of pectin is found in fruit that is slightly underripe. As underripe fruit is more tart and less flavorful, it is suggested that a combination of slightly underripe and ripe fruit be used when making jelly. When fruit is heated with a small amount of water, the pectin is extracted and will form a gel when the proper proportions of sugar and acid are present. Pectin is also made from apples or citrus fruits and sold commercially in liquid or powdered form.

Some fruits, such as crab apples, grapes, and citrus fruits, contain enough pectin and acid in the proper proportions so that when the right amount of sugar and heat is present, a gel is formed. Other fruits need the addition of lemon juice or citric acid and a commercial pectin to form a satisfactory gel. Tested recipes

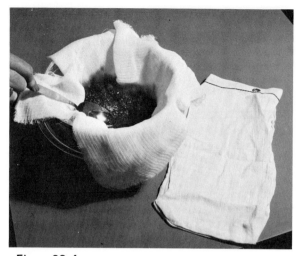

Figure 22-4.
One way of extracting juice for jelly is to pour the pulp mixture into a colander lined with cheese cloth.

will show what ingredients and proportions to use to make jellies from various fruits.

To obtain the juice from fruit, the fruit is first washed and blemishes, cores, and stems are removed. The fruit is cut into chunks or soft fruits such as berries are crushed. Firm fruits, such as apples, need the addition of 1 cup of water to 1 pound of fruit when cooking. Soft fruits and berries need no additional water unless they are not juicy; then the addition of 1/4 cup of water is advisable. Too much liquid will weaken the gel. The fruit is boiled for 2 to 3 minutes for soft fruit, but firmer fruits will take 10 to 20 minutes. Excessive boiling destroys the jellying strength and destroys the flavor of the fruit.

To remove the fruit pulp and to obtain a clear juice, the mixture is poured into a colander in which four layers of cheesecloth have been spread as shown in Figure 22-4, into a wet jelly bag, or into a food press. The cloth or bag is gently twisted to press out the juice as shown in Figure 22-5. The next step depends on the recipe chosen. It is best to make jelly in small batches and not to attempt to double a recipe.

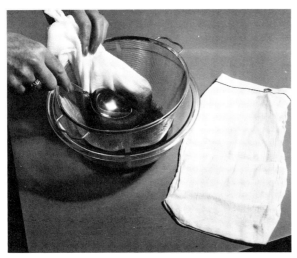

Figure 22-5.
Gently twisting the cheese cloth and/or pressing with a spoon aids in extracting the juice.

Jelly is basically a sugar-fruit mixture. As the mixture boils, it becomes concentrated and reaches a jellying point. Three tests can be used to determine when this point has been reached.

1. A candy, deep-fat, or jelly thermometer should show a temperature of 8° F (4.4° C) above the boiling point of water, 212° F (100° C).

2. A metal spoon, dipped into the mixture, and held 12 inches above the pan, out of the steam, will run off in two drops as the mixture is reaching the jellying point. When the jellying point has been reached, the drops will slide together and drop off the spoon in a sheet.

3. The jellying point can also be checked by placing a small amount on a plate and setting it in the refrigerator. If the jelly gels in a few minutes, it is ready.

After the jelly has gelled, it is immediately removed from the heat. It should stand for 1 minute to allow a film to form on the surface. The jelly is then ladled into hot jars and sealed

or covered with paraffin. Table 22-1 lists some of the causes and solutions to problems that may arise in jelly making.

Jam

Jam is a thickened mixture of small fruits or fruits that have been cut into small pieces or crushed. Fruits that have no juice require the addition of 1/2 cup to 1 cup of water. Sugar is used in a proportion of 3/4 pound of sugar to 1 pound of fruit. The fruit and water are mixed and cooked in an open, large pan until most of the water has evaporated. Tested recipes will give exact directions. The sugar is then added and the mixture is brought to a full boil. The same tests for jellying can be applied to the thickening of jam. It is best to stir and skim jam for 5 minutes after it is removed from the heat so that the pieces of fruit are evenly dispersed throughout the mixture. Jam is ladled into hot, sterilized jars and sealed according to the manufacturer's directions.

Preserves

Preserves are made from small fruits such as strawberries or cherries, or from fruits such as peaches or pears that have been cut into uniform pieces. A high-quality preserve should have plump fruit that is evenly distributed throughout the syrup. This is attained by allowing soft fruits such as berries combined with the sugar to stand until the juices start to flow. The mixture is then cooked. Hard fruit such as apples can be precooked in water until it is barely tender before the sugar is added. Preserves are ladled into hot, sterilized jars and the same sealing procedure is followed as for making jams.

Uncooked Jams and Jellies

Recipe directions for uncooked jams and jellies, as with the cooked versions, need to be

Table 22-1

Problems and Solutions in Jelly Making

Jelly did not set.	Too much sugar; mixture cooked too slowly and too long.
Jelly is too soft.	Mixture lacked acid or pectin. Wrong proportions of juice and sugar and not enough acid. Too short a cooking time.
Jelly has a gummy texture.	Jelly mixture was overcooked.
Jelly is tough.	Mixture contained too little sugar. Had to be cooked too long to reach the jellying point.
Jelly is cloudy.	Juice was not extracted properly. Mixture stood too long before being ladled into the jars.
Jelly has mold on the surface.	Jars were not properly sterilized. Seal was imperfect. Storage area was damp.

followed exactly and the ingredients must be carefully measured. Liquid or powdered commercial pectins are always used in the making of these products, but one type should not be substituted for the other. Uncooked jams and jellies are packed in clean, freezer containers and should be allowed to set before they are stored at $0°$ F ($-18°$ C). This is best done by refrigeration that may take 1 to 2 days. The uncooked jams and jellies will keep 3 weeks in the refrigerator or up to 6 months in the refrigerator.

Freezing

The preservation of food by freezing is not only the fastest method of food preservation but freezing also produces the least changes in the nutritive, chemical, and physical characteristics of food. Although freezing, by the cold temperature, decreases the microorganisms that are present in food, microbial growth can take place when food is thawing and some foods will show a definite change in texture.

Freezing is a quick way to preserve food, but it may not always to be the most economical

way when consideration is given to the initial cash outlay for the purchase of a freezer and to the fact that large quantities of food should only be frozen when there is an economical saving. The amounts of food that are frozen should be related to the quantity of food that can be eaten within a certain period of time. Frozen foods do not keep indefinitely, and the longer they are stored the greater will be the loss of nutrients, flavor, and texture. The proper packaging of frozen foods is presented in Chapter 3, "Food Safety."

Fruits

Fruits to be frozen should be "eating ripe." Immature or green fruits do not have the flavor or texture of ripe fruits. Fruits are washed in cold water and should be prepared for freezing in the form in which they will be served. There are three ways to pack fruit for freezing:

1. Sugar Syrup Pack. The basic proportions for a light, medium, and heavy sugar syrup are shown in Table 22-2. The sugar is stirred into the water to dissolve. It is not heated but it should be chilled before

Table 22-2
Proportions for Sugar-Syrup Pack in Freezing Fruit

	Water	Sugar	Yield	Approximate Coverage
Light	4 cups	2 cups	5 cups	7 pints
Medium	4 cups	3 cups	5-1/2 cups	8 pints
Heavy	4 cups	4 cups	4-1/4 cups	9 pints

it is poured over the fruit. Approximately 2/3 cup of syrup should be allowed for each pint of fruit.

2. Sugar Pack. Sugar is sprinkled over a small amount of fruit in a bowl and mixed in carefully. Ripe berries that are delicate and soft are more easily coated by spreading in a shallow pan; the sugar is sprinkled on and mixed in gently. The approximate proportions are 3 pounds of fruit to 1 pound of sugar.

3. Unsweetened Pack. The fruit may be packed dry or with water. Small fruits such as berries and cherries freeze best when they are spread in a shallow container and allowed to freeze before they are packed in a container. Fruit packed without sugar will collapse and lose flavor more quickly. The packing of frozen fruit is shown in Figure 22-6.

Fruits, such as peaches and apricots, that tend to darken because of enzymatic action need to be dipped in an ascorbic acid solution or the ascorbic acid may be added to the sugar syrup. One half teaspoon of ascorbic acid powder or crystal form is added to each quart of syrup, or for a sugar pack, a small amount is sprinkled over the fruit before adding the sugar.

Frozen fruits should thaw in their original, sealed container at room temperature or in the refrigerator, and they should be served just at the end of thawing while a few crystals remain. Completely thawed fruits will have a mushy texture. Frozen fruits can also be cooked and used for making jams and jellies.

Vegetables

Most vegetables freeze satisfactorily except for those that are usually eaten raw or have a high water content, such as lettuce, celery, radishes, and tomatoes. Vegetables must be blanched before they are frozen to stop enzymatic action and to slightly shrink them. Vegetables will have their best flavor when they are frozen as soon as possible after being harvested. The following steps are used in blanching vegetables.

1. The vegetables are washed, and any undesired portions such as tough stems and blemishes are removed. The vegetables are then cut into the desired size.

2. The prepared vegetables are then placed in a wire basket or colander and submerged in a pan of boiling water. One gallon of boiling water is needed to blanch 1 pound of vegetables. The time for blanching is measured from the time the vegetables are submerged in the boiling water. The blanching time needs to be exact to avoid soft texture, loss of nutrients, and inferior flavors. The use of a timer helps to facilitate the timing process.

3. After blanching, the vegetables are immediately submerged in icy cold water. This rapid chilling stops the cooking, saves the nutrients, and provides a top-quality

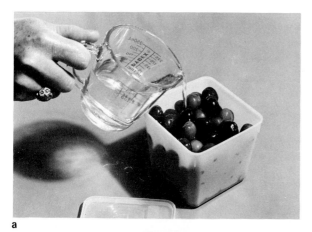

a

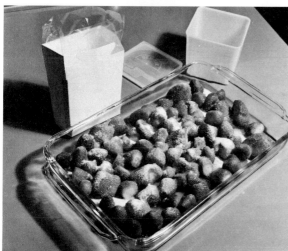

b

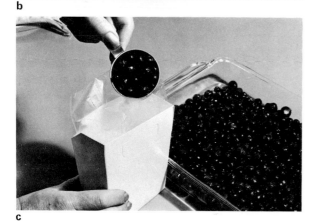

c

product. The length of time for chilling will be approximately the same as for blanching.

4. The vegetables are then drained immediately and packaged for freezing. The steps to freezing vegetables are shown in Figure 22-7.

Frozen vegetables are cooked in rapidly boiling water and served immediately.

Meats, Poultry, and Fish

It is best to freeze meat, poultry, and fish in amounts that will be needed for one meal. Cut-up poultry and meat frozen without the bone will take less freezer space.

Precooked Foods

The freezing of precooked foods is discussed in Chapter 3, on "Food Safety."

Dehydration

Dehydration is the most ancient method of food preservation known to man, dating back to the ancient Egyptian culture. In recent years dehydration has again become a popular means of home food preservation, as a result of the introduction of food-drying equipment to the marketplace and the increased use of dehydrated foods for hiking and camping. The food

Figure 22-6.

(a) Fruits frozen in a sugar-syrup pack such as pitted fresh cherries are covered with a sugar syrup before being frozen. (b) Fruit that is sugar coated before being frozen is easily done so in a shallow pan. (c) Fruits are sometimes frozen in their natural state without the addition of sugar or a syrup as shown here with blueberries.

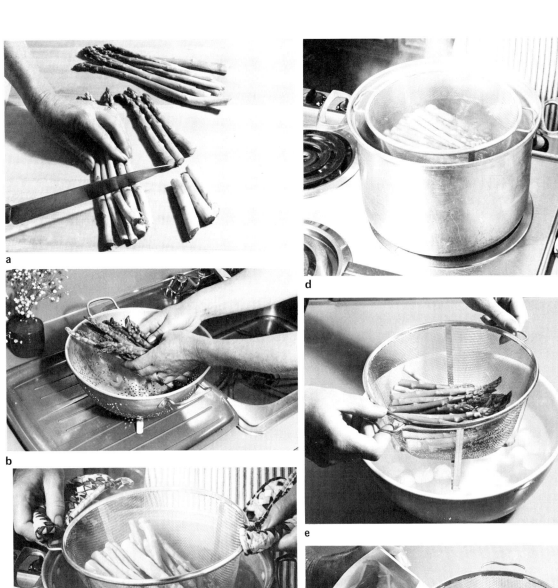

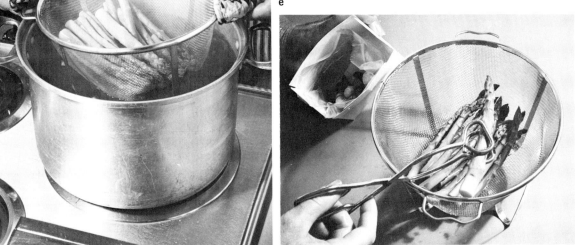

a

b

c

d

e

f

industry uses many refined methods of dehydration to produce such foods as dry milk, instant-mashed potatoes, and instant coffee.

A dehydrated food is one from which most of the water has been removed. Food dehydration done in the home is usually accomplished by some type of heated air with or without a blower. Some food dehydration is accomplished by sun drying but this is very dependent upon the geographical location. Dehydration will not stop the enzymatic reactions that occur naturally in food without certain steps being taken prior to the dehydration process.

Fruits

Only ripe fruits that do not show signs of bruising or decay should be used for drying. Overripe fruits may be used for making fruit leathers. All fruits must be washed and the inedible portions such as the stem and blossom removed before drying. Fruits with seeds must be pitted, but it is not necessary to peel fruits. Fruits for dehydration may be coarsely shredded or cut into uniform pieces of 1/8 inch- to 1/4-inch thickness. Whole fruits, such as blueberries and grapes, need to be dipped in boiling water until the skin splits.

Because of enzymatic reactions, certain fruits such as pears, apples, and bananas will turn brown if they are not pretreated. To pretreat, the fruits are dipped in a solution of sodium bisulfite (1 to 3 tablespoons per gallon of water). The fruits should not touch metal while they are dehydrating, and fruits treated with sodium bisulfite will taste better if they are stored for several months before they are eaten. Some manufacturers of home dehydrators suggest the use of ascorbic acid to prevent discoloration. The suggested proportion is 1 teaspoon of ascorbic acid to 1 quart of water. These foods do not need extended storage before being eaten.

Fruit leathers are made of ripe fruit and resemble taffy. The directions for making fruit leathers are given in the recipe section of this chapter.

Vegetables

Vegetables need to be thoroughly cleaned and the unedible portions removed before they are dried. Personal preference will determine whether vegetables are peeled or not, but nutrient retention is greater when they are not peeled. Vegetables are coarsely shredded or cut into slices, strips, or cubes. For even dehydrating, the pieces should be of the same size.

With the exception of celery, garlic, herbs, mushrooms, onions, peppers, and tomatoes, vegetables need to be blanched or steamed to eliminate enzymatic activity that will change the flavor, color, and texture of vegetables during storage. The specific time required for steaming and blanching vegetables for dehydration is the same as that required for preparing vegetables for freezing. Vegetable leathers may also be made by cooking the vegetables in a small amount of water, pureeing, and dehydrating. The leather is then broken into pieces or powdered in a blender and used as a flavorful addition to many food dishes.

Meats

Meats selected for dehydration should have a minimum of connective tissue and marbling. Poultry and fish must be fresh. Meat with the

Figure 22-7. [Opposite]

(a) Vegetables that are to be frozen are first trimmed to remove undesirable blemishes, tough stems, etc. (b) They are then washed. (c) The cleaned and trimmed vegetables are then placed in a colander and (d) submerged in boiling water for the specified time period. (e) The vegetables are then submerged in icy cold water. (f) Vegetables are drained immediately and packaged for freezing.

exception of beef jerky is braised before being dehydrated; fish and poultry will be more palatable if they are cooked by steaming before dehydration. Meat, poultry, and fish are best cut into cubes for drying.

Storage of Dehydrated Foods

Dehydrated fruits and vegetables take up a minimum of storage space. They are protected from insect manifestation when stored in small plastic bags and then placed in a larger container with a lid. Before the bags are closed, excess air is removed by squeezing the bags. With the exception of melons, dehydrated fruits and vegetables will keep for 2 years when stored in a cool, dry, dark place. Meats will keep best for any lengthy period of time when stored under refrigeration.

Reconstituting Dehydrated Foods

Dehydrated foods may be eaten as is or reconstituted. To reconstitute, an equal part of the dried food is mixed with an equal amount of water. To obtain the fresh food portion needed, one half of the dried food is reconstituted. More water may be needed during reconstituting, but it is better to add more water than to drain off water and lose precious nutrients.

Approximately 2 hours is needed to reconstitute food at room temperature or overnight in the refrigerator. The process may be hastened by bringing the water and dried food to a boil, removing from the heat, and allowing to stand. Shreds will take less time to reconstitute than halved or whole pieces of food.

When eating dehydrated foods that have not been reconstituted, it must be remembered that it is easy to consume more than is needed for an adequate diet. When dehydrated foods are consumed, ample water needs to be ingested to aid the digestive process.

RECIPES

No canning recipes are provided in this chapter. It is recommended that tested recipes be followed for the foods available and the equipment being used.

1. Wash the plums, cover with water, add the oranges and lemons, and cook until the plums are soft.
2. Extract juice by pressing through a jelly bag, in a colander, or a food press.
3. For each 4 cups of juice, add 3-1/2 cups of sugar. Boil rapidly to the jelly stage.
4. Ladle into hot sterilized jars; seal.

Yield: eight 8-ounce jars

———— Plum-Orange Jelly ————

	Standard	Metric
Plums, 5 pounds, chopped	10 cups	2500 mL
Water	5 cups	1250 mL
Oranges, sliced thin	6	6
Lemon, sliced thin	1	1
Sugar, amount determined by juice		

———— Orange Jelly ————

	Standard	Metric
Water	2 cups	500 mL
Powdered fruit pectin	1 pkg.	1 pkg.

	Standard	Metric
Sugar	3-1/2 cups	825 mL
Frozen orange juice concentrate, thawed	1-6 oz. can	1-6 oz. can

1. Mix together in a saucepan the water and pectin and bring quickly to a full rolling boil; boil hard for 1 minute.
2. Add the sugar and thawed orange juice concentrate; stir until dissolved (do not boil).
3. Remove from the heat; pour into hot sterilized glasses; seal.

Yield: 5-1/2 pints

---------------- Apple Jelly ----------------

	Standard	Metric
Bottled or canned apple juice	1 quart	1000 mL
Powdered fruit pectin	1 pkg.	1 pkg.
Sugar	5-1/2 cups	1,375 mL

1. Combine the apple juice and pectin in a large saucepan; bring to a full boil.
2. Add the sugar; stir until dissolved. Boil for 2 minutes.
3. Remove from heat; let stand for 1 minute; skim for 1 minute.
4. Ladle into hot sterilized jars; seal.

Yield: 14-1/2 pints

---------------- Peach Pear Jam ----------------

	Standard	Metric
Mashed peaches	1-3/4 cups	430 mL
Mashed pears	1-3/4 cups	430 mL
Lemon juice	1/2 cup	125 mL
Cinnamon	1/2 tsp.	2 mL
Nutmeg	1/2 tsp.	2 mL
Liquid fruit pectin	1/2 bottle	1/2 bottle

1. Combine the peaches, pears, lemon juice, cinnamon, and nutmeg in a large pan. Bring to a full

rolling boil and boil hard for 1 minute, stirring constantly.
2. Remove from heat and stir in the pectin.
3. Stir and skim for 5 minutes.
4. Ladle into hot jars; seal.

Yield: 8-1/2 pints

---------------- Strawberry Jam ----------------

	Standard	Metric
Strawberries	8 cups	2000 mL
Sugar	6 cups	1500 mL
Lemon juice	1/2 cup	125 mL

(Use lemon juice only if the berries are very ripe.)

1. Remove the stems from the berries, wash, and drain.
2. Crush the berries and add the lemon juice if the berries are very ripe.
3. Combine the berries and sugar in a large saucepan and cook slowly, stirring constantly, until the sugar dissolves.
4. Bring quickly to a boil and boil rapidly until the jelling point is reached.
5. Ladle into hot jars; seal.

Yield: 6-1/2 pints

---------------- Uncooked Raspberry Jam ----------------

	Standard	Metric
Frozen raspberries, thawed and pureed	3-10 oz. pkg.	3-10 oz. pkg.
Sugar	4 cups	1000 mL
Powdered fruit pectin	1 pkg.	1 pkg.
Water	1 cup	250 mL

1. Combine the pureed raspberries and sugar in a large bowl and mix thoroughly. Let stand for 20 minutes, stirring occasionally.
2. Combine the powdered pectin and water and boil rapidly for 1 minute, stirring constantly.

3. Remove from the heat and add the fruit to the pectin; stir for 2 minutes.
4. Ladle into clean containers and cover with tight-fitting lids.
5. Let stand at room temperature for 24 hours. If the jam does not set, refrigerate until it does. Freeze at 0° F (–18° C).

Yield: 4 to 5 1/2 pints

--------------- Uncooked Fresh Peach Jam ---------------

	Standard	Metric
Finely mashed peaches	3 cups	750 mL
Powdered ascorbic acid	1 tsp.	5 mL
Sugar	6 cups	1500 mL
Powdered pectin	1 pkg.	1 pkg.
Water	1 cup	250 mL

1. Mix together the peaches and ascorbic acid; combine with the sugar and let stand for 20 minutes, stirring occasionally.
2. Combine the powdered pectin and water and boil rapidly for 1 minute, stirring constantly.
3. Remove from the heat and add the fruit to the pectin; stir for 2 minutes.
4. Ladle into clean containers and cover with tight-fitting lids.
5. Let stand at room temperature for 24 hours. If the jam does not set, refrigerate until it does.
6. Freeze at 0° F (–18° C) or store in the refrigerator.

Yield: 9-1/2 pints

--------------- Cantaloupe Preserves ---------------

	Standard	Metric
Firm and ripe cantaloupe	2 lbs.	908 gms
Sugar	4 cups	1000 mL
Lemon juice	1/4 cup	60 mL

1. Pare the cantaloupe and cut into thin slices 1-inch long.

2. Mix the cantaloupe and sugar and let stand overnight.
3. Add the lemon juice to the cantaloupe mixture and cook until clear, stirring gently.
4. Ladle into hot, sterilized jars; seal.

Yield: 4-1/2 pints

--------------- Apple Preserves ---------------

	Standard	Metric
Sugar	2 cups	500 mL
Hot water	1 cup	250 mL
Apples, pared, cored, and cut into 1/4 inch slices	4 cups	1000 mL

1. Combine the sugar and water in a saucepan. Bring to a boil, stirring constantly, until when tested it forms a hard ball in cold water or reaches a temperature of 265° F (130° C).
2. Add the apples and cook at a simmer, stirring constantly, until they are transparent.
3. Ladle into hot, sterilized jars; seal.

Yield: 6-1/2 pints

--------------- Fruit Leathers ---------------

	Standard	Metric
Overripe fruit, any combination	2-1/2 cups	625 mL
Honey or corn syrup	2 Tbsp.	30 mL

1. Wash the fruits and remove any seeds, pits, stems, and blossoms. Fruit, with the exception of bananas, does not need to be peeled.
2. Puree the fruit in a food blender, adding 2 tablespoons of honey or corn syrup.
3. Cover a drying tray with plastic wrap and tape down the edges of the wrap underneath the tray.
4. Pour the puree onto the tray, spreading evenly almost to the edge.
5. Dry the leather in a dehydrator on medium heat

until the middle of the leather is no longer spongy. Turn the leather, peel off the plastic wrap, and dry until the leather feels dry when touched.

6. Fruit leathers will dry in 12 to 24 hours depending on the type of fruit combinations used.

7. Fruit leathers may be dried in oven at 140° F (60° C) for 4 to 5 hours.

--------------------- Beef Jerky ---------------------

	Standard	Metric
Lean beef	3 pounds	1362 gms
Onion powder	1 tsp.	5 mL
Garlic powder	1 tsp.	5 mL
Pepper	1/2 tsp.	2 mL
Worcestershire sauce	1/3 cup	75 mL
Soy sauce	1/4 cup	60 mL
Catsup	3 Tbsp.	45 mL
Hickory smoke salt	1/2 tsp.	2 mL

1. Trim all fat, skin, gristle, and bone from the meat and cut into pieces of approximately 4 inches by 8 inches.

2. Partially freeze the meat so that it will be easier to slice.

3. Slice the meat, across the grain, into 1/8-inch slices.

4. Combine the onion powder, garlic powder, pepper, Worcestershire sauce, soy sauce, catsup, and hickory smoke salt in a bowl and mix thoroughly.

5. Place the meat strips in a shallow baking dish and pour the marinade over the strips. Marinate the beef for 1 hour, turning the strips several times. Drain the marinade.

6. Place the beef strips on a tray and dehydrate them until the strips are hard and leathery; for approximately 8 to 12 hours.

LEARNING ACTIVITIES

1. Contact the local country extension agent to find what seasonal fruits and vegetables are available in your area. Find out where any u-pick fields and roadside stands are located.

2. Investigate the cost of the equipment needed for canning, listed in this chapter, and make a report to the class.

3. Select a fruit in season and preserve it by using both the hot-pack and raw-pack methods. Determine if there is any difference in flavor, texture, and shrinkage obtained by the two methods.

4. Can and freeze the same vegetable and evaluate the difference in the texture and flavor. Keep a chart of the time expended in each preparation.

5. Prepare a jelly using a commercial pec-tin and one with a fruit high in pectin. Analyze the difference in the gel of the two products and the time of preparation.

6. If possible, dehydrate several fruits and vegetables. Compare the taste of the dehydrated food with the same fresh food and a reconstituted food.

7. Plan a 3-day camper or hiker menu using dehydrated foods.

8. Prepare a jam, using a fruit in season, and compare the cost and flavor with the same commercial product.

9. Make a list of vegetables that could be economically grown in your area, considering the local soil and climate conditions.

REVIEW QUESTIONS

1. Why is food preserved?
2. What are the four methods of home food preservation?
3. What is the maximum storage time for most preserved foods?
4. Why may it be unwise to preserve food at home?
5. How are the reasons in question number 4 outweighed?
6. How are microorganisms or enzymes inactivated by canning?
7. What foods must be cooked in a pressure canner and why?
8. Why should jars in which other foods have been purchased not be used in canning?
9. What is the proper preparation of jars for canning?
10. What is meant by the terms *raw-pack* and *hot-pack?*
11. Why are fruits usually packed in a sugar syrup for canning?
12. How are jars checked for a proper seal?
13. What ingredients contribute to gel formation?
14. How is juice extracted from fruit for making jelly?
15. What three methods can be used to determine the jellying point?
16. What is the difference between a jam and a preserve?
17. What is meant by the term dehydration?
18. Why are vegetables blanched before they are frozen or dehydrated?
19. What are three ways to pack fruit for freezing?
20. Why is it important to follow sanitary procedures when preparing foods for preservation?
21. Why should food that has been pressure-canned not be tasted before it is cooked.

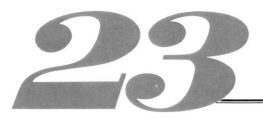

Meal Planning

Meal planning involves the development of aesthetic and nutritionally balanced menus and a program for preparing the food, serving the meal, and cleaning up after the meal.

Throughout this text, nutritional factors, menu-planning points, and food-purchasing tips have been discussed in relation to specific foods. It is now important to learn how various menus can be planned to meet individual needs, and how time schedules can be organized for meal preparation.

Planning of Menus

A menu plan is the first stage of meal preparation. It tells what foods are going to be included in a meal and gives assurance that a portion of the daily nutrient needs will be met and that the meal will be aesthetically appealing. A menu plan also makes it easier to work out a time schedule for meal preparation.

Menus may be planned in detail for each day between shopping intervals so that the shopping list can be developed from the menus. Menus that are planned in detail state the specific foods to be served at a meal, and sometimes include the method of food preparation and recipes to be used.

Detailed menu planning is helpful in incorporating a variety of foods into a meal. Because the planning is carefully thought out, it encourages the use of a variety of recipes and different methods of food preparation. Menu planning is also helpful in developing a time schedule for meal preparation because the exact foods to be prepared are specified in the menu. However, individual and family time schedules may be so erratic that detailed menus will not be practical or even possible. For example, if a menu has been planned that takes 2 hours of preparation, but because of interruptions only 30 minutes are available for cooking, a more flexible plan that involves available foods must be used.

Another and more flexible way to plan menus is to select a variety of foods that meet general needs while shopping for food. For example, if shopping is done at 7-day intervals, then enough meat, vegetables, fruits, dairy products, breads, and cereals should be purchased to last that length of time. These foods can then be mixed and matched for individual meals, but the meals should still be planned at least one day in advance. Some individuals combine these two forms of planning; breakfast, lunch, and snacks are partially planned, but menus for dinner and entertaining are detailed.

One way to develop a menu-planning program is to write down menus on file cards as the menus are used. The file cards are then arranged in some type of order. The cards may be categorized by entrees, such as beef, fish, or chicken, or they may be further classified as 30-minute meals, oven meals, or meals for entertaining. Prior to each shopping trip, several of the menu cards can be chosen for the next week's meals. With a little effort, a complete year of menu cards can be developed.

When menus are planned on paper, they are written in the order that the food is to be served, with the beverage being the last item. The first letter of all words is capitalized, with the exception of conjunctions and prepositions. Menus will be easier to read when each line of the menu is balanced in proportion to the succeeding lines, as in the following dinner menu for entertaining.

Chilled Fresh Fruit Cup

Baked Chicken Legs à la Sour Cream

Parsleyed Rice

Glazed Carrots

Lettuce and Tomatoes with French Dressing

French Bread   Buttter

Chocolate Ice Cream Pie

Coffee   Tea

Specific Menu-Planning Factors

Most individuals consume three meals plus snacks during a 24-hour period. These meals may be light, moderately heavy, or heavy in calorie value, depending on the age and physical activity of the individual. However, all meals, with the exception of snacks, are composed of a main dish or entrée around which the rest of the meal is planned, and each meal needs to be planned for food variety and a balance of the daily nutrient needs. When meals are not planned, they become monotonous and are either skipped, causing a deficiency in nutrients, or filled in with empty-calorie foods. The following discussion relates to specific menu-planning points for the major meals and snacks that are eaten during the day.

Breakfast

Breakfast, the first meal of the day, is the beginning supplier of nutrients and energy for the body and should thus be planned with great care. Hurried time schedules may cause an individual to skip breakfast, and instead eat a high-calorie snack at midmorning to replace this important meal. However, a little time spent the night before in planning the next day's breakfast, setting out the nonperishable food items and equipment such as a toaster or fry pan, and setting the table can make breakfast a more pleasant and unhurried experience.

Breakfast menus should include a fruit or juice, a protein food, an energy food, and a beverage. The most common protein foods eaten for breakfast are eggs, meat, or a combination of cereal and milk. However, some individuals do not like these foods in the morning, and there is nothing wrong with a breakfast menu that includes foods not usually considered breakfast foods, such as chili, a hamburger, a milkshake, a serving of cereal with ice cream, cheese, or a bowl of soup.

The energy foods commonly eaten for breakfast are whole-grain or enriched breads and cereals. Some protein foods, such as bacon or sausage, are also high in fat, which is also an energy-providing nutrient. The choice of what beverage to drink with breakfast depends on individual likes and nutrient needs; children should have milk, but many adults prefer tea or coffee.

Lunch

Lunch is most often a lighter meal than dinner. It is usually eaten at midday, but may be interchanged with dinner and eaten in the evening. Lunches should be planned to contain a protein food, an energy food, a fruit and/or vegetable, and a beverage. An energy food at midday is particularly important for the person who is doing heavy physical work.

A family often must plan several lunches. Children going to school may either take a lunch from home or purchase lunch at school. School lunches are carefully planned to meet the nutrient needs of children. However, some schools also offer a variety of food-vending machines, and children should be carefully educated to select the proper foods before they are allowed to purchase food from vending machines. Children are often responsible for preparing their own lunches, but preplanning must be done so that adequate lunch supplies are available for them.

Many working men and women also take a carried lunch, which requires careful planning to meet the nutritional requirements and taste preferences of individuals and to break the monotony of the same foods day after day. Carried lunches are often not eaten or much of the food is wasted because the food becomes unappetizing as a result of a lack of variety. Keeping some foods hot in an insulated container and using a variety of breads and rolls, together with different sandwich fillings, all help to keep lunch interesting. Table 23-1 is a list of varied sandwich fillings that may be used in a carried lunch. Many surprise treats can be added to a carried lunch to make it more appealing, such as crackers and cheese, carrot and celery sticks, popcorn, canned foods, such as sardines or sausages, or fruits or milk puddings. It is important to store carried lunches in as cool an area as is available to prevent the growth of microorganisms.

Individuals who eat lunch at home must also plan to have interesting foods available so that snacking does not replace lunch. Those who eat lunch at restaurants and fast-food outlets need to carefully plan their food selections.

Dinner

Dinner is the largest meal of the day and should include a protein food, an energy food, one or two servings of fruits and/or vegetables, and a beverage. This meal should be used to round out the needed daily nutrient requirements that have been consumed at other meals during the day, so that food choices for dinner will vary. Dinner will often include a dessert and may contain an appetizer course, such as a soup or a juice. Desserts served at dinner should be planned that contribute to the nutrient needs of the day—fruit or milk pudding are good choices for dessert.

In busy families the dinner meal is often eaten in shifts. Menus need to be planned in which the major food preparation is done only once. Soups and stews are particularly good for those evenings when dinner may extend over 1-1/2 hours. However, certain foods such as meat or casserole dishes containing meat, cheese, or milk, will taste better and be more nutritious if they are cooled and reheated for eating at another time.

Snacking

With the advent of television, busy schedules, and increased leisure time, snacking has become a favorite American way of eating and

Table 23-1

Fillings for Sandwiches

Liverwurst with chopped, stuffed olives or dill pickles mixed in to season.

Peanut Butter with orange marmalade and honey added for spreading consistency.

Bacon cooked crisp and crumbled, in peanut butter.

Cheese and Dates, ground in equal parts, moistened for spreading consistency with orange juice. Point up flavor with a dash of grated orange peel. Add finely chopped nuts for variety.

Brown Bread, spread with butter and then with prepared mustard. Top with mashed baked beans, or omit mustard and add finely chopped mustard pickles to the beans.

Ground Cooked Chicken and cream cheese, mixed and moistened with a little lemon juice.

Dried Beef, about six slices, chopped fine and mixed with one (3 oz.) package cream cheese. Season with a bit of prepared horseradish if desired.

Sardines, canned in oil, drained, bones and skin removed, mashed with hard-cooked egg yolk. Add a dash of lemon juice.

Ham, cooked, chopped, and mixed with pickle relish and a little salad dressing.

Roast Beef, left over, chopped and mixed with a little chopped pickle and salad dressing.

Chicken, cooked, ground, with chopped pimiento added and just enough salad dressing for spreading consistency.

Ham, cooked, chopped, and mixed with cream cheese and finely chopped stuffed olives or dill pickles.

Salmon or Tuna, canned, drained, and mashed with pickle relish and a little salad dressing.

Cream Cheese, softened at room temperature and whipped until very light and fluffy. Use food color to tint the cheese with delicate pastel colors.

Chicken Liver Paté, spread on bread and garnished with strips or cutouts of pimientos.

Peanut Butter mixed with chopped dates with orange marmalade added for spreading consistency.

Cheese Tuna, one cup grated cheddar cheese mixed with 1/2 cup of tuna, drained. Add finely chopped dill pickle and a little salad dressing.

Cheese Olive, one (3 oz.) package cream cheese mixed with eight ripe olives pitted and finely chopped. Point up flavor with lemon juice.

Deviled Ham, mixed with finely chopped nuts and spread on rye bread. Use canned ham. Add a little horseradish if desired.

Bacon-cheese, crumbled, crisp bacon mixed into cream cheese with a little grated orange peel added.

directly influences the types of food that are selected. There are good snack foods and there are snack foods that are a poor choice for a healthful diet. Many convenience foods, which are classified as "snack foods," require little or no preparation; however, they can be both expensive and contain mainly *empty calories.* This term refers to foods that contain mainly calories with only few, if any, of the needed nutrients. Snacking on "empty calorie" foods can be extremely detrimental to an individual's health, because when nutrient-loaded foods are offered, the individual who has snacked on "empty-calorie" foods is no longer hungry. Examples of good snacks include milk and other dairy products, vegetables, and fruits, whereas, empty-calorie foods include soft drinks, potato chips, and candy.

Menu-Planning Points to Consider

This topic has been considered in each chapter in which specific foods were discussed. In planning meals from a variety of food choices, these factors must be considered as a composite group.

Internal Factors

Balance. A meal is balanced when approximately one-third of the human nutrient requirements are provided and the aesthetic factors of color, shape, flavor, and texture create a pleasing food combination. However, a meal is not balanced if too many foods are prepared in the same way for one meal, such as more than one food being fried or prepared in a cream sauce. Other factors that cause a lack of balance include having no entrée or more than one entrée, duplicating the same food in a meal, such as serving an apple salad and apple pie, or including more than one food of similar nutrient content in a meal. For example, a meal that contains corn or squash does not also need potatoes, because these foods are all high in the starch form of carbohydrate.

Color. All foods contribute color to a meal, but foods should be combined that do not clash, create an unpleasant color scheme, or provide no contrast by being all of the same color. For example, a menu including a cream soup, cottage cheese salad, and baked custard is likely to be unappetizing because of its lack of color.

Shape

Shape means the size and form of a food when it is served. All foods offer form to a meal, but too many small pieces of the same size and shape or too many similar shapes are not pleasing to look at. For example, a meal that includes cut green beans, chopped pieces of chicken in a sauce, and chopped carrot and celery pieces as the salad does not offer much variety in shape.

Flavor. The flavor of food adds to the enjoyment of eating. Meals should be composed of contrasting flavors that are neither too strong, too tart, too sweet, or too sour, but rather are a pleasing combination of some of these flavors. A meal that consists of all bland flavors is also not enjoyable.

Texture. The texture of a food is its composition. Some foods are soft, some are chewy, and other foods are crisp and crunchy. A pleasing meal has a variety of textures.

External Factors

Age. The ages of individuals for whom meals are planned have a direct effect on the types and amounts of food that are served and their methods of preparation. Young children and senior citizens are most affected, since both of these age groups need smaller amounts of foods that often are cut into smaller pieces, minced, or ground. Many fruits and vegetables that are usually eaten raw by other individuals need to be soft-cooked and diced, chopped, or mashed for these age groups.

Strongly flavored foods, such as cabbage or Brussels sprouts and legumes, many times can not be tolerated by young children or by senior citizens. Some persons develop allergic reactions toward certain foods at various ages, and this also affects meal planning.

Culture. For individuals who have strong cultural reasons for not eating certain foods, other foods of similar nutrient quality can usually be substituted.

Food Availability. Most foods are available in some form the year around in the United States. However, items such as fresh fruits and vegetables are more available and less costly at their seasonal peaks; veal and lamb are more plentiful and sold at a lower price during the spring months.

Economics. Economics refers to the cost of food. It is important to understand that the higher cost of some foods does not improve their nutrient quality, and that many expensive foods in a menu can be replaced by less costly food.

Meals must be planned around the amount of money that is available to spend on food. Some meals are more costly than others, but the average cost of meals over a 5-day period should be about the same. Meal costs are always dependent on the geographical location of residence, the foods selected, the amount of convenience foods used in meal preparation, and the importance placed on foods in relation to other activities. For example, some families or individuals prefer to eat less expensive foods and use the money saved for a special trip, whereas others enjoy eating more costly food.

Space and Equipment. Meals can only be planned that adapt to the space and equipment available. For example, a meal that requires different oven temperatures cannot be planned unless two ovens are available, deep-fried foods cannot be included in meals if the kitchen equipment does not include either a deep fryer or a heavy deep pan and thermometer, and a frozen dessert cannot be planned if a freezer is not available. Meals will be very limited in food choices if all that is available for cooking is a single burner and one or two pans. Meals should also not be planned that require excessive counter space if the kitchen is tiny, nor should advance preparation be planned unless sufficient storage space is available.

All meal planning and preparation can be greatly facilitated by good kitchen organization. Equipment should be placed at the site of its first use, and drawer dividers, lazy susans, and pegboards for hanging equipment should be provided to eliminate kitchen clutter. Many storage organizers are available to fit individual kitchen needs.

Unless the kitchen is very small, it should be organized into several work centers, and necessary food and equipment for certain preparations should be stored at these centers. The mix center is the area where ingredients are mixed for baking, and the clean-up and washing center is located at the sink and is also the area where fresh vegetables are cleaned and water is added to certain equipment, such as the coffee pot. The cooking and serving center is located at the range, and cooking utensils and serving dishes should both be stored here.

Time Scheduling. The ultimate purpose in time scheduling is to have all foods for a meal ready to serve at a specified hour and to reduce the time spent in the kitchen. Schedules for menu plans are developed by first deciding which foods can be prepared ahead of time without affecting food quality or proper serving temperatures and which preparation jobs can be combined into one operation. A decision is then made as to how and when the jobs will be performed, and if there is more than one individual preparing a meal, job assignments should also be made. A schedule must also include time for table setting and for cleaning up, as well as time for getting appropriately dressed. Table 23-2 shows a time schedule for a meal plan.

Individuals who have only a limited amount of time for food preparation cannot plan meals that take 3 to 4 hours of cooking (unless partial preparation can be done the day before). Many individuals find it helpful to plan meals that can be partially prepared the day before and then completed the day of serving. Others plan meals that can be completely cooked in the oven, using the automatic timing device, or prepared during the day in a slow cooker or a pressure cooker. A microwave oven is a great time saver. The use of convenience foods is also helpful in shortening food preparation time, although this increases the cost of most food.

With the busy schedules that most people have today it is important to think two meals ahead and plan to do all work that can be done ahead of time. For example, if a dinner meal plan calls for a ground beef casserole, a molded salad, and a milk pudding, the casserole and salad can be prepared the evening before, and the milk pudding can be prepared in the morning. Most refrigerated dishes that are to be

Table 23-2

Menu

Meat Loaf
Baked Potatoes with Sour Cream
Buttered Broccoli Spears
Individual Tomato Aspic
Bread   Butter
Angel Food Cake with Fruit Topping
Coffee   Milk

Serving Time: 6:30

Preparation	Time Started	Time Ended
1. Evening before: make cake and tomato aspic	Sometime	
2. Day of serving: Preheat oven and mix meat loaf ingredients; scrub potatoes.	5:00	5:15
3. Place meat loaf and potatoes in oven.	5:15	6:30
4. Unmold aspic; place on lettuce leaves and refrigerate.	5:20	5:30
5. Slice cake; prepare fruit topping.	5:30	5:45
6. Set table.	5:45	6:00
7. Make coffee; pour milk and refrigerate.	6:00	6:10
8. Wash broccoli if fresh; place in pan.	6:10	6:15
9. Cook broccoli.	6:15	6:25
10. Melt butter; place salads on table.	6:20	6:25
11. Serve dinner.	6:30	
12. Clean up.	7:00	

cooked will take slightly longer cooking times.

Using time intelligently when preparing food can save hours of time needed for food preparation at a later date. If a freezer is available, it is just as simple to prepare several batches of spaghetti sauce or several casseroles at one time for freezing for later use as it is to make one batch or one casserole.

Special Types of Menus

Some menus require special considerations to meet different needs. Special types of menus include planned-over menus, low-cost menus, low-calorie menus, and emergency menus.

Planned-Over Menus

Planned-over menus use foods previously cooked for a meal that was served 1 or 2 days earlier. Planned-overs differ from leftovers in that a planned-over results from cooking a larger portion of food the first time, such as a roast. Planned-overs should not be refrigerated for longer than 1 or 2 days, because the food loses its quality and there is the danger of microorganism growth. Just reheating foods is sometimes an unappetizing way to use planned-overs. However, planned-over meats and vegetables can be made more appealing by serving them in a sauce or in a soup, or by using them as a supplement to various casserole dishes. Fresh fruits that have been cut can be cooked and served alone, as a topping for ice cream, or as a special ingredient in cake, such as an apple sauce cake.

Low-Cost Menus

Many individuals find it necessary to plan low-cost menus; others do so simply to keep their food costs down. There are several ways to plan low-cost menus, including the use of lower-priced canned items, the purchase of economical cuts of meat that yield a high count of servings per pound, and the use of nonfat dry milk whenever possible. Purchasing day-old breads is also a cost saving, and many bakeries have a special section of day-old items. Home-prepared mixes are a good cost saving over commercially prepared mixes. Empty-calorie foods are expensive and should be avoided.

Weekly menus for low-cost meals may be planned that include one or two meatless meals per week. High-quality protein substitutes for meat include eggs, cheese, legumes, and peanut butter. Cereal and pasta products can also be used as meat extenders so that a smaller portion of meat is required. Home-cooked cereals are a better buy than the dry cereals; bulk products, such as a box of cereal, are always a saving over single serving items. Fresh fruits and vegetables should be purchased only when they are in abundant supply. Chapter 1 provides additional shopping guides that can be used to plan low-cost menus.

Low-Calorie Menus

In planning low-calorie menus, the most important consideration is to make sure that all the important nutrients are included in each day's food and then to understand that the most sensible program of weight reduction is the loss of 1 to 2 pounds a week. There are 3,500 calories in a pound of body fat and a reduction of 500 calories per day can lead to a loss of 1 pound per week. No single food is fattening, but the amounts served can lead to excess body weight. Low-calorie menus are those that offer a lesser amount of food, with the exception of vegetables. The standard 1/2 cup of vegetables should be maintained or increased, and meat servings should be reduced to approximate 3-ounce servings. Low-calorie menus should include few foods that are high in sugar, including fruits which are canned in heavy syrup. There should also be an absence of foods that are fried or served in rich sauces and gravies, as well as alcoholic beverages.

It is important that low-calorie menus offer a wide variety of foods, including some low-calorie desserts. If low-calorie menus are not varied and interesting, the individual will revert to old and higher-calorie eating patterns.

Emergency Menus

In most households emergencies arise: perhaps the food that was to be cooked cannot be readied in the time available, additional people may have to be served, or a power outage may occur. An emergency meal-planning shelf can help to relieve the situation if it contains foods that can be quickly prepared, some even without heating, to allow for these unexpected situations. Examples of foods that could be kept on the emergency shelf in case of a power outage include canned meats that need no further cooking, canned and marinated vegetables, canned mixed fruits, and instant puddings.

LEARNING ACTIVITIES

1. Plan 3 days of detailed menus for breakfast, lunch, dinner, and afternoon and evening snacks, making sure to meet the daily nutrient requirements and aesthetic factors of menu planning.
2. Make a shopping list from the nine menus and calculate the average daily cost from looking at prices at a local market.
3. Exchange foods in the nine menus, if possible, to meet the food needs of an individual on a limited income.
4. Prepare a grocery list for 5 days from the basic food groups that include approximate amounts of food needed for a single individual or a family of four.
5. Plan nine menus from the foods purchased that differ from the menus planned in number 1.
6. Begin a year menu-planning file, using

the menus that have been planned throughout the use of this text, choosing file headings that will be appropriate to needs.

7. Plan three separate breakfast menus and list the preparation potential of each of them.
8. Interview three teenagers to find out what they would like to eat for breakfast if they were given a choice. If their suggestions are nutrient-qualifying, plan three menus around their choices.
9. Plan a carried lunch for a schoolchild, working man, and working woman that are suitable to both their likes and nutrient needs; include a nutritious surprise in each of them.
10. Plan three desserts that are low in calories, high in nutrients, and acceptable as part of a dinner menu.
11. Plan a dinner menu that would maintain its quality if held 1 hour.
12. Do a research paper on the geographical areas that average the highest cost for food. Present your findings to the class.
13. Reorganize your kitchen so that all foods and equipment are available in the three major work centers. Over a 1-week period, determine if this has helped to reduce food preparation time.
14. Plan a breakfast and a dinner menu and develop a time schedule for each. Prepare the meals and analyze the effects of your time schedule.
15. Plan a menu for which most of the preparation could be done the night before.
16. Prepare a planned-over menu, a low-income menu, and a low-calorie menu utilizing all the suggestions given in this chapter.
17. Prepare a list of foods that you feel are necessary to keep on an emergency shelf; from these foods plan a menu for a power outage.

REVIEW QUESTIONS

1. What five factors are involved in meal-planning?
2. What are the advantages and disadvantages of detailed menu planning?
3. What is a more flexible program for planning meals than detailed menu planning? How is shopping done for this plan?
4. What may happen when meals are not planned?
5. Why is breakfast such an important meal?
6. What types of preparation can make breakfast a more enjoyable eating experience?
7. What types of food should be included in a breakfast?
8. What are some ways that lunches can be varied to make them more interesting?
9. What types of foods hold particularly well when dinner is being served over several hours?
10. What are four factors that contribute to an unbalanced meal?
11. Why would creamed cauliflower and creamed eggs not be considered good partners in a meal?
12. What are the shapes of three foods that would give good contrast to a meal?
13. What types of flavors would be pleasing

combinations with a dish such as sweet and sour pork?

14. What difference in food preparation may need to be made for young children and for senior citizens?

15. What four factors may increase or decrease the cost of food?

16. Around which three work centers should the average kitchen be organized?

17. Why are time schedules important in meal planning?

18. What are the organizational steps in planning a time schedule?

19. How can meals be partially prepared or the meal be cooked quickly?

20. What are the characteristics of a planned-over menu?

21. What foods can be substituted for meat in a meal?

22. What are four ways to keep the cost of food down?

23. What is the most important consideration in planning low-calorie menus?

24. What foods should be used sparingly in low-calorie menus?

25. What foods could be considered suitable emergency shelf items?

24

Table Service and Settings

The final phase of a creative meal, table service and settings, involves the decision of how to serve the food after it is cooked. As discussed in Chapter 1, the changing of American lifestyles in recent years has greatly influenced the way food is served. Changes in housing has also had a great impact on table service and settings. In the past, many people lived in large or medium-sized homes in which the dining area was an important room in the home. Today many homes and apartments do not have a separate dining area; many have only a snack bar or space for a small table. Thus, the table service and setting for most dining have changed from the traditional, formal style to one that is informal and casual.

The attitude toward entertaining has also changed. In the past, guests came to dinner only by written invitation and the meal was planned and prepared in advance; today it is common to ask people for dinner on the same day the meal is planned and cooked. All of these changes have evolved into a more casual and relaxed form of entertaining. However, it is still important to be knowledgeable of the amenities that make the serving of food and the setting of a table a gracious and beautiful art.

Table Service

Table service means the manner in which food is served to people. It varies from extremely informal to very formal, depending on the kinds of food served, the time schedules of the individuals involved, the type of dining facilities, the dishes and flatware available, and the occasion. Most meals are served informally, but all are more interesting when the type of table service and the selection of where to eat are varied. A meal can be eaten in many places, including a kitchen table or snack bar, a dining room table, on trays, outdoors, or at a low table with people seated on floor cushions. Five major types of table service are used, and each may be altered or combined with another to fit individual needs.

Plate Service

Plate service is the type most used with people who are on hurried schedules. The food is served onto the plates at the cook center and is then taken to the eating area either by a designated person or by individuals carrying their own plates. Plate service is advantageous because no extra serving dishes are used, leftovers need not be transferred several times in the steps leading to food storage, and if individuals are eating at various times during the meal, the food is more easily kept warm.

The disadvantage of this type of service is that persons are often not given the opportunity to serve themselves the amount of food their appetites require, and children may not develop the ability to choose proper portions of food, which is important in the adult years. In addition, there is often not a designated place for sitting, which disrupts the important social significance of eating.

Family Service

With this type of service, all food is placed on the table in serving dishes and each individual helps himself or herself to the food as it is passed from left to right. The advantages and disadvantages of this type of service are the opposite of those in plate service. This service is most often used in the traditional family life-style, but because of busy time schedules it may be limited to only special occasions, such as weekend or holiday meals.

Combination

Combination service uses both a form of plate and family service. The entrée portion of the meal is served at the table, family style, but other courses, including appetizers, soup, salad, or dessert are served in individual portions in the kitchen and placed on the table. Appetizers and soup are eaten prior to the main course, and the salad may be eaten with the main course or before or after it. Dessert is the last course of the meal. When the courses are eaten separately, the dishes for one course are cleared before the next course is brought to the table.

English

English service is more formal than plate, family, or combination service, and is most often reserved for entertaining or for special occasions. With this type of service, which is most adaptable to groups of six to ten, the host and hostess are both assigned duties. The main course is always served by the host at the table. If a meat is being served that requires carving, this is most often done at the table before the food is served onto the plates. However, some hosts prefer to do the carving in the kitchen prior to serving the guests. The plates, main course foods, and proper serving utensils are placed in front of the host. If space is limited, some of the food, or the plates, may be placed on a small table or on a serving cart next to the host. At a meal that includes several foods for the main course, or where many people are to be served, the person seated to the left of the host may assist in the serving.

Other courses served prior to the main course, including an appetizer, soup, or salad, may be served by the host or the hostess. Plate service may also be used for these courses. Another variation is for guests to help themselves to these preliminary courses at a side bar, and then be seated at the table. Dessert and beverage are served by the hostess after the main course has been cleared.

With this type of service it is important to follow a specified procedure for the passing of the filled plates: it is the duty of the host or hostess, depending on the course, to designate for whom the plate is intended. When the host is serving, the first plate is passed to the hostess, and if possible, the last plate before the host serves himself should be for a guest of honor if one is present. In this way the hostess has an opportunity to look at the food and make silently sure that everything is satisfactory, and that the guest has the warmest plate of food. After the hostess is served, the plates are passed down the side of the table to her right, and then down the left side. When the hostess serves the dessert and beverage, the guest of honor or the first person on the hostess' left receives the first dessert and service then continues on the left side to the host and is completed on the right side. A male guest is seated to the right of the hostess and a female guest is seated to the right of the host.

Buffet

Buffet service is characterized by people helping themselves to food that has been set out on a table, and is a popular form of table service to use when six or more persons are being served. Although the atmosphere of a buffet service is basically casual, the service may be formal or informal.

An informal buffet has no designated area where persons are to eat except perhaps a specific room area. All food and flatware are picked up from the buffet. The table appointments may be made extremely informal by using paper plates and plastic flatware, as at a picnic, or they may be more formal. If possible, paper cups or mugs should be used for the beverage, because the balancing of a cup and saucer, a plate of food, flatware, and a napkin is sometimes difficult to do.

The menu for an informal buffet should include foods that are simple to serve and eat, since the plates are usually held on the lap while eating. Foods should not be served that require a knife for cutting, such as a slice of roast beef or ham, and breads should always be served buttered. A simple informal buffet includes a main dish, a salad, bread, and a simple dessert. Molded salads are not a wise choice at a buffet because they tend to melt when placed next to warm foods, and at an informal buffet all food is placed on one dinner plate. The dessert is usually a finger-type food such as cookies, small cakes, tarts, or fruits and cheese that does not require additional flatware.

Menus for a formal buffet can have greater flexibility because the food is eaten at a large table or at smaller tables, which have been preset with the flatware, glasses, and linen.

Food is arranged on a buffet table so that the guests can serve themselves in the easiest way possible. In an informal buffet, the stack of plates is placed between the main course and the salad so that both foods may be served onto the plate before the plate is picked up. Although there may be more than one food served as part of the main course at a formal buffet, a similar procedure should be followed as much as possible. With an informal buffet, the flatware, napkins, and beverage are placed on the table after the food so that these items do not have to be managed while serving food onto the plate. It is helpful to have the flatware rolled in the napkin.

Figure 24-1 illustrates the setting of an informal buffet.

The beverage may also be placed at a side table so that people may help themselves when they desire without disrupting the main buffet line. The beverage is most often served to individuals after they are seated at a formal buffet. With an informal buffet, the dessert may be on the table with the main course, but it is usually placed on the buffet table after

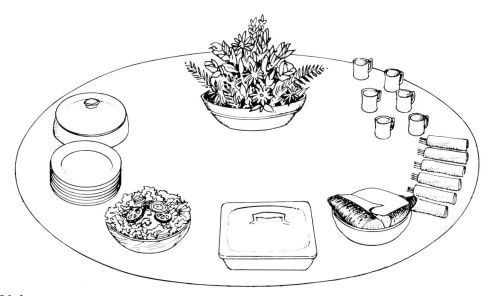

Figure 24-1.
The most convenient way to serve food at an informal buffet is shown here.

the main course serving dishes and the plates have been cleared. In this case, small plates are needed for the dessert, which may also be passed while the guests are seated.

A buffet table should be placed in an area where a good traffic flow can be maintained. If many people are being served, it is advisable to have duplicate foods on either side of the table, and two buffet lines.

Serving Food

In family, combination, and English forms of table service, some or all of the food is passed at the table. The rule for passing and receiving food from another person is to receive with the right hand and pass with the left hand, going in a counterclockwise direction. However, in close spaces it is also acceptable to receive with the left hand. Whatever the direction is for passing food, food should all go in one direction and should not be passed across the table.

If plates or portions of food are served to individuals seated at the table, the acceptable procedure is to serve food on the person's right side. If hot beverages such as coffee are being poured, it is wise to remove the cup and saucer from the cover and pour away from the individual. Water glasses should be filled while they are on the table.

Clearing the Table

The hostess is responsible for designating who will clear the table. All others should remain seated until the clearing has been completed. If a meal has separate courses, the dishes from each course should be removed before the next course is served, and the table should always be cleared before dessert is served.

The order for clearing the table is to remove the serving dishes first, then the soiled plates, followed by the removal of any unused flatware and other items that will not be used for the dessert course. Individual plates are removed from the left side. If more than one plate is to be removed, the dinner plate is removed first and transferred to the right hand;

then the salad and/or bread and butter plate is removed and placed on top of the dinner plate. These plates are then placed on a tray or taken to the kitchen before the next cover or individual place setting is cleared. Soiled plates should never be scraped and stacked at the table.

Because the buffet service is used for serving large groups of people, it is helpful to have several individuals assist in clearing. The dishes may be taken directly to the kitchen or they may be placed on a tray near the kitchen, which is removed when it is full. For informal buffets, using paper plates, individuals may place their own plates in a receptacle provided and put the flatware on a nearby tray. The biggest disadvantage to using this method is that some flatware is often lost.

Table Settings

A table setting presents the theme for a meal, and if the setting creates an attractive and harmonious background, the meal is more enjoyable. More variety and interest are created in meals when the settings are varied to suit the type of meal being served and the occasion. The flatware, dishes, linens, and centerpiece are included in a table setting. The items used are called table appointments. Although some inventories of these items may not be large, there are many inexpensive ways to change the appearance of the table.

Linen

Linen, although a fabric itself, is used in table settings to refer to all the various types of table coverings and napkins. Table coverings are used not only to protect the eating surface but to add warmth, textural depth, and color interest to a meal. Table coverings include the cloth that completely covers the table, place mats, and table runners. A table runner may extend the full length of both sides of the table, or it may be used down the center as a decorative addition, with place mats used for the individual covers. Occasionally, a tablecloth may be used with the runner.

Additional variety is added to a meal by varying the shapes of place mats and the textures of all linens. Place mat shapes include round, oval, and rectangular. The fabrics used include linen, cotton, and synthetic fabrics, together with burlap, wood, and natural fibers. Paper and plastic coverings are the most timesaving because they can be wiped off or, as with paper, discarded. Many plastic coverings have impregnated designs that add interest to the table.

An eating surface made of a plastic material is not easily damaged by warm temperatures and moisture, but wood is easily marred. To protect the table, an additional cloth or a pad may be placed under the tablecloth. The undercover also adds to a more pleasant eating environment by eliminating the noises caused by the moving of dishes.

All meals should be served with a napkin for each individual. Most homes use paper napkins for everyday service, but the atmosphere for formal meals is enhanced when cloth napkins are used. Napkins come in three sizes, including the cocktail napkin used when serving appetizers before the meal, the dinner napkin, and the banquet napkin. The dinner size is the size of napkin that is most often used.

Dinnerware

Dinnerware refers to the dishes on which food is served. It may be an expensive variety, but it should be of good design and color. Poor color and design can make the best-tasting food unappetizing. Dinnerware is often sold as a place setting, which includes a dinner plate, salad plate, and cup and saucer or mug. Other pieces of dinnerware that are commonly used include the soup bowl, bread and butter plate, luncheon plate, and small sauce dish. Although it is nice to have a complete setting of one style of dishes, it is not mandatory because many of the different types of dinnerware can be interchanged for a meal.

Five types of dinnerware are used today, including earthenware, stoneware, china, porcelain, and plastic. Each type of dinnerware has its merits and with the exception of plastic, all are made from clay.

Earthenware. Earthenware, sometimes called "ironstone" ware, is a coarse-textured dishware that is sometimes elaborately decorated. Because it is fired at a low temperature, it easily chips and cracks and is not recommended for oven use.

Stoneware. Stoneware is more durable than earthenware and is ovenproof. Its warm, earthy colors make it an attractive food container.

China. China is made from refined clay and is translucent in appearance. There are varying grades of china. A certain type called "bone china" includes bone ash as an ingredient and is very translucent and expensive.

Porcelain. Porcelain is similar to china in translucency, but because of its manufacturing process, it can be used in the oven.

Plastic. There are varying grades of plastic dinnerware on the market. The less expensive plastics are more susceptible to staining, and some are not dishwasher-safe. Plastics, in general, however, are ideal to use with young children because they are so resistant to breakage.

Glassware

Many types of dinnerware are available in glass. Some glassware is treated to withstand heat, whereas other glassware can only be used for cool foods and beverages. Some expensive glass is hand-blown, but equally high-quality glass can be purchased that is machine-made. Machine-made glass comes in varying price ranges, some of which is aesthetically pleasing. Glassware can also be colored or colorless.

Glassware that is used for beverages is divided into two categories. Stemware has a stem and pedestal or foot; water goblets and various wine glasses belong to this category. Glasses without a stem are called tumblers.

Flatware

Flatware is the name given to utensils used for eating and serving food. Although there are many different types of flatware, the pieces that are most often used for eating include the knife, spoon, fork, and salad fork. Flatware is made from stainless steel, sterling silver or silverplate, and plastic. Some types of flatware use different material in the handles, such as wood or plastic. Stainless steel, which is often used for everyday meals, is a highly durable ware made from chromium alloy steel. Sterling silver is silver with copper added to give it strength. Silverplate, which is made by coating items of a nonprecious metal with silver, is not as expensive as silver and is equally attractive.

Holloware

Holloware is the term used by manufacturers when referring to such items as teapots, bowls, trays, and candleholders that are made from a metal substance, such as silver, silverplate, stainless steel, or pewter.

Centerpieces

A centerpiece is some type of decorative item that is placed in the center of the table to further create a pleasant environment for the food that is to be served. Centerpieces are usually thought of as flowers, but many decorative arrangements can be made from fruits, vegetables, bricks and rocks, pieces of wood, candles of various shapes and heights, or decorative art pieces. Two rules apply to centerpieces. First, the centerpiece should not be so large that it overpowers the table and food; second, it should be low enough to allow people across the table to be seen.

Setting the Table

After the menu has been planned, the meal is cooking, the type of table service to be used has been selected, and the table appointments chosen, the table must be set. Except for informal buffets, the table should be set before food is brought to it. The method for setting up a buffet table is discussed under table service, and the following discussion relates to those meals that are served informally or formally with the other types of service.

An individual place setting is called a cover and requires a width of 20 to 24 inches and a depth of approximately 12 to 16 inches. The area of a cover is also determined by the size of the table or the place mat if one is used. The flatware used in setting the table is determined by the kinds of food being served and whether the service is formal or informal, but no more flatware items should be used than are necessary. Everyday meals usually include only a knife, fork, spoon, napkin, and perhaps a salad fork.

The following points are helpful to know when setting the table:

1. Flatware is placed 1 inch from the edge of the table.
2. The knife is placed to the right of the plate with the blade turned toward the plate.
3. The spoon is placed next to the knife.
4. The fork is placed to the left of the plate with the tines up.
5. If a salad fork is used, it is placed to the left of the dinner fork if the salad is served before the main course or as part of the main course. If the salad is served after the main course, or if the salad fork is intended as a dessert fork, it is placed next to the plate, before the dinner fork. Dessert flatware may also be served with the dessert.
6. The napkin is placed to the left of the flatware on the left-hand side of the plate, with the fold to the outer edge and the corners at the lower right-hand edge. Napkins may also be decoratively folded and placed on the cover dinner plate or attractively arranged in a water goblet.
7. If the salad is not served as a separate course, the salad plate is placed above the dinner fork.
8. The bread and butter plate is placed further toward the center of the cover, with the bread and butter knife lying across the upper edge of the plate.
9. Water goblets are placed directly above the tip of the knife.
10. The coffee cup and saucer are placed at an area level with the tip of the spoon on the right-hand side of the plate, with the handle of the cup in a horizontal line.
11. A soup spoon is placed to the right of the teaspoon. Figure 24-2 illustrates the proper ways to set individual covers for attractive meal service and Figure 24-3 shows a more complete formal table setting for 4 people.

Table Etiquette

Table etiquette means the use of acceptable manners when eating food. The many rules of table etiquette vary in their application, depending on the type of table service used, what is acceptable to individual groups, and where

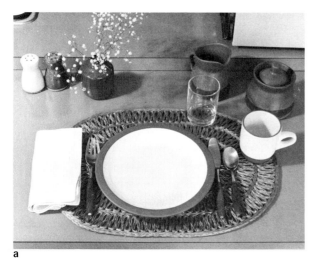

a

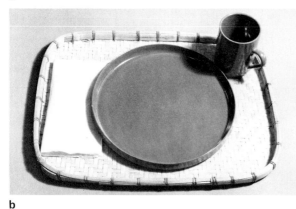

b

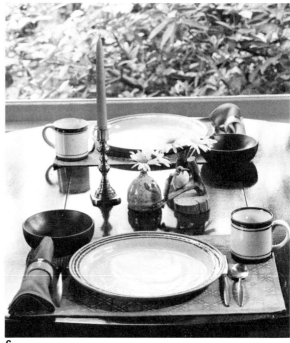

c

Figure 24-2.

(a) Breakfast is more attractive when a pleasant, informal table cover is arranged. (b) Trays provide an informal base for a table cover. Trays are particularly convenient for meals such as lunches that require no eating utensils. (c) Attractive table settings can be arranged with a mixture of tablewares and a few flowers.

the meal is served. This section discusses general table etiquette that should be acceptable to all members of American society.

At many meals there is a designated or understood host and hostess; the hostess is female and the host is male. Either one or both may be responsible for the preparation and serving of the meal. It is the responsibility of the hostess to announce that a meal is ready to be served and, when there are guests, to tell them where they are to be seated. If it is a formal type of meal service, the host and other males assist the females in being seated at the dinner table.

The hostess may request that a blessing be said before people are seated or before any activity is begun after people are seated. Once the hostess places the napkin on her lap, it is a sign for others to do the same. The hostess is also responsible for giving the signal that eating may begin, either by taking the first bite or by placing her fork or spoon, depending on the course, on the plate. If a person must leave the table during the meal, that person's napkin is placed on the chair during his or her absence. The sign that a meal has been completed is the hostess' placing her napkin casually folded to the left of the plate. Others at the table then follow this procedure.

The hostess also provides the signal for

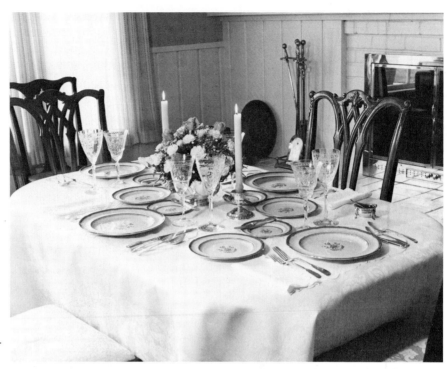

Figure 24-3.
Formal table settings for entertaining are elegant.

which flatware should be used for specific courses. If there is no hostess, the best rule to follow is to use flatware starting from the outside and working inward toward the plate.

Once flatware has been used, it should not be placed on the tablecloth or cover, but on the plate or dish with which it is used. Table knives and forks are always kept on the dinner plate, with the cutting edge of the knife turned toward the center of the plate. Butter knives are kept on the bread plate, if one is provided, or on the dinner plate; salad forks are kept on the salad plate; and soup spoons are placed on the cover plate beneath the soup bowl. When eating is completed, the knife and fork are placed near the center of the plate as illustrated in Figure 24-4.

Proper eating is also a part of table etiquette. The hand that is not being used to carry food to the mouth is kept on the lap; it is never proper to rest an elbow on the table. Individual bites of food are cut as they are to be eaten,

and bread is broken into small pieces before it is buttered or eaten. Soup is eaten by dipping the spoon toward the outer edge of the bowl, away from the person, but soft desserts are eaten by scooping the food toward the person. Beverages should never be drunk when the mouth is full, nor should they be gulped. Talking should be done only when the mouth is empty of food, and chewing is done only with the mouth closed.

Figure 24-4.
It is proper etiquette for flatware to be properly placed on the plate when eating is completed.

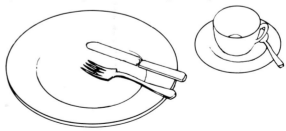

Pleasant conversation at mealtime is most important to good table etiquette; both the host and hostess should endeavor to include all at the table in amiable talk. Loud, boisterous, and argumentative discussions are not a part of good conversation.

Distinctive Tables

A distinctive table is a special one created for a special occasion. Ideas for setting a table are limitless and are bounded only by the imagination. Table settings do take planning and preparation but the effort is always worth it. The following are some ideas to spark the imagination.

1. The color of a tablecloth is the starting point for creating many distinctive tables.

    a. A lime-colored cloth could use as the centerpiece an arrangement of eggplant, limes, and lemons with a base of shiny green leaves, such as magnolia or laurel.

    b. A yellow cloth may use as a centerpiece a pyramid of artichokes and green grapes on a base of shiny green leaves.

    c. A deep royal-blue cloth could feature white candles and individual bouquets of white flowers, such as daisies, at each cover.

    d. A black tablecloth can be stunning with white china dishware and a pewter centerpiece or painted white rocks.

2. A green or red felt table cover can be used as an undercover for a lace tablecloth, and the color can be further enhanced by using the same colored candles and flowers.

3. When linens are in short supply and the meal is casual, newspapers used as a table cover can add interesting table conversation. Wallpaper may also be used as a table cover.

4. A red-and-white checked fabric is a festive cloth to use when serving a meal with an Italian theme.

5. A fishnet over a tablecloth, shells, cork buoys, and paper cutouts add gaiety to a meal featuring seafood.

6. Travel posters as individual place mats may set the theme for a meal featuring foreign foods.

7. Chinese characters painted black on white paper can add an international flavor.

8. A meal featuring a stew may use potatoes as holders for candles surrounding a pyramid of fresh vegetables.

9. Many interesting decorations can be hung from a branch to add fun for holidays, such as Valentine's day, Easter, or St. Patricks Day.

10. A pumpkin shell is a good container for flowers or fall leaves, and the table cover could be crepe paper.

LEARNING ACTIVITIES

1. If possible, interview a couple living in a home with a formal dining room, one living in a home with a dining room table in the living room area, and one with no eating table, to discover what the differences are in their table service. Present your findings to the class.

2. Using one of the five major types of meal service, plan a menu that could be eaten outdoors, at a snack bar, or at a dining room table.

3. Interview 20 people to determine which of the five types of meal service they most often use. Make an analysis of

why this type of meal service is chosen, according to what seems to be their life style.

4. Interview 10 people different from those used in number 2 and find out on what occasions the family service is most often used.

5. Plan a menu that uses the combination form of meal service.

6. Act out for the class the serving procedure for a menu that would use the English type of table service. Discuss appropriate table etiquette for this type of service.

7. Plan an informal buffet menu, diagram the table setting, and plan how you would serve dessert and clear the table and plates.

8. At a meal prepared in class, practice the proper form for serving food family style and clearing the table.

9. Prepare a list of 10 inexpensive linens that could be made to complete a set of linens for eight people.

10. Investigate at one or more department stores and through catalogs the types of dishes that would be interchangeable, have good design, and be functional for eight place settings. Prepare a list of costs and reasons for the particular choices made.

11. Compare the cost of stoneware, earthenware, and plastic and considering their advantages and disadvantages, determine which would be the best buy.

12. Investigate at a low-cost store the types of glassware that appear to be free of defects, are of good design, and are low in cost. Compare this with the cost of more expensive glassware and determine which type of glassware would be the best buy for your available funds.

13. Check the cost of eight four-piece place settings of stainless steel, silver, and silverplate. Make a list of the reasons why you would purchase one of these based on cost and value.

14. Plan five menus for special occasions, which include a centerpiece that helps to create the theme for the meal.

15. Do a demonstration on the proper way to set the table for both an informal and a more formal meal.

16. Observe in a public eating area the number of table etiquette rules that are broken, and do a skit for the class which shows incorrect and correct table etiquette.

REVIEW QUESTIONS

1. How have changes in home construction affected the way food is served in homes?

2. Identify five factors that influence the way food is served.

3. What are the advantages and disadvantages of using plate service?

4. What are the advantages and disadvantages of using family service?

5. What is meant by combination service?

6. What are the duties of the host in the English style of service?

7. What are the duties of the hostess in serving by English service?

8. Who is served first and last when the English style of service is used?

9. What is the general meaning of buffet service?

10. What would be the characteristics of a good menu for an informal style of buffet service? Where would the guests eat?
11. How is food appropriately placed on a buffet table to facilitate the serving of food?
12. What is the purpose of having a side table for the serving of a beverage at a buffet table?
13. How is food properly passed from one person to another at a table?
14. How is a plate of food or portions of food served to a person who is seated at a table?
15. Who designates the clearing of the table?
16. What is the order for clearing the table?
17. What are three methods by which plates may be cleared after a buffet meal?
18. What aesthetic factors should be considered when choosing items for a table setting?
19. What are three types of table covering that may be used for a table?
20. How can textural quality and warmth be added to a table setting?
21. What are the characteristic differences between the five types of dinnerware?
22. What is the difference in design between a water goblet and a water tumbler?
23. What is the difference between sterling silver and silverplate?
24. What is a "cover"?
25. What is the proper arrangement of flatware and napkin for an individual cover?
26. Where are the salad plate, bread and butter plate, water goblet, and cup and saucer placed on a table?

Bibliography

Bennion, Marion, and O. Hughes. *Introductory Foods*, 7th ed. New York: Macmillan Publishing Co. Inc., 1980.

Composition of Food. Handbook #8 Series. U.S. Department of Agriculture, Superintendent of Documents, Washington D.C., 20402.
  #8-1, Dairy and Egg Products, Raw, Processed and Prepared, 1976.
  #8-2, Spices and Herbs, Raw, Processed and Prepared, 1977.
  #8-3, Baby Food, Raw, Processed and Prepared, 1978.
  #8-4, Fats and Oils, Raw, Processed and Prepared, 1979.
  #8-5, Poultry Products, Raw, Processed and Prepared, 1979.
  #8-6, Soups, Sauces and Gravies, Raw, Processed and Prepared, 1980.
  (Further series to be published.)

Eberkrand, Florence, and Lydia Inman. *Equipment in the Home*, Third ed. New York: Harper & Row Publishers, Inc., 1973.

Fleck, Henrietta. *Introduction to Nutrition*, 4th ed. New York: Macmillan Publishing Co. Inc., 1981.

Food for Us All. U.S. Department of Agriculture, Superintendent of Documents, Washington, D.C. 20402, 1969.

Handbook of Food Preparation. 7th ed. American Home Economics Association, 2010 Massachusetts Avenue, N.W., Washington, D.C. 20036.

Handbook of Household Equipment Terminology, rev. ed. American Home Economics Association, 2010 Massachusetts Avenue, N.W., Washington, D.C. 20036.

Handbook for Metric Usage. American Home Economics Association, 2010 Massachusetts Avenue, N.W., Washington, D.C. 20036.

McWilliams, Margaret. *Food Fundamentals*, 2nd ed. New York: John Wiley & Sons, 1974.

Niles, Kathryn, and H. Streufert. *Family Table Service: for Today's Living*, 2nd ed. Minneapolis, Minn. Burgess Publishing Company, 1967.

Nutritive Value of American Foods in Common Units. Agriculture Handbook No. 456. U.S. Department of Agriculture, Superintendent of Documents, Washington, D.C., 20402, 1975.

Peckham, Gladys C. and Jeanne Freelund-Graves: *Foundations of Food Preparation*, 4th ed. New York: Macmillan Publishing Co. Inc., 1979.

Protecting Our Food. U.S. Department of Agriculture, Superintendent of Documents, Washington, D.C. 20402, 1966.

Rainey, Jean. *How to Shop for Food*, New York: Barnes and Noble Books, Div. of Harper & Row, 1972.

Robinson, Corinne H. *Fundamentals of Normal Nutrition*, 3rd ed. New York: Macmillan Publishing Co., Inc., 1978.

Runyan, Thora J. *Nutrition for Today.* New York: Harper & Row Publishers, 1976.

Stare, Frederick J. and M. McWilliams. *Living Nutrition.* 2nd ed. New York: John Wiley & Sons, Inc. 1977.

That We May Eat. U.S. Department of Agriculture, Superintendent of Documents, Washington, D.C. 20402, 1975.

The Shopper's Guide. U.S. Department of Agriculture, Superintendent of Documents, Washington, D.C. 20402, 1974.

Vail, Gladys E., Jean A. Phillips, Lucile Osborn Rust, Ruth M. Griswold, and Margaret M. Justin. *Foods*, 6th ed. Boston: Houghton Mifflin Company, 1978.

Vester, Kelly G. *Food-Borne Illness, Cause and Prevention*, 3rd ed. Food Service Guides, P.O. Box 709, Rocky Mount, N.C., 27801, 1970.

What's to Eat. U.S. Department of Agriculture, Superintendent of Documents, Washington, D.C. 20402, 1979.

Wilson, Patricia. *Household Equipment, Selection and Management.* Boston: Houghton Mifflin Company, 1976.

Recipe Index

Subject Index